Molecular Pathology of Breast Cancer

Molecular Pathology of Breast Cancer

Editor: Dominik Barker

MURPHY & MOORE
www.murphy-moorepublishing.com

www.murphy-moorepublishing.com

MURPHY & MOORE

Cataloging-in-Publication Data

Molecular pathology of breast cancer / edited by Dominik Barker.
p. cm.
Includes bibliographical references and index.
ISBN 978-1-63987-375-3
1. Breast--Cancer--Molecular aspects. 2. Breast--Cancer. 3. Pathology, Molecular.
4. Cancer--Molecular diagnosis. I. Barker, Dominik.
RC280.B8 M65 2022
616.994 49--dc23

Murphy & Moore Publishing,
1 Rockefeller Plaza,
New York City, NY 10020, USA

ISBN 978-1-63987-375-3 (Hardback)

Contents

Preface

It is often said that books are a boon to mankind. They document every progress and pass on the knowledge from one generation to the other. They play a crucial role in our lives. Thus I was both excited and nervous while editing this book. I was pleased by the thought of being able to make a mark but I was also nervous to do it right because the future of students depends upon it. Hence, I took a few months to research further into the discipline, revise my knowledge and also explore some more aspects. Post this process, I begun with the editing of this book.

The branch of pathology which deals with the research and diagnosis of disease by studying the molecules inside organ, tissues and bodily fluids is termed as molecular pathology. It is generally used to diagnose infectious diseases and cancer. Breast cancer is a type of cancer in which the breast cells grow abnormally. Such cancerous cells divide faster than healthy cells. Breast cancer mostly develops in cells from the lining of milk ducts and the lobules which supply milk to these ducts. The progression of breast cancer from the perspective of molecular pathology views it as a linear process with different steps. It begins as flat epithelial atypia (FEA), progresses to atypical ductal hyperplasia (ADH), transforms into DCIS and finally results in the potentially lethal stage of invasive ductal carcinoma. This book attempts to understand the molecular pathology of breast cancer. It is an upcoming area of research that has undergone rapid development over the past few decades. Those with an interest in this field would find this book helpful.

I thank my publisher with all my heart for considering me worthy of this unparalleled opportunity and for showing unwavering faith in my skills. I would also like to thank the editorial team who worked closely with me at every step and contributed immensely towards the successful completion of this book. Last but not the least, I wish to thank my friends and colleagues for their support.

Editor

1

MicroRNA in Breast Cancer — Gene Regulators and Targets for Novel Therapies

Yunus A. Luqmani and Maitham A. Khajah

1. Introduction

MicroRNAs (miRNAs) are a recently discovered class of endogenously expressed, single stranded, non-protein coding RNAs of about 19-25 nucleotides in length, that bind to the 3` un-translated regions (UTR) of target messenger RNAs (mRNAs) through complementarity with the first 2-8 nucleotides at the 5` end of the miRNA. They play important roles in diverse biological and pathological processes, through the regulation of gene expression at both transcriptional and post-transcriptional level [1,2]. The miRNA-mediated gene regulation is part of a larger mechanism known as RNA interference which involves other regulatory RNAs; small interfering RNAs (siRNA), which induce silencing of specific mRNA through complementary nucleotide sequences, and piwi-interfering RNAs (piRNAs) which, through similar mechanisms, induce silencing of active mobile elements to maintain germ line integrity and fertility. To date, over 1000 miRNAs and 16,228,619 predicted mRNA target sites have been identified, affecting over 30% of the human genome [3]. What makes them important players in regulating protein expression is the ability of a single miRNA to interact with more than one target gene (due to the imperfect matching between miRNA and its target which still produces a functional effect). In addition, a single gene can be regulated by multiple miRNAs. Currently, around 200 human transcription factor-miRNA relationships have been described and collated into the TransmiR database [4]. These include transcription factors such as Nanog and Oct3/4, [5], hormones such as estradiol [6], and tumor suppressor genes such as p53 [7]. Since the initial reports of the miRNAs *lin-4* and *let-7* as developmental regulators of *Caenorhabditis elegans* (*C. elegans*) [8,9], there have been numerous studies describing the involvement of miRNAs in normal cellular function as well as in various disease conditions, such as cardiac arrhythmias [10,11], fibrosis [12,13], remodeling [14,15], metabolic disorders [16], diabetes [17],

Alzheimer and Parkinson`s disease [18], autoimmune disorders (e.g. systemic lupus erythematous, rheumatoid arthritis and multiple sclerosis) [19], stroke [20] and schizophrenia [21].

This chapter will summarise and discuss recent evidence elucidating the role of these newly discovered regulators of gene expression in cancer pathogenesis, with particular emphasis on breast cancer.

1.1. Biogenesis of miRNAs

The biogenesis of mature miRNA is a multistep process which requires the contribution of various enzymes, binding proteins and transporters. In the nucleus, miRNAs are transcribed from either intra-or inter-genic regions by RNA polymerase II to form the primary miRNAs (pri-miRNAs), structures of approximately 1-3 kb in length [22]. These are initially cleaved by RNase III enzyme Drosha, and the double-stranded RNA-binding partner protein Pasha (DiGeorge Syndrome Critical Region 8 Protein), into stem-loop structures of approximately 50-70 nucleotides, with a 3` overhang of a few nucleotides, termed precursor-miRNAs (pre-miRNAs) [23,24]. These pre-miRNAs are then transported into the cytoplasm by a nuclear exporter protein termed Exportin-5 (RanGTP-dependent dsRNA-binding protein) [25]. Once in the cytoplasm, the pre-miRNAs are further cleaved from their terminal loops into double-stranded oligonucleotides of approximately 18-24 bp in length into mature miRNA, by RNase-III Dicer: miRNA* duplexes [26]. These strands are then separated and one of them becomes a mature miRNA molecule to be incorporated with several argonaute (AGO) and other proteins into an RNA-induced silencing complex (RISC) which either perfectly or imperfectly hybridises with its target mRNA. In case of near-perfect to perfect matching, this results in mRNA cleavage and degradation by the action of mRNA processing bodies [27,28,29,30], while translational inhibition or sequestration of mRNA from the translational machinery results in the case of imperfect matching [27,31]. In either event, the end result is ultimately reduced protein levels. In vertebrates, most of the miRNA-mRNA interactions are of imperfect complementarity at the 5` end seed sequence [32], unlike the plant miRNA-mRNA interactions which generally target via perfect complementarity [33]. It has been suggested that the miRNA star strand is often degraded, but some evidence suggests that it plays a role in the regulation of miRNA homeostasis and other downstream effects [34,35]. For example, ectopic expression of miRNA-24-2 star strand in the estrogen receptor (ER) positive breast cancer cell line MCF-7, results in suppression of cell survival, through the targeted suppression of protein kinase Cα (PKCα), and decreased tumor formation when injected into nude mice [36]. Recent evidence suggests the existence of alternative miRNA biogenesis pathways not involving Drosha activity, from introns that bear hairpin structures similar to Drosha processed pre-miRNAs. These miRNAs are termed mitrons [37,38,39]. Both pathways merge at the point of cytoplasmic transfer via Exportin-5. In addition, another new group of miRNAs (termed smitrons) has been described as splicing-independent mitron-like miRNA, which require Drosha activity but not splicing, DGCR8 or Dicer activity [40,41,42,43]. Their subsequent mechanism of processing into the RISC is unclear. These events are illustrated in Figure 1.

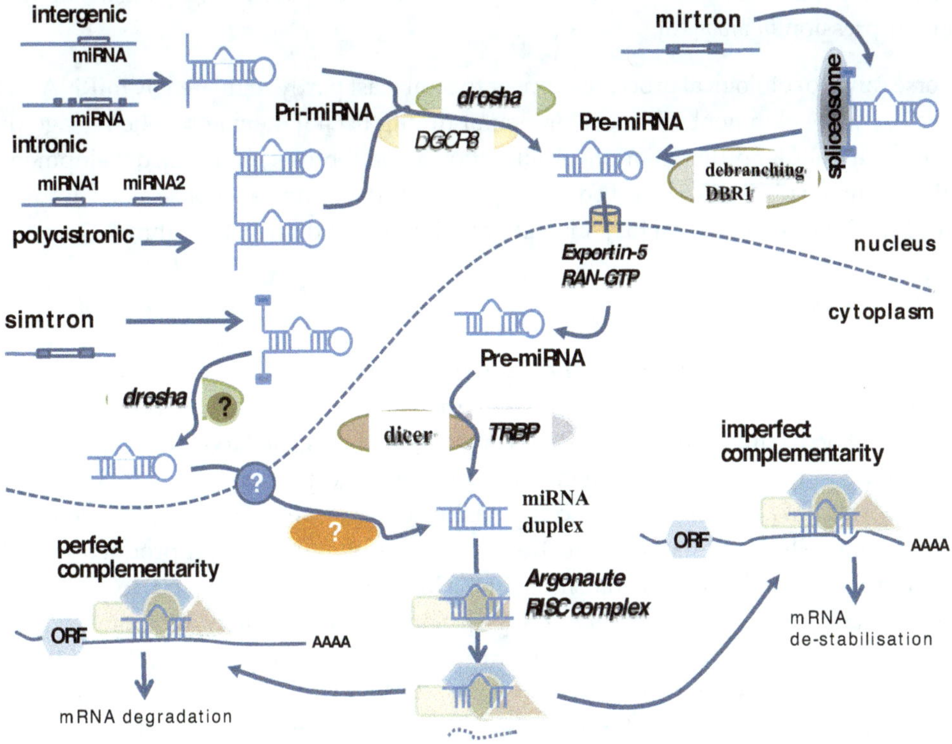

Figure 1. miRNA biogenesis. Following transcription by RNA polymerase II from intergenic, intronic or polycistronic regions, the primary transcripts (pri-miRNA) are processed by drosha/DGCR8 enzyme complex into approximately 70 nucleotide pre-miRNA hairpin structures. Two other pathways involving short intronic hairpins have been described; mirtrons that are spliced and processed via a debranching enzyme (DRB1), and simtrons that are processed by drosha in cooperation with an unknown factor. All enter the cytoplasm through Exportin-5/RAN-GTP activity (except for the simtron-derived molecule which is processed by other undefined mechanisms) and are further processed by dicer/TRBP into a duplex form which then associates into an RNA induced silencing complex (RISC). Within this, RNase H activity degrades the passenger strand and the antisense strand guides the complex to its target mRNA sequence in the 3′ UTR sequence downstream of the open reading frame (ORF). Perfect base pairing results in mRNA degradation, and permitted imperfect matching, in mRNA de-stabilisation, both of which result in translational blockade.

1.2. Physiological role of miRNAs

Aside from their major function of inducing mRNA target gene degradation or translational inhibition, several specific actions of miRNAs have been reported. One such is in senescence-associated transcriptional gene silencing; an event triggered by cancer-initiating or promoting events, through repression of proliferation promoting genes regulated by a retinoblastoma protein (RB)/E2F repressor complex. For example, AGO2, RB1 and *let-7* interact to repress RB1/E2F-target genes in senescence in premalignant cancer cell lines, which may contribute to tumor suppression [44]. In addition, miRNA can *positively* regulate gene expression by targeting promoter elements of protein coding genes, a phenomenon known as RNA activation (RNAa). For example, transfection of miRNA-373 and its precursor (pre-miRNA-373) into the prostate cancer cell line PC-3, resulted in the induction of E-cadherin and cold-shock domain-containing protein C2 (CSDC2) expression [45]. Also, miRNA-744,-1186 and-466d-3p can induce the expression of cyclin B1 in mouse cell lines and lead to chromosomal instability and tumor suppression *in vivo* [46].

A diverse range of biological processes appear to be at least partly regulated by miRNAs. These include early development and developmental timing [47,48], hematopoietic lineage differentiation [49], cellular differentiation, proliferation and apoptosis [50,51,52], development and function of innate [53,54,55,56] and adaptive [57,58,59,60] immune response, neurotransmitter synthesis [61], viral replication [62], insulin secretion [63] and cardiac rhythm [64].

1.2.1. Development

Genetic deletion studies indicate that some developmental processes are absolutely dependent on miRNAs. In *C. elegans,* miRNAs play a role in locomotion, body size and egg laying [65]. For example, *lin-4* and *let-7* control the timing of larva development [8,66]; severe defects in germline development and embryonic morphogenesis was evident in *dcr-1* mutant worms [67]. In Drosophila, cell division defects were evident in *dicer-1* mutant germline stem cells, with marked reduction in the rate of germline cyst production and cell cycle control (delayed G1 to S transition) [68]. Mice null in Direc-1 and AGO-2, did not survive beyond embryonic day (ED) 7.5 [69]. Some miRNAs show temporal expression profiles during mouse prenatal development (at ED 9.5, 10.5 and 11.5); miRNA-2 and-193 showed specific expression in mouse embryo at ED 10.5 suggesting a role in developmental transitions [70]. In human embryonic stem cells, about 14 miRNAs were found to interact with developmental transcription factors such as POU class 5 homeobox 1 (OCT4), sex determining region Y (SRY)-Box 2 (SOX2), and Nanog Homeobox (NANOG) [70]. Some miRNAs, such as 142 and 181, were shown to be specifically expressed in hematopoietic tissues, suggesting a role in morphogenesis [71], while Dicer and AGO gene family (mainly AGO-1 and 2) transcripts were restrictively expressed at ED 11.5 and 14.5 in specific organs including brain, neural tube, limb, lungs and hair follicles, with significant expression in lung tissues undergoing branching morphogenesis [72]. Dicer-1 deficient mouse lungs exhibit defective morphology, with significant apoptosis in the epithelium [73].

Involvement of miRNAs in the development of the cardiovascular system [74] is reflected by variable expression/activity of miRNAs such as-126,-143,-145, and-218 [75]. miRNA-1 has a unique expression profile in cardiac myocytes and plays a critical role in heart development, by influencing cardiac morphogenesis, electrical conduction and cell-cycle control [76]. It is strongly expressed during heart development between ED 8.5-11.5 and represses the expression of heart and neural crest derivatives expressed-2 (Hand-2) transcription factors, which are responsible for ventricular cardiomyocyte differentiation [77]. In the nervous system, Dicer deficient zebra fish show defects in neuronal cell differentiation and development [78]. In mammals, miRNA-124 and-128 are highly expressed in neuronal progenitor cells and mature neurons, and are considered to be the main regulators of neuronal development [79,80,81]. miRNA-124a is thought to constitute 25-50% of the total brain miRNA population, and is implicated in switching brain progenitor cells into a neuron lineage [82]. miRNA-134 plays a role in central synaptic function [83,84]. miRNAs are also implicated in the development of skeletal muscles; miRNA-1 is abundantly expressed in the muscle progenitor cells and differentiating muscle [77], and facilitates myotube formation [85] by interacting with muscle differentiating factors such as serum response factor (SRF), myocyte enhancer factor-2 (MEF-2) and myogenic regulatory factors (MRFs) [77].

1.2.2. Differentiation

miRNAs have been shown to play an important role in the differentiation of pluripotent embryonic stem (ES) cells which gives rise to more than 200 cell types in the adult body. Differential expression has been observed during ES cell differentiation, with decrease in miRNA 290-295 cluster and-296, and increase in miRNA-21 and-22 [86]. Mice oocytes with targeted deletion of Dicer, failed to produce any miRNA, resulting in failure of cell division, in part due to disorganized spindle formation, reflecting the importance of maternal miRNAs in the earliest stages of embryonic development [87]. Over-expression of miRNAs 290-295/302 could overcome the proliferation defects of Dgcr8 mutant mouse ES cells, whereas over-expression of *Let-7* could rescue them from their differentiation defects [79]. Reduced expression of *Let-7* was seen in breast tumor initiating cells (BT-IC), and its forced expression markedly reduced BT-IC proliferation and the proportion of undifferentiated cells, with subsequent reduction in tumor size and metastasis through reduced expression of its targets, H-RAS and HMGA2 [88].

2. Involvement of miRNAs in etiology of cancer

Numerous miRNAs are involved in controlling the activity of intracellular signaling molecules (e.g. MAPK, PI3K/PTEN, NFκB, TGFβ, Notch, and Hedgehog) which are critical in regulating multiple processes linked to cancer pathogenesis such as proliferation, apoptosis, angiogenesis and immune function, emphasizing their potential value in cancer classification, as diagnostic biomarkers for staging, predictive markers of prognosis and response to therapy, and as therapeutic targets [89,90,91]. For example, miRNA-21 is described as a positive-feedback regulator of MAPK/ERK1/2 pathways. Its own expression is induced by the activation of ERK1/2, whose activity it then increases by repressing negative regulators of ERK/MAPK. Stimulation of HER2/neu signaling enhances MAPK/ERK phosphorylation, which results in enhanced miRNA-21 levels and increased invasive capacity of HER2/neu expressing breast cancer cells, by repression of the metastasis suppressor protein; programmed cell death 4 (PDCD4) [92]. The miRNA-200 family have been reported to target the downstream mediators of the TGF-β pathway, ZEB-1 and-2, resulting in inhibition of the epithelial to mesenchymal transition process (EMT), with subsequent suppression of metastasis in various cancer cell lines including those of the breast [93,94]. Interestingly, ZEB1 reduces the expression of the miRNA-200 cluster and hence promotes EMT in a feed-forward manner [95]. *Let-7* directly targets the Ras proto-oncogene which plays a major role in cancer pathogenesis [96]. Phosphatase and tensin homolog (PTEN), considered one of the main negative regulators of the phosphatidylinositol-4,5-bisphosphate 3-kinase (PI3K) pathway, is targeted by various miRNAs including miRNA-21,-26a,-221, and-222 [90]. miRNA-21 enhances proliferation, survival and migration in cancer cells through targeting of PTEN, leading to enhanced PI3K activity [97]. The role of the transcription factor, NFκB, is well established in cancer pathogenesis, and some evidence suggests that several miRNAs, such as-301,-146,-155, and-9, indirectly activate it by inhibiting the NFκB repressing factor (NKRF) [98,99].

A multiplicity of factors, that include chromosomal instability, genomic mutations and polymorphisms, epigenetic changes, alterations in synthetic pathways, promoter methylation, or changes in the activity of their transcriptional factors, modify the expression of miRNAs [29,86]. For example, single nucleotide polymorphism (SNP) type mutations in miRNA-146a can predispose for development of various tumors [100,101,102] including those of the breast [103]. Specific G/C polymorphisms (rs2910164) in miRNA-146a precursor leads to increased production of the mature form, which binds to and modulates the BRCA1 and BRCA2 genes, whose activity is a predisposing factor for early onset familial breast cancer [103].

Although miRNAs have been found to be both over-as well as under-expressed in cancer cells as compared with normal tissues, the more frequent observation is one of decreased expression. For example, whereas miRNA-21 is elevated, miRNAs-126,-143, and-145 are all decreased in most (~ 80%) types of tumors [104]. This means that miRNAs can function both as oncogenes (e.g.-9,-17-92 cluster,-21,-27a,-103,-106,-107,-125b, and-155) or more often, as tumor suppressor genes (e.g. *let-7*,-15a, 16-1, 23b, 29a/b/c, 34a, 124, 133, 137, 143, 145, 192, and 215) [102,105,106,107,108,109,110,111].

Analysis of dysregulated miRNA expression may also have prognostic relevance in many cancers; for example, metastatic breast tumors show elevated miRNA-10b and reduced miRNA-126,-206, and-335 levels [112,113]. A recent report suggested that higher expression of miRNA-126 and-10a in breast cancer patients was associated with longer relapse-free survival [114]. The detection of circulating miRNA in plasma and serum also presents these molecules as potential novel biomarkers for cancer and other diseases. A pilot study showed that miRNA-155 serum levels could be a significant index to distinguish patients with breast cancer from healthy individuals, and serum levels of miRNA-34 could indicate disease prognosis [115]. Another report [116] suggested that four miRNAs,-215,-299-5p,-411, and-452, that were differentially expressed between serum samples from patients with metastatic breast cancer and healthy volunteers, could be used as biomarkers for detection and staging; requiring only a blood sample. Heneghan *et al* [117] demonstrated increased serum levels of miRNA-195 in breast cancer patients (as compared with healthy control subjects), which were then decreased (together with *let-7a*) after curative tumor resection. Molecular classification of non-BRCA1/2 hereditary breast tumors into four distinct subgroups, on the basis of their miRNA expression profiles, was used in a recent report to search for novel susceptibility pathways in hereditary breast cancer [118]. Furthermore, high expression of *let-7*, miRNAs-21,-23, and-27a has been linked with drug resistance in ovarian cancer [119]. miRNA-452 was shown to be significantly down-regulated in adriamycin-resistant, as compared with the parental MCF-7 breast cancer cells; modulating its level partially reversed the adriamycin-resistance, by targeting insulin-like growth factor-1 receptor (IGF-1R) [120].

3. Role of miRNAs in EMT

3.1. Pathways of the EMT process

Cellular transition from epithelial to mesenchymal phenotype (EMT) and *vice versa* (MET) was first identified as a physiological event occurring during embryonic development [121]. Currently, it is well established that the EMT process is a hallmark event occurring in a number of disease conditions including breast cancer [122]. In our laboratory, it has been demonstrated that EMT can be induced in breast cells *in vitro,* in parallel with development of endocrine resistance induced by blockade of ERα function, and this results in enhanced cellular proliferative and invasive capacity [123,124]. During the EMT process *in vivo,* individual epithelial cells lose their cell-cell and cell-matrix contacts and apico-basolateral polarity, and gain a mesenchymal phenotype which enables them to dissociate from the tumour mass, invade into and interact with the extracellular matrix (ECM) before entering blood and lymphatic vessels. Many phenotypic changes occur during this process; these include loss of cell-cell adhesion as a result of reduced E-cadherin and catenins expression in adherens junctions, reduced claudins and occludins expression at tight junctions and reduced expression of various epithelial cytokeratins such as KRT8, 18 and 19, which presumably aids in disruption of cytoskeletal connections that maintain tissue architecture [123]. Various transcription factors such as WNT, NOTCH, TWIST, ZEB1/TCF8, ZEB2, SNAIL, SLUG, GOOSECOID, FOXC1/2, E12/E47 and TCF3, and downstream mediators of several growth factor receptors such as TGFβ, IGF1R, epidermal growth factor receptor (EGFR), platelet derived growth factor receptor (PDGFR), fibroblast growth factor receptor (FGFR), and signaling molecules PI3K/AKT, mTOR, ERK/MEK, and MAPK all play important roles in the EMT process, which has been described in detail previously [122,123,125]. In addition, the stroma of neoplastic tissues and hypoxia can also induce EMT through the production of hypoxia induced factor (HIF-1α) [123].

3.2. miRNAs implicated in the EMT process in breast cancer

miRNA can either induce or inhibit the EMT process by modulating various target genes (Figure 2)

3.2.1. Inducers of EMT

miRNA-9: miRNA-9 is up-regulated in breast cancers relative to normal tissues [126]. It showed a thousand-fold increase seen in c-*myc*-induced mouse mammary tumours [127], and its level was significantly elevated in primary breast tumours from patients with diagnosed metastases, in comparison with those from metastasis-free patients [128]. This is consistent with its higher expression in HER2+and triple-negative (ERα-ve/progesterone receptor (PR)-ve and HER2-ve) tumours, in comparison to luminal subtypes, and in tumours with advanced T stage, high histologic grade, p53 over-expression and high proliferation index, as well as in tumors with mesenchymal-like phenotype (high vimentin, low E-cadherin) [129]. Ectopic expression of miRNA-9 leads to an EMT-like conversion in human mammary epithelial cells *in vitro*. These become scattered with spindle-like morphology and exhibit a significant decrease in E-cadherin and increase in vimentin [128].

miRNA-24: TGF-β acts both as a tumor suppressor in early-stage adenomas, through its ability to inhibit cell growth and, as an important promoter of the EMT process during late stages of cancer progression [130]. Expression of miRNA-24 was significantly increased in breast cancer cell lines which had undergone TGF-β-induced EMT through targeting the guanine nucleotide exchange factor Net1A; an important activator of Rho kinase [131,132]. In addition, Papadimitriou *et al* [131] showed that miRNA-24 levels are up-regulated in metastatic compared with primary breast tumor samples with mesenchymal phenotype.

miRNA-29: N-myc interactor (NMI) is a cytokine-inducible protein that interacts with several transcription factors important in tumour progression such as STATs, myc, BRCA1, TIP60 and SOX10 [133,134], and loss of NMI expression promotes EMT by the activation of TGFβ signaling pathway [135]. A recent report by Rostas *et al* [136] showed increased levels of miRNA-29 in the highly invasive mesenchymal-like breast cancer cell lines, and its over-expression in breast cancer cells expressing robust level of NMI resulted in decreased NMI expression and increased invasion, whereas treating cells with miRNA-29 antagonist increased NMI expression, reversed EMT, and decreased invasion, suggesting a novel inverse regulatory relationship of NMI and miRNA-29 in breast cancer.

miRNA-29a: enhanced miRNA-29a and reduced tristetraprolin (TTP, a protein involved in the degradation of mRNAs with AU-rich 3' UTRs) was observed in breast cancer patient samples with invasive phenotype. Over-expression of miRNA-29a induced EMT and metastasis in Ras-transformed mouse mammary epithelial cells through suppression of TTP [137].

miRNA-103/107: enhanced miRNA-103/107, and reduced expression of the RNase III endonuclease Dicer, was observed in breast cancer cell lines with highly invasive mesenchymal phenotype. Over-expression of miRNA103/107 induced Dicer down-regulation and induction of EMT, with subsequent enhancement in invasive capacity. Furthermore, miRNA103/107 could induce EMT by decreasing miRNA-200 (which negatively regulates EMT), and controlling the levels of ZEB1/2 in a miRNA-200-dependent manner [138,139].

miRNA-106b-25 cluster: the expression profile of this miRNA cluster in human breast cancer patients significantly correlates with metastatic phenotype and shorter relapse free survival. Over-expression induced EMT in breast cancer cell lines, with reduced E-cadherin and increased expression of mesenchymal markers such as β-catenin, Jag1, MMP-9 and vimentin, as well as increasing the percentage of cells with tumor initiating characteristics ($CD24^{low}$ $CD44^{+}$); typical of mesenchymal cells. This cluster also induced EMT by enhancing the action of the metastatic regulator Six1 (a major mediator of the TGF-β-initiated EMT promoting pathway) and by targeting the inhibitory Smad7 protein, which results in increased levels of the TGF-β type I receptor and downstream activation of TGF-β signaling [140].

miRNA-155: Johansson *et al* [141] have demonstrated that miRNA-155 could mediate a switch in TGFβ effect, from tumor suppression to induction of EMT both, in breast cancer cell lines, and in MMTV-PyMT mice. Treatment of mouse mammary gland epithelial cells with a synthetic miRNA-155 mimic repressed the level of the mammary epithelium differentiation factor CCAAT-enhancer binding protein beta (C/EBPβ) and induced EMT in response to TGFβ treatment; loss of E-cadherin expression, induction of vimentin, and enhanced metastasis and invasion, both *in vitro* and *in vivo*.

miRNA 221/222: miRNA-221/222 induces EMT and subsequent enhancement in invasion by decreasing expression of epithelial-specific genes while increasing expression of mesenchymal-specific genes, in part through stimulation of the transcription factor FOSL1 (Fra-1) and reduction of adiponectin receptor 1 (ADIPOR1). miRNA-221/222-mediated reduction of E-cadherin was effected through targeting of the 3' UTR of the GATA family transcriptional repressor TRPS1 (tricho-rhino-phalangeal syndrome type 1), and modulating ZEB2 levels [142,143,144]. Lambertini *et al* [145] showed that miRNA-221can induce EMT in MDA-MB-231 cells by directly targeting SLUG, a master regulator of the EMT process. Another recent report showed that the secreted form of miRNA221/222 serves as a signaling molecule which plays a pivotal role in the induction of tamoxifen resistance in the ER+ve breast cancer cell line MCF-7; this can be blocked by anti-miR221/222 treatment [146].

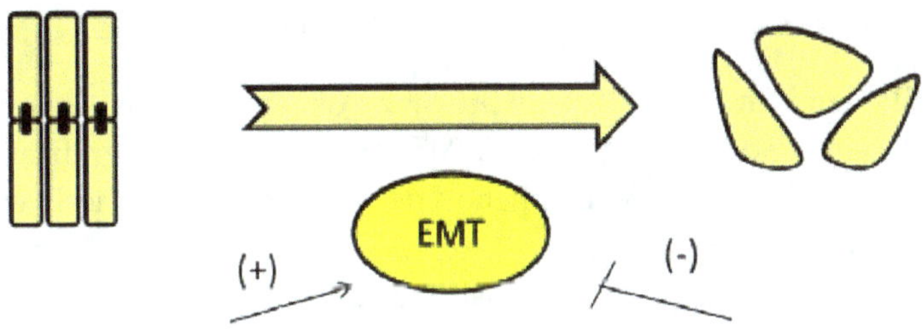

miRNA	Target (s)
9	E-cadherin, vimentin
24	TGFβ, Net1A, Rho
29	NMI
29a	TTP, dicer
103/107	dicer, miRNA-200, ZEB1/2
106b-25 cluster	E-cadherin, β-catenin, Jag1, MMP-9, vimentin, TGFβ, Six1
155	E-cadherin, C/EBPβ, vimentin
221/222	E-cadherin, Fra-1, ZEB2/Slug

miRNA	Target (s)
7	SETDB1, STAT3
124	Slug, vimentin, fibronectin, E-cadherin
145	Snail, ZEB1/2, OCT4, fibronectin, E-cadherin
200 family & 205	ZEB1/2, PI3K/AKT
206	IL-6, NFkB, Notch3
375	MTDH
448	SATB1, amphiregulin, Twist, NFkB

Figure 2. Regulation of EMT in breast cancer cells. miRNAs can act as either inducers or inhibitors of EMT by increasing (blue) or decreasing (red) the expression of various target genes as indicated.

3.2.2. Inhibitors of EMT

miRNA-7: Zhang *et al* [147] showed that miRNA-7 expression was significantly reduced in cancer stem cells isolated from MDA-MB-231 and MCF-7 cell lines, and down-regulates the oncogene SETDB1 by targeting the 3`UTR of the mRNA. Over-expression of miRNA-7 suppressed the EMT-like characteristics of MDA-MB-231 cells, as reflected in the observation that these cells became less scattered and lost their spindle-like morphology, increased E-cadherin and reduced vimentin expression. This was in part due to reduced expression and activity of STAT3.

miRNA-124: as mentioned previously, this miRNA is highly expressed in the brain and plays a crucial role in neural development. Recent evidence suggests that it is also involved in cancer pathogenesis, with reduced expression seen in various cancers, including the breast. Its expression was inversely correlated to histological grade. Its over-expression could repress many of the mesenchymal characteristics of highly metastatic breast cancer cell lines (e.g. MDA-MB-231 and B-549) [148] by reducing SLUG expression, through direct interaction with its 3′-UTR region.

miRNA-145: Hu *et al* [149] have demonstrated that the expression of miRNA-145 was decreased in breast tumor tissues with invasive phenotype, and its over-expression in various breast cancer cell lines leads to enhanced E-cadherin expression, reduced expression of fibronectin, ZEB1/2 and SNAIL, and inhibition of EMT by targeting Oct4.

miRNA-200 family and miRNA-205: expression of the miRNA-200 family (miRNA-200a,-200b,-200c,-141 and-429) and miRNA-205 were found to be significantly reduced in breast cancer cell lines with mesenchymal phenotype, but high in E-cadherin expressing cells with epithelial characteristics. Similarly, their expression was lost in regions of metaplastic breast tumours with mesenchymal characteristics and lacking E-cadherin expression [94]. Enforced expression of miRNA-200 alone was sufficient to prevent EMT induced by TGFβ stimulation [94]. ZEB-1 (TCF8/deltaEF1) and ZEB-2 (SMAD-interacting protein 1 [SIP1]/ZFXH1B), which are able to initiate EMT by binding to E-boxes within the E-cadherin promoter, repressing its transcription, were the main target genes for these miRNAs [150]. Over-expression of miRNA-200 could induce MET in both normal and cancer cell lines and reduce the motility and invasiveness of MDA-MB-231 by enhancing E-cadherin expression [151,152]. Chen *et al* [153] demonstrated that the loss of miRNA-200c in breast cancer cells was correlated with both EMT and acquired resistance to doxorubicin. In addition, decreased levels of E-cadherin and PTEN, and increased levels of ZEB1 and phospho-Akt were seen in these cells, which correlated with loss of miRNA-200c. Ectopic expression of miRNA-200c reversed all of these changes, suggesting that miRNA-200c inhibits the acquired resistance of breast cancer cells against doxorubicin through inactivation of the PI3K/Akt signaling pathway.

miRNA-375: this was reported to be significantly down-regulated in tamoxifen-resistant (TamR) MCF-7 cells which had acquired a mesenchymal phenotype. Its re-expression re-sensitized the TamR cells to tamoxifen, reversed the EMT process, and reduced invasiveness by targeting the metadherin (MTDH) gene [154].

miRNA-448: suppression of miRNA-448 induced EMT in MCF7 cells, with characteristic acquisition of a fibroblast-like cell morphology, dissolution of tight junctions (ZO-1), formation of F-actin stress fibers, severe E-cadherin suppression and enhanced vimentin expression. In addition, enhanced invasive capacity was also observed upon miRNA-448 inhibition *in vitro*.

These effects were due to direct targeting of specific AT-rich sequence-binding protein-1 (SATB1) mRNA, leading to elevated levels of amphiregulin and EGFR-mediated TWIST1 expression, as well as NF-κB activation through the MAPK and PI3K/Akt pathways. On the other hand, over-expression of miRNA-448 in MDA-MB-231 cells (which otherwise express very low levels), leads to MET and decreases cell migration and invasion. Similar effects were also observed *in vivo* where miRNA-448-silenced MCF-7 cells (which are usually poorly invasive) showed a spindle-like morphology, with islands of cancer cells that had invaded the muscle and lung tissues when injected into the left flank of nude mice [155].

3.2.3. Role of p53 in EMT and miRNA expression

Deletions and/or mutations in p53 are frequently involved in the pathogenesis of many human cancers including those of the breast (mutated in 25-30% of breast cancers) [156,157]. Kim *et al* [158] observed that p53 prevented EMT in primary hepatocellular carcinomas by repressing ZEB1 and 2 in a 3′UTR-dependent manner. Furthermore, p53-induced ZEB1/2 repression was mediated through up-regulation of various miRNAs; -141, -192, -193b, -194, -200b, -200c, -215, -224, and -34a). p53 is able to positively modulate miRNA-205 expression in triple negative breast cancer cell lines, through regulation of two newly identified target genes, E2F1 and LAMC1, resulting in reduced cellular proliferation [159]. In addition, p53 knockdown can increase proliferation of both luminal and basal-like breast cancer cell lines, in part through up-regulation of miRNA-134,-146a, and-181b. Over-expression of miRNA-146a leads to decreased NF-kB expression and inhibition of the NF-kB-dependent extrinsic apoptotic pathway (TNF, FADD, and TRADD) in basal-like cells expressing mutant p53, suggesting that targeting miR-146a expression may have potential therapeutic value for reducing the aggressiveness of such tumors [160].

4. ER signalling, EMT and miRNA

Estrogen (E_2), acting through ERα, plays a major role in controlling the normal growth and development of mammary epithelial cells, as well as in the pathogenesis of breast cancer. E_2 binding induces ERα activation by the dissociation of the inactive ER-heat shock protein complex, leading to conformational changes, dimerization and autophosphorylation. The activated dimer complex binds to either estrogen response elements (EREs) or to other promoters such as the AP1/SP1 sites in target genes, to initiate events culminating in cellular proliferation. Other target genes may include transcriptional repressors or initiate anti-proliferative or pro-apoptotic function [161].

The mammary ducts are composed of an inner layer of luminal epithelial cells and an outer layer of basal or myoepithelial cells. The majority of breast cancers arise from the luminal epithelium of small mammary ducts, and are classified as luminal-A subtype, characterized as low grade, weakly proliferative and invasive. These express ERα, PR, luminal associated transcription factors such as GATA-3 and FOXA1, and epithelial markers such as E-cadherin [162]. Luminal-A cancers can progress into more aggressive and metastatic forms through the

EMT process. Although ERα plays a critical role in enhancing cellular proliferation, where anti-estrogen therapy (e.g. tamoxifen) are the preferred treatment options, E_2/ERα signaling also promotes the differentiation of mammary epithelial cells along the luminal/epithelial lineage and thereby *opposes* the EMT process. ERα stimulates the transcription factors required for luminal differentiation such as GATA-3 and FOXA1 [163,164]. In fact, forced GATA-3 expression in mesenchymal-like breast cancer cells reduces their metastatic capabilities by inducing MET [165]. ER signaling also suppresses EMT-promoting transcription factors such as SLUG and SNAIL [166,167]. Furthermore, ER antagonizes signaling pathways that lead to EMT, such as those of TGFβ and NFκB. E_2/ERα signaling has been shown to oppose the action of TGFβ in promoting EMT, by initiating formation of ternary complexes of Smad2/3 and SmadE3 ubiquitin ligase smurf, thereby increasing the proteosomal degradation of Smad proteins [168]. The NFκB subunit, RELB, is needed to maintain the mesenchymal phenotype; ectopic expression of ERα in the presence of E_2 was shown to decrease RELB expression in ER-ve cell lines [169,170].

In our laboratory, we have established several endocrine resistant breast cancer cell lines that exhibit an ERα-depleted phenotype induced by shRNA transfection of the ER+ve MCF-7 cells. Such cells have all gained estrogen independence and exhibit a series of changes in morphology and enhanced motility and invasiveness accompanied by a modified gene expression profile indicative of EMT. Microarray and real time-PCR analysis have confirmed the loss of genes associated with epithelial cells such as E-cadherin, catenin, occludins, claudins, and enhanced gene expression associated with mesenchymal cells such as N-cadherin, vimentin, fibronectin, integrin β4 and α5, and various metalloproteinases [124,171,172]. This model of endocrine resistance induced by ERα loss was also confirmed by others. Moreover, ectopic ERα over-expression in ER–ve breast cancer cell lines reverses the EMT process through enhanced E-cadherin and reduced SLUG expression [173].

The ERα mRNA has a long 3' UTR of about 4.3 kb which has been reported to reduce mRNA stability and which bears evolutionarily conserved miRNA target sites, suggesting that it might be regulated by miRNAs. Overall, ER–ve cells display generally lower levels of miRNA expression. Of the miRNAs that are up-regulated there are distinct differences between ER-ve and ER+ve cells (Figure 3).

Of note, miRNA-10b,-125, and-145 were significantly down-regulated in the majority of breast cancer samples and cell lines, whereas miRNA-21,-17-5b,-29b-2,-146,-155, and 181b-1 were up-regulated [126,174]. Estrogen has been shown to induce Dicer expression; loss of ERα may contribute to reduced Dicer and consequently lower miRNAs levels in ER–ve cells. In addition, some miRNA such as miRNA-29a, 103/107 and-200c, and *let-7* inhibit Dicer expression and thereby promote the EMT process [175,176,177,178]. Restoration of miRNA-200c in triple negative breast cancer cells causes an increase in Dicer levels [176]. The expression of both AGO-1 and-2 was reported to be significantly elevated in ER–ve cells [179]; forced expression of AGO-2 enhanced breast cancer cell motility through reduced E-cadherin expression [180]. Understanding how miRNAs modulate ERα and its signaling pathway may offer new therapeutic approaches to restore endocrine sensitivity and responsiveness to anti-estrogen therapies, and reverse the EMT process, thereby reducing metastasis. The following section

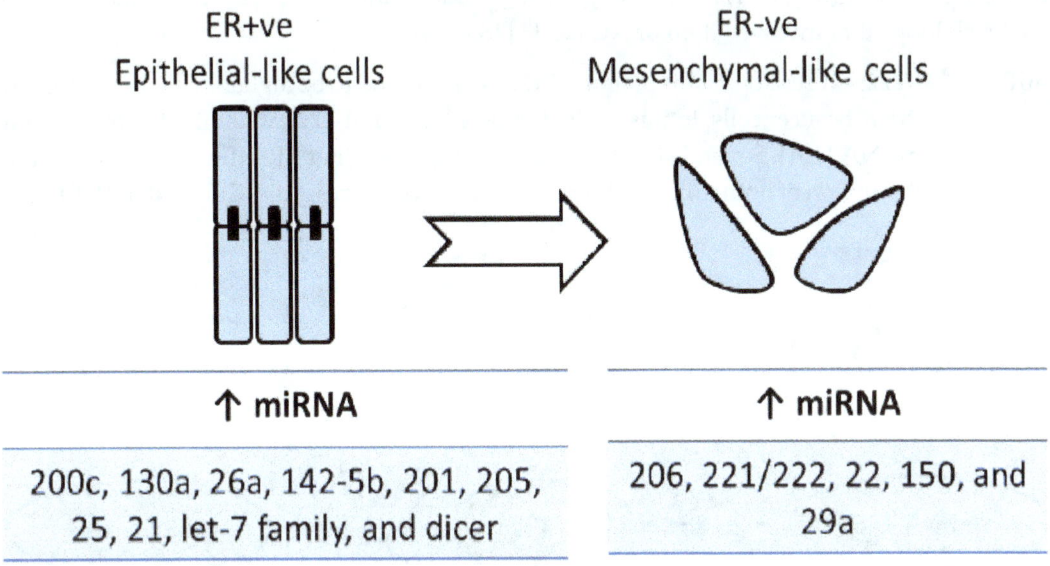

Figure 3. Up-regulation of miRNA expression in relation to ER status of breast tumours

describes individual miRNAs that have been shown to modulate ERα expression and hence the EMT process (Figure 4).

miRNA-22: over-expression of miRNA-22 represses ERα expression through the 3`UTR leading to reduction in estrogen signaling. This also leads to impaired estrogen-induced proliferation of MCF7 breast cancer cells to an extent similar to that of shRNA directed at the ERα mRNA [181]. Similar findings were also reported by Xiong *et al* [182].

miRNA-145: transfection of miRNA-145 into ER+ve breast cancer cells significantly reduced ERα protein levels through interaction of two miRNA-145 target sites within the coding region of ERα mRNA, reducing the levels of its downstream target cyclin D1 [183].

miRNA-206: E_2/ERα directly suppresses miRNA-206 levels [184], while the miRNA-206 itself directly targets the mRNAs encoding components of ERα signaling molecules such as the nuclear receptor co-activator proteins steroid receptor co-activator-1 (SRC-1) and-3 as well as GATA-3 [184,185]. In addition, ectopic expression of miRNA-206 in ER+ve breast cancer cells reduces endogenous ERα at both mRNA and protein levels and leads to enhanced invasive capacity [186,187]. Moreover, miRNA-206 can also decrease the expression of DNA polymerase A1 subunits as well as the oncogenic receptor c-MET, while increasing the expression of the tumor suppressor forkhead box O3 (FOXO3). Consequently, this leads to the inhibition of cell proliferation, suggesting a role for miRNA-206 in repressing proliferation of ER+ve breast cancer by enhancing myoepithelial differentiation and ERα silencing [30,184,188]. Enhanced level/activity of EGF add its receptor (EGFR/HER1) is seen in mesenchymal type breast cancer cells and may contribute to ER silencing though enhancement of miRNA-206 levels [184]. Ectopic expression of miRNA-206 in MCF-7 cells enhances IL-6 expression, which is known to induce EMT through STAT signaling. Also, it maintains its level by autocrine positive feedback loops that involve NFκB or NOTCH3 [189,190].

miRNA-221/222: expression of this pair of miRNAs was found to be higher in ER-ve compared with ER+ve breast cancer cells. In this context, miRNA-221 and-222 can inhibit the translation of the ERα mRNA [191]. Several studies have also suggested that ERα directly represses the gene promoter region of both miRNAs by recruiting the co-repressors NCoR and SMRT [187].

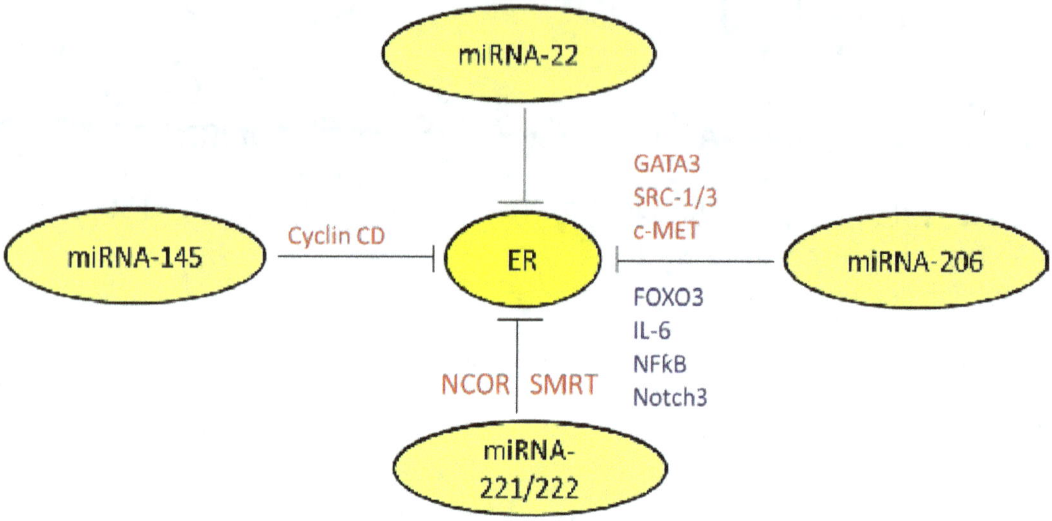

Figure 4. miRNAs that negatively regulate ER expression in breast cancer. These act either directly (miRNA-22), or through up-(blue) or down-(red) regulation of other target mRNAs.

5. miRNAs and cell invasion

Cancer cell invasion is a multi-step process which involves dissociation of extracellular matrix components by the action of various proteases and the subsequent movement of detached tumor cells from the original tumor site to distinct organs, and is associated with poor clinical outcome and reduced survival rates. Several miRNAs have been implicated in either enhancing or reducing cellular invasion by targeting various mRNAs that encode proteins crucial to the process (Figure 5).

5.1. miRNAs with anti-metastatic actions

miRNA-7: expression of miRNA-7 was significantly reduced in cancer stem cells (CSCs) isolated from breast cancer cell lines which demonstrated significant metastatic migration to the bone and the brain. It attenuated the invasion and self-renewal of CSCs by enhancing the expression of KLF4 [192]. A recent report also confirmed the anti-metastatic properties of miRNA-7 both *in vitro* and *in vivo* by targeting the oncogene SETDB1 and showing decrease in expression and activity of STAT3 in MDA-MB-231 cells [147].

miRNA-18a: a recent report showed that over-expression of miRNA-18a in MDA-MB-231 cells reduced cell invasiveness and sensitivity to anoikis and hypoxia *in vitro*, and primary tumor growth and lung metastasis *in vivo*. On the other hand, its inhibition leads to a pro-metastatic effect by targeting of the HIF1A gene [193].

miRNA-31: expression of miRNA-31 is reduced in several metastatic breast cancer cell lines, and correlates inversely with metastasis in human breast cancer patients. Over-expression of this miRNA in otherwise-aggressive breast tumor cells suppresses metastasis, whereas inhibition of miRNA-31, by miRNA sponge strategy, induced metastasis in non-aggressive breast cancer cells both *in vitro* and *in vivo* by enhancing the expression of several metastasis-promoting genes including Fzd3, ITGA5, RDX, and RhoA [194].

miRNA-107: over-expression of this miRNA in MDA-MB-231 cells significantly inhibited cell migration and invasion by targeting of the cyclin-dependent kinase 8 (CDK8) gene [195].

miRNA-124: expression of miRNA-124 was significantly reduced in MDA-MB-231 compared to MCF-7 cells. Induced over-expression in MDA-MB-231 significantly inhibited cell migration and invasion *in vitro*, in part through reduced SLUG and enhanced E-cadherin expression [148,196]. In addition, reduced tumor formation and lung metastasis was seen in MDA-MB-231 cells over-expressing miRNA-124 when injected into the tail vein of nude mice [148]. Another report confirmed its anti-metastatic role through its ectopic expression in MDA-MB-231 and T47D cells, which significantly reduced their invasive capacity through targeting of flotillin-1 (FLOT1) [197]. Other evidence suggests that its anti-metastatic properties are exerted through the suppression of several pro-metastatic genes such as connective tissue growth factor (CTGF), Ras homolog family member G (RhoG), ITGB1 and ROCK1 [196].

miRNA-145: the expression of miRNA-145 was found to be reduced in breast cancer cells compared to normal tissue, and its over-expression in various breast cancer cell lines (MDA-MB-231, MCF-7, MDA-MB-468 and SK-BR-3) significantly reduced motility and invasiveness. This effect was due to down-regulation of the cell–cell adhesion protein JAM-A and the actin bundling protein fascin [198], and silencing of the metastasis gene mucin 1 (MUC1), with subsequent reduction of beta-catenin as well as the oncogenic cadherin 11 [199].

miRNA-146a/b: over-expression of miRNA146a/b in MDA-MB-231 resulted in marked inhibition of migration and invasion due to reduced NF-κB activity. This was through miRNA146a/b-induced down-regulation of two key regulators of this signaling pathway; interleukin (IL)-1 receptor-associated kinase and TNF receptor-associated factor 6 [200].

miRNA-149: a recent report [201], showed reduced expression of miRNA-149 in basal compared with luminal A/B, erbB2/HER2 positive and normal-like cancers and cell lines. It was also found to be inversely correlated with higher tumor stage. Over-expression of a mature miRNA-149 mimic in MDA-MB-231 cells significantly reduced their spreading in culture; the cells exhibited a depolarized actin cytoskeleton and failed to establish prominent cell protrusions and lamellipodia. Moreover, significant reduction in migration and invasion towards a serum plus EGF gradient was observed in cells over-expressing miRNA-149. These effects were due to decreased phosphorylation levels of src and rac, and to targeting of the small GTPases rap1a and rap1b, the downstream effectors of the integrin receptor.

miRNA-195-5p: a recent study demonstrated that over-expression of miRNA-195-5p significantly inhibited MDA-MB-231 and MCF-7 breast cancer cell invasion by targeting cyclin E1 and *raf*-1/Ccdn1 genes respectively [202,203].

miRNA-223: over-expression of miRNA-223 in MDA-MB-231 significantly decreased cell migration and invasion by down-regulating STAT5A [204].

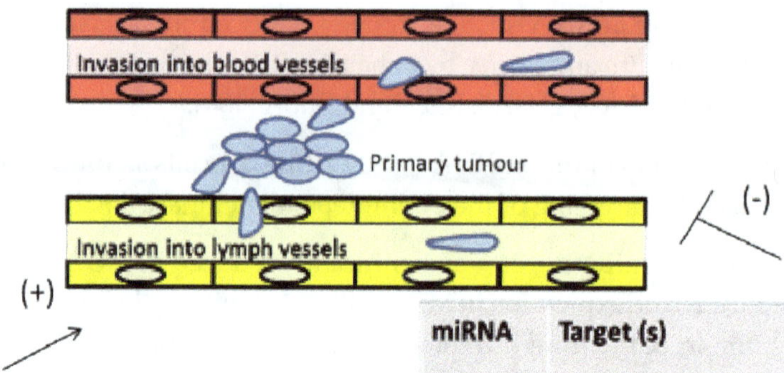

miRNA	Target (s)
9	E-cadherin, β-catenin, VGEFA
10b	RHOC, TIAM1
18b	NLRP7, KLK3, OLFM3, POSTN, MAGED4B, KIR3DL3, CRX, SEMG1, CEACAM5
21	PDCD4, TPM1, TIMP3, PTEN, PI3K, MARK, ERK1/2
24	TGFβ, Net1A
Has-30c	NOV, CCN3
155	C/CBPβ
221/222	E-cadherin, Fra-1, uPA
301a	PTEN, Wnt, PI3K, β-catenin
373/520	E-cadherin, CD44
495	JAM-A

miRNA	Target (s)
7	STAT3, SETDB1
18a	HIF1A
31	Fzd3, ITGA5, RDX, RhoA
107	CDK8
124	Slug, FLOT1, CTGF, RhoG, ROCK1, E-cadherin
145	JAM-A, fascin, MUC1, cadherin-11, β-catenin
146a/b	NFkB, IRAK, TRAF6
149	SRC, Rac, Rap1 a/b
195-5p	cyclin E1, Raf1, Ccdn1
200	ZEB1/2
223	STAT5
302	CXCR4
335	SOX4, tenascin-C, MERTK, PTPRN2
448	STAB1, amphiregulin, Twist, NFkB

Figure 5. miRNAs involved in breast cancer cell invasion. miRNAs can act as either inducers or inhibitors of invasion by increasing (blue) or decreasing (red) the expression of various target genes as indicated.

miRNA-302a: expression levels of this miRNA was significantly decreased in metastatic breast cancer cell lines and tumor tissues, and enforced expression of miRNA302a significantly inhibited both *in vitro* and *in vivo* cell invasion, by inhibiting the CXCR4 gene [205].

miRNA-335: the expression of miRNA-335 and-126 was lost in human breast cancer tissues from patients who developed metastasis and relapse. Restoring miRNA-335 expression in highly metastatic breast cancer cell lines suppresses lung and bone metastasis *in vivo* through targeting of the progenitor cell transcription factor SOX4, the extracellular matrix component tenascin C, the c-Mer tyrosine kinase MERTK, and the receptor protein tyrosine phosphatase PTPRN2 [112].

5.2. miRNAs with pro-metastatic actions

miRNA-9: over-expression of miRNA-9 in human mammary epithelial cells and the human breast cancer cell line SUM149 resulted in significant increase in their motility and invasiveness *in vitro*, through E-cadherin suppression. In addition, it led to increased β-catenin activity as well as vascular endothelial growth factor (VEGFA) expression in MCF7-RAS breast carcinoma cells, with subsequent enhancement in their invasive capacity. Furthermore, miRNA-9 knockdown in the highly metastatic 4T1 mouse mammary tumour cells, inhibited lung metastasis formation when injected into the mammary fat pads of syngeneic immunocompetent mice *in vivo* [128].

miRNA-10b: the transcription factor TWIST induces the expression of miRNA-10b [206], which is highly expressed in metastatic breast cancer cells and correlates with poor clinical progression in patients with breast cancer. Transfection of the antisense inhibitor for miRNA-10b in MDA-MB-231 cells caused a significant reduction in the invasive properties of these cells. Moreover, over-expression of this miRNA in otherwise non-metastatic breast tumour cells (SUM149) initiates robust invasion and lung metastasis *in vivo* when injected into the mammary fat pads of immunodeficient mice, by enhancing the expression of the pro-metastatic gene RHOC [113]. In addition, miRNA-10b also targets another pro-metastatic gene which influences breast cancer cells; the guanidine exchanger factor for rac activation [T-lymphoma invasion and metastasis (TIAM1)] [207]. Furthermore, Ahmad *et al* [208] demonstrated increased expression of miRNA-10b in the primary breast cancer specimens of patients who subsequently developed brain metastasis compared to those who did not, suggesting that miRNA-10b could serve as a prognostic factor for brain metastasis in breast cancer patients and a potential target for anti-metastatic therapy.

miRNA-18b: expression of miRNA-18b was shown to be up-regulated in various breast cancer cell lines and in clinical specimens of breast tumors. Inhibition of miRNA18b in breast cancer cell lines significantly suppressed their invasive capacity by modulating several target genes including NLRP7, KLK3, OLFM3, POSTN, MAGED4B, KIR3DL3, CRX, SEMG1, and CEACAM5 [209].

miRNA-21: suppression of the oncogenic miRNA-21 in MDA-MB-231 significantly reduced invasion *in vitro* and lung metastasis *in vivo* through targeting of the tumour suppressor gene tropomyosin 1 (TPM1), maspin, tissue inhibitor of metalloproteinase 3 (TIMP3), and the programmed cell death 4 (PDCD4) [92,210,211]. In addition, miRNA-21 is involved in HER2/neu-induced cell invasion, which is mediated by the MAPK pathway [92].

miRNA-24: TGF-β treatment of breast cancer cell lines results in EMT and enhanced invasive capacity. Down-regulation of miRNA-24 expression resulted in suppression of the TGF-β-induced cell invasiveness through Net1A regulation [131].

Has-miRNA-30c: enhanced expression of has-miRNA-30c was observed in MDA-MB-231 compared to the poorly metastatic MCF-7 cells. Transfection of has-miRNA-30c into MDA-MB-231 cells significantly enhanced their invasive capacity towards conditioned osteoblast media, while transfection with anti-miRNA-30c had the opposite effect. This effect was due to targeting and inhibiting of NOV/CCN3, which has been described as an inhibitor of invasion [212].

miRNA-221/222: up-regulation of miRNA-221/222 in breast cancer is associated with malignancy and poor clinical outcome, while down-regulation of this miRNA is inversely correlated with metastasis [112,213,214,215]. Falkenberg *et al* [216] reported that miRN-221/222 is a significant prognostic marker for distinguishing sub-groups, particularly in advanced nodal (LN+) and HER2+breast tumors, and its over-expression in T47D, MDA-MB-231 and SKBR3 cell lines markedly enhanced their invasive capacity through targeting of the serine protease urokinase-type plasminogen activator (uPA).

miRNA-301a: a study by Ma *et al* [217] demonstrated that miRNA-301a was significantly up-regulated in primary tumor samples with a metastatic phenotype, as well as in metastatic breast cancer cell lines. *In vitro* over-expression of miRNA-301a in the non-invasive MCF-7 cells leads to significant enhancement in migration and invasion through targeting of PTEN and activation of the wnt/β-catenin signaling pathway, while its inhibition in the invasive MDA-MB-231 significantly decreased cell invasion. Furthermore, mice injected with miRNA-103a over-expressing MCF-7 cells displayed prominent lung metastasis, while mice injected with MDA-MB-231 cells pre-treated with miRNA-103a inhibitor reduced the degree of lung metastasis.

miRNA-373 and-520c: the expression of both these miRNAs (which are members of the same family and share similar seed sequence [218]) was significantly up-regulated in clinical breast cancer metastasis samples. Stable over-expression of miRNA-373 and-520c stimulated breast cancer cell migration *in vitro* and *in vivo* by the suppression of the cell surface glycoprotein CD44 through binding to the 3` UTR region of its mRNA [219]. In addition, miRNA-373 promotes cell invasion through targeting of sites in the promoter of E-cadherin mRNA [45].

miRNA-495: expression of miRNA-495 was significantly increased in both clinical breast cancer tissue samples compared to adjacent normal breast tissue as well as in MDA-MB-231 compared to MCF-7. Over-expression of miRNA-495 significantly enhanced invasive capacity of both cell lines, while its knockdown by miRNA-495 inhibitor showed the opposite effects. Its pro-metastatic effect was due to targeting and inhibiting of the JAM-A gene [220].

6. miRNAs implicated in breast cancer proliferation

Several miRNAs have been implicated in either enhancing or reducing cellular proliferation by targeting various mRNAs that encode proteins crucial to the process (Figure 6).

miRNA-21: this was found to be highly expressed in breast tumors compared to normal breast tissue biopsies. Suppression of miRNA-21 levels (using anti-miR-21 oligonucleotides) in MCF-7 suppressed cell growth in vitro as well as the tumor growth in the xenograft mouse model *in vivo*. This effect was associated with increased apoptosis, down-regulation of the anti-apoptotic protein bcl-2 [221], and modulation of several survival-related genes including ACTA2, APAF1, BTG2, FAS, p21, PDCD4, and SESN1 [211].

miRNA-22: it is highly expressed in ER-ve breast cancer cell lines and in clinical samples with mesenchymal phenotype. miRNA-22-mediates growth repression of ER+ve breast cancer cells and it might serve as a potential therapeutic agent in the treatment of ER+ve cancers [182].

miRNA-26a/b: a recent study by Tan *et al* [222] demonstrated that forced expression of miRNA-26a/b markedly inhibited E_2-stimulated proliferation of ER+ve breast cancer cells *in vitro* by modulating CHD1, GREB1 and KPNA2 target genes. miRNA26a/b depletion enhanced their proliferative capacity. In addition, injecting miRNA26a or by over-expressing MCF-7 breast cancer cells into nude mice, resulted in the formation of slower growing and significantly smaller tumors compared with tumors derived from untreated MCF-7 injected mice.

miRNA-27a: it has been suggested that miRNA-27a enhances the proliferation of breast cancer cell lines through targeting of genes that regulate the specificity protein transcription factors (Sp) which are often over-expressed in tumors and associated with enhanced proliferative and angiogenic capacity. Suppression of miRNA-27a (using anti-sense miRNA-27a) in MDA-MB-231 resulted in growth suppression through increased expression of Myt-1 and the zinc finger ZBTB10 gene (a putative Sp repressor), and increased levels of Sp1, Sp3, and Sp4. In addition, decreased expression of Sp-dependent survival and angiogenic genes, including survivin, VEGF and VEGF receptor 1 (VEGFR1) was also seen after miRNA-27a suppression [65].

miRNA-34c: the expression of miRNA-34c was significantly decreased in basal-like breast cancer cells (MDA-MB-231, MDA-MB-468 and BT-549) and was associated with poor prognosis. Its over-expression resulted in suppressed proliferation and increased cell death by influencing the cell cycle mainly by inducing an arrest in the G2/M phase and down-regulation of various cell cycle-regulators such as CCND1, CDK4 and CDK6. Furthermore, CDC23 was identified as an miRNA-34c-regulated target that could be responsible for the induction of cell cycle arrest [223].

miRNA-93: this miRNA induced MET in claudin-low SUM159 cells, and reduced their proliferation level through down-regulation of TGFβ signaling and multiple stem cell regulatory genes such as JAK1, STAT3, AKT3, SOX4, EZH1, and HMGA2. On the other hand, it enhanced the CSC population in MCF7 cultures that display a more differentiated phenotype, suggesting different effects based on cellular differentiation state [224].

miRNA-107: the expression of miRNA-107 was decreased in breast cancer specimens compared with adjacent normal tissues, and its over-expression significantly suppressed proliferative capacity, and induced arrest at G0/G1 phase in MDA-MB-231 cells. These effects were due to down-regulation of CDK8 target gene by miRNA-107 [195].

miRNA-124: expression of miRNA-124 was reduced in breast cancer tissues and inversely correlated with TNM stage and lymph node metastasis. Its over-expression in MDA-MB-231 and T47D cells significantly inhibited their growth and proliferative capacity. This was due to increased number of cells in the G0 and G1 phase and decreased number in the S, G2 and M phases [197]. The anti-proliferative function of miRNA-124 in MDA-MB-231 and MCF-7 cells was seen as a consequence of targeting and inhibiting the E26 transformation specific-1 (Ets-1) gene [225].

miRNA-145: expression of this miRNA was significantly lower in breast cancer cell lines, as well as in primary human breast tumors as compared with normal breast tissues. Transfection with a synthetic miRNA-145 precursor into several breast cancer cell lines produced a pro-apoptotic effect, which was dependent on p53-mediated transactivation of PUMA [183].

miRNA-195-5p: this miRNA was significantly down-regulated in breast cancer tissues compared to adjacent normal tissues, and over-expression of miRNA-195-5p in MDA-MB-231 cells inhibited their proliferative capacity and ability to form colonies, and caused G1 phase arrest by targeting of cyclin E1 (CCNE1) [202]. In addition, its over-expression also inhibited the proliferative capacity of MCF-7 cells by targeting of raf-1 and Ccdn1 genes [203].

miRNA-196a: over-expression of miRNA196a in various breast cancer cell lines led to reduction in their proliferative capacity by suppressing annexin A1 (ANXA1), a mediator of apoptosis and inhibitor of cell proliferation [226].

miRNA-206: introduction of miRNA-206 into MCF-7 cells inhibited cell growth in a dose-and time-dependent manner [188], in part through inducing a significant block in G1phase [191].

miRNA-221/222: by targeting the cell cycle inhibitor p27(Kip1) [216,227], miRNA-221/222 enhanced ER–ve breast cancer cell proliferation. In addition, it also increased ER+ve cell proliferation by stimulating cell transition from G1 to S phase [191]. Other reports have suggested that miRNA-221/222 is involved in the EGFR-RAS-RAF-MEK signaling pathway and down-regulates PTEN, leading to enhanced cell proliferation [228,229].

miRNA-486-5p: expression of miRNA-486-5p was reduced in breast cancer biopsies compared to adjacent non-neoplastic tissues, as well as in various breast cancer cell lines. Its over-expression in MDA-MB-231 and T47D significantly reduced their proliferative capacity *in vitro* by inducing G0/G1 arrest and promotion of apoptosis. Furthermore, its over-expression in MDA-MB-231 cells significantly inhibited xenograft tumor growth when injected subcutaneously into the right flank of nude mice. The oncogene PIM-1 was identified as a direct target of miRN-486-5p, suggesting that the miRNA-486-5p/PIM-1 axis might be a useful therapeutic target for prevention or treatment of breast cancer [230]. Zhao *et al* [231] demonstrated that over-expression of miRNA-486-5p in SKBR3 cells inhibits HER3 expression and lowers its downstream mediators, inhibits clonogenic potential, and enhances their sensitivity to trastuzumab or doxorubicin by repressing proliferative signal pathways mediated by HER3/HER2/PI3K/AKT.

miRNA-769-3p: Luo *et al* (2014a) have shown that culturing MCF-7 cells under hypoxic conditions followed by re-oxygenation enhanced the expression levels of various miRNAs such as miRNA-769-3p,-501-3p,-2276, and-1282. Over-expression of miRNA-769-3p significantly inhibited cell proliferation and enhanced apoptosis by targeting and inhibiting the expression of the NDRG1 gene, suggesting that miRNA-769-3p can functionally regulate NDRG1 during changes in oxygen concentration in breast cancer cells.

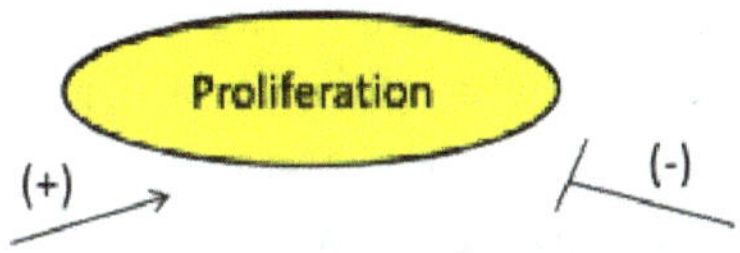

miRNA	Target (s)
21	PTEN, PI3K, Bcl2, ACTA2, APAF1, BTG2, Fas, p21, PDCD4, SESN1
27a	SP, myt-1, ZBTB10, survivin, VGED, VGEFR1
221/222	Kip1, PTEN, EGFR, RAS, RAF, MEK

miRNA	Target (s)
22	
24-2* strand	PCKα
26a/b	CHD1, GREB1, KPNA2
34c	CCND1, CDK4/6, CDC23
93	TGFβ, JAK1, STAT3, AKT3, SOX3, EZH1, HMGA2
107	CDK8
124	Ets-1
145	PUMA
195-5p	CCNE1, Raf1, Ccdn1
196a	ANXA1
206	G1-phase
486-5p	PIM1, HER2/3, PI3K/AKT
769-3p	NDRG1
Let-7	RB1, E2F, HRAS, HMGA2

Figure 6. miRNAs involved in breast cancer cell proliferation. miRNAs can act as either inducers or inhibitors of proliferation by increasing (blue) or decreasing (red) the expression of various target genes as indicated.

7. miRNAs controlling the biosynthesis of other miRNAs

An example of miRNAs regulating the expression levels of other miRNAs was reported by Martello *et al* [139]. They showed that miRNA-103/107 attenuated the global biosynthesis of other miRNAs through targeting of the RNase-III Dicer. miRNA103-107 also specifically down-regulated miRNA-200, which led to EMT, and subsequent enhancement in breast cancer cell invasion, but without major impact on primary tumor growth.

8. miRNAs as therapeutic agents

Several studies, as outlined above, have highlighted the contribution of various miRNAs in multiple processes of tumor pathogenesis (proliferation, invasion, EMT and endocrine/chemotherapy resistance), making them potential tools for applications as indicators in breast cancer diagnosis and staging, as markers of response to therapy and as therapeutic agents/targets for treatment. Unlike mRNAs, miRNAs (presumably due to their smaller size) are relatively stable in formalin fixed tissue specimens and in the blood stream, which facilitates their detection/measurement. There is opportunity to develop miRNA-based drugs that target specific oncomiRs or replace down-regulated miRNAs which have tumor suppressor properties. Unlike other nucleic acid, protein or small molecule drugs, many miRNAs (such as miRNA-31) have pleiotropic actions by which they can affect several related target genes; this can have a desirable cumulative effect that has obvious advantages in treating multifactorial diseases like cancer [194]. Of course it could also produce deleterious effects, so it is important to identify all the potential targets of particular miRNAs.

The value of using miRNAs as diagnostic and/or prognostic signature in breast cancer is currently receiving some attention. For example, miRNA-7,-128a, 210, and 516-3p can be used as markers for distant metastases of ER+ve, lymph node-ve breast cancer cases [214], while miRNA-210 can be used as marker for distant metastasis in triple –ve breast tumours [214,232,233]. Some miRNAs could be used as markers for disease survival in ER+ve (e.g. miRNA-128a,-135a, 767-3p) [234], ER–ve (e.g. miRNA-27b,-30c,-144,-150,-210,-342) [234], as well as in triple negative breast tumours (e.g. miRNA-21,-205,-210,-221,-222) [235,236]. Also, some miRNA such as-30a-3p,-30c, and-182 can be used as markers for response to adjuvant tamoxifen treatment in advanced ER+ve cases [237], while miRNA-21can predict the response to neoadjuvant trastuzumab treatment in breast cancer [213,238,239].

8.1. miRNA mimics

miRNA mimics, or replacement therapy, aims to restore normal levels of certain miRNAs that are down-regulated. They usually carry the same sequence as the missing or deficient naturally occurring miRNA. Introduction would be via viral or liposomal delivery [240].

8.2. Antagomirs

These are oligonucleotides that are chemically engineered to bind to a specific miRNA to prevent it from interacting with its mRNA target. To increase their stability, they can be chemically modified through the inclusion of 2′-O-methyl modified ribose sugars, 2′-O-methyl ribose sugars with the addition of an extra 2′-O, 4′C methylene bridge sugar [241,242,243,244]. An example of an important miRNA in breast cancer pathogenesis is miRNA-21, which is significantly up-regulated in breast tumors compared to normal tissue. Treatment of both ER +ve and ER-ve breast cancer cells with anti-miRNA-21 oligonucleotides suppressed both cell growth and migration *in vitro* and tumor growth in the xenograft mouse model *in vivo* [213,221]. Furthermore, miRNA-21 has the capacity to sensitize breast cancer cells to some anti-cancer agents such as topotecan and taxol [221]. Combination treatment of taxol with miR-

NA-21 inhibitor significantly decreased the 50% inhibitory concentration (IC50) of taxol in breast cancer cells when compared with taxol monotherapy. In addition, treatment of the miRNA-21 inhibitor-transfected cells with taxol resulted in significantly reduced cell viability and invasiveness compared with control cells [213]. Of note, the most developed miRNA-based agent to date is the miRNA-122 inhibitor for the treatment of hepatitis C virus [245], but before reaching clinical usage its interaction with other clinically used drugs should be extensively studied.

8.3. miR masks

Another range of compounds that are under development are known as target masks [246], of which there are several types. A target mask is conceptually an oligonucleotide whose sequence has been designed to bind either to an endogenous miRNA (miR sponge) or to its target on the mRNA (sponge miR mask). Whilst the binding of the sponge miR mask will prevent the binding of all miRNA belonging to the same seed family [247], (and is therefore miRNA seed specific and not gene specific), the miR mask blocks only a particular miRNA from interacting with its target mRNA.

These interactions are illustrated in Figure 7.

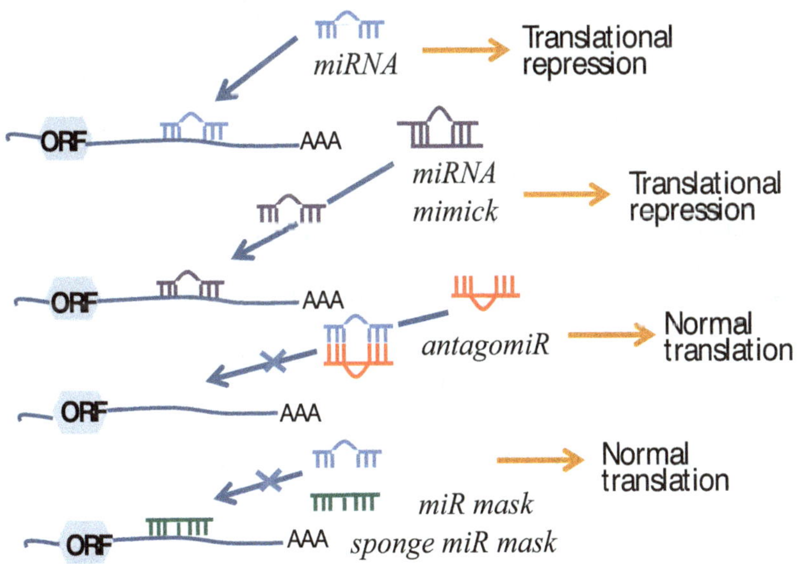

Figure 7. Manipulation of miRNA function. Endogenous miRNAs bind to target sequences in the 3′ UTR regions of their target mRNA, downstream of the open reading frame (ORF), to produce translational arrest. miRNA mimics are synthetic oligonucleotide duplexes that have the same sequence as the endogenous miRNA and also produce the same effect. Antagomirs (also called antimiRs) are oligonucleotides that have complementarity with the miRNA and bind to it, preventing it from interacting with its target mRNA, thereby allowing normal mRNA translation. An miR mask is a construct that is complementary to a sequence in the mRNA; this binding does not initiate mRNA degradation or translational inhibition but prevents the endogenous miRNA from binding. The sponge miR mask differs from the miR mask in that it binds to any mRNA with a similar target sequence and is therefore miRNA seed specific and not gene specific.

9. Summary

- miRNAs are endogenously synthesized single stranded RNA molecules that are 19-25 nucleotides in length, which play a vital role in the regulation of gene expression.
- Their exact mechanism of regulating gene expression is determined by the degree of complementarity with their target mRNAs; perfect complementarity usually results in mRNA degradation while permitted imperfect complementarity results in translational inhibition.
- miRNA biogenesis takes place in two phases; nuclear and cytoplasmic, both of which include events mainly carried out by Drosha, Argonaute and Dicer.
- The expression level of miRNA is mostly found to be down-regulated in cancers, and miRNA-155 was the first to be found to actually induce tumorigenesis.
- miRNAs are differently expressed in ER-ve *vs* ER+ve breast cancer cells; enhanced expression of miRNA-206,-221/222,-22, 150, and-29a was seen in ER-ve cells while enhanced expression of miRNA-200c,-130a-26a,-142-5b,-201,-205,-25,-21 and *let-7* family was seen in ER+ve cells.
- miRNA-221/222 targets and down-regulates ERα, induces EMT, and enhances breast cancer cell invasion and proliferation.
- miRNA-9,-24, and-155 induce EMT and enhance cell invasion.
- miRNA-7 and-44 inhibit EMT and decrease cell invasion.
- miRNA-124 and-145 inhibit EMT, and decrease cell invasion and proliferation.
- miRNAs could be used as non-invasive biomarkers for the diagnosis and prognosis, and as a promising therapeutic target for breast cancer.
- miRNA mimicks, antagomiRs and miR masks are being developed as new ways to interfere with miRNA regulation of gene translation in cancer cells.

Author details

Yunus A. Luqmani* and Maitham A. Khajah

*Address all correspondence to: yunus@hsc.edu.kw

Faculty of Pharmacy, Kuwait University, Safat, Kuwait

References

[1] Bartel DP (2004) MicroRNAs: genomics, biogenesis, mechanism, and function. Cell 116: 281-297.

[2] He L, Hannon GJ (2004) MicroRNAs: small RNAs with a big role in gene regulation. Nat Rev Genet 5: 522-531.

[3] Betel D, Koppal A, Agius P, Sander C, Leslie C (2010) Comprehensive modeling of microRNA targets predicts functional non-conserved and non-canonical sites. Genome Biol 11: 2010-2011.

[4] Wang J, Lu M, Qiu C, Cui Q (2010) TransmiR: a transcription factor-microRNA regulation database. Nucleic Acids Res 38: 28.

[5] Barroso-del Jesus A, Lucena-Aguilar G, Menendez P (2009) The miR-302-367 cluster as a potential stemness regulator in ESCs. Cell Cycle 8: 394-398.

[6] Klinge CM (2012) miRNAs and estrogen action. Trends Endocrinol Metab 23: 223-233.

[7] Yamakuchi M, Lowenstein CJ (2009) MiR-34, SIRT1 and p53: the feedback loop. Cell Cycle 8: 712-715.

[8] Lee RC, Feinbaum RL, Ambros V (1993) The C. elegans heterochronic gene lin-4 encodes small RNAs with antisense complementarity to lin-14. Cell 75: 843-854.

[9] Wightman B, Ha I, Ruvkun G (1993) Posttranscriptional regulation of the heterochronic gene lin-14 by lin-4 mediates temporal pattern formation in C. elegans. Cell 75: 855-862.

[10] Yang B, Lin H, Xiao J, Lu Y, Luo X, et al. (2007) The muscle-specific microRNA miR-1 regulates cardiac arrhythmogenic potential by targeting GJA1 and KCNJ2. Nat Med 13: 486-491.

[11] Luo X, Lin H, Pan Z, Xiao J, Zhang Y, et al. (2008) Down-regulation of miR-1/miR-133 contributes to re-expression of pacemaker channel genes HCN2 and HCN4 in hypertrophic heart. J Biol Chem 283: 20045-20052.

[12] Thum T, Gross C, Fiedler J, Fischer T, Kissler S, et al. (2008) MicroRNA-21 contributes to myocardial disease by stimulating MAP kinase signalling in fibroblasts. Nature 456: 980-984.

[13] van Rooij E, Sutherland LB, Thatcher JE, DiMaio JM, Naseem RH, et al. (2008) Dysregulation of microRNAs after myocardial infarction reveals a role of miR-29 in cardiac fibrosis. Proc Natl Acad Sci U S A 105: 13027-13032.

[14] van Rooij E, Sutherland LB, Qi X, Richardson JA, Hill J, et al. (2007) Control of stress-dependent cardiac growth and gene expression by a microRNA. Science 316: 575-579.

[15] Care A, Catalucci D, Felicetti F, Bonci D, Addario A, et al. (2007) MicroRNA-133 controls cardiac hypertrophy. Nat Med 13: 613-618.

[16] Najafi-Shoushtari SH, Kristo F, Li Y, Shioda T, Cohen DE, et al. (2010) MicroRNA-33 and the SREBP host genes cooperate to control cholesterol homeostasis. Science 328: 1566-1569.

[17] Xiao J, Luo X, Lin H, Zhang Y, Lu Y, et al. (2007) MicroRNA miR-133 represses HERG K+channel expression contributing to QT prolongation in diabetic hearts. J Biol Chem 282: 12363-12367.

[18] Fiore R, Siegel G, Schratt G (2008) MicroRNA function in neuronal development, plasticity and disease. Biochim Biophys Acta 8: 471-478.

[19] Furer V, Greenberg JD, Attur M, Abramson SB, Pillinger MH (2010) The role of microRNA in rheumatoid arthritis and other autoimmune diseases. Clin Immunol 136: 1-15.

[20] Zeng L, Liu J, Wang Y, Wang L, Weng S, et al. (2011) MicroRNA-210 as a novel blood biomarker in acute cerebral ischemia. Front Biosci 3: 1265-1272.

[21] Forero DA, van der Ven K, Callaerts P, Del-Favero J (2010) miRNA genes and the brain: implications for psychiatric disorders. Hum Mutat 31: 1195-1204.

[22] Lee Y, Kim M, Han J, Yeom KH, Lee S, et al. (2004) MicroRNA genes are transcribed by RNA polymerase II. Embo J 23: 4051-4060.

[23] Gregory RI, Yan KP, Amuthan G, Chendrimada T, Doratotaj B, et al. (2004) The Microprocessor complex mediates the genesis of microRNAs. Nature 432: 235-240.

[24] Lee Y, Ahn C, Han J, Choi H, Kim J, et al. (2003) The nuclear RNase III Drosha initiates microRNA processing. Nature 425: 415-419.

[25] Bohnsack MT, Czaplinski K, Gorlich D (2004) Exportin 5 is a RanGTP-dependent dsRNA-binding protein that mediates nuclear export of pre-miRNAs. Rna 10: 185-191.

[26] Hammond SM, Bernstein E, Beach D, Hannon GJ (2000) An RNA-directed nuclease mediates post-transcriptional gene silencing in Drosophila cells. Nature 404: 293-296.

[27] Liu J, Valencia-Sanchez MA, Hannon GJ, Parker R (2005) MicroRNA-dependent localization of targeted mRNAs to mammalian P-bodies. Nat Cell Biol 7: 719-723.

[28] Sen GL, Blau HM (2005) Argonaute 2/RISC resides in sites of mammalian mRNA decay known as cytoplasmic bodies. Nat Cell Biol 7: 633-636.

[29] Lee YS, Dutta A (2009) MicroRNAs in cancer. Annu Rev Pathol 4: 199-227.

[30] Di Leva G, Croce CM (2010) Roles of small RNAs in tumor formation. Trends Mol Med 16: 257-267.

[31] Olsen PH, Ambros V (1999) The lin-4 regulatory RNA controls developmental timing in Caenorhabditis elegans by blocking LIN-14 protein synthesis after the initiation of translation. Dev Biol 216: 671-680.

[32] Doench JG, Sharp PA (2004) Specificity of microRNA target selection in translational repression. Genes Dev 18: 504-511.

[33] Rhoades MW, Reinhart BJ, Lim LP, Burge CB, Bartel B, et al. (2002) Prediction of plant microRNA targets. Cell 110: 513-520.

[34] Bartel DP (2009) MicroRNAs: target recognition and regulatory functions. Cell 136: 215-233.

[35] Suzuki HI, Miyazono K (2011) Emerging complexity of microRNA generation cascades. J Biochem 149: 15-25.

[36] Martin EC, Elliott S, Rhodes LV, Antoon JW, Fewell C, et al. (2014) Preferential star strand biogenesis of pre-miR-24-2 targets PKC-alpha and suppresses cell survival in MCF-7 breast cancer cells. Mol Carcinog 53: 38-48.

[37] Ruby JG, Jan CH, Bartel DP (2007) Intronic microRNA precursors that bypass Drosha processing. Nature 448: 83-86.

[38] Okamura K, Hagen JW, Duan H, Tyler DM, Lai EC (2007) The mirtron pathway generates microRNA-class regulatory RNAs in Drosophila. Cell 130: 89-100.

[39] Curtis HJ, Sibley CR, Wood MJ (2012) Mirtrons, an emerging class of atypical miRNA. Wiley Interdiscip Rev RNA 3: 617-632.

[40] Diederichs S, Haber DA (2007) Dual role for argonautes in microRNA processing and posttranscriptional regulation of microRNA expression. Cell 131: 1097-1108.

[41] Yang JS, Lai EC (2010) Dicer-independent, Ago2-mediated microRNA biogenesis in vertebrates. Cell Cycle 9: 4455-4460.

[42] Ender C, Krek A, Friedlander MR, Beitzinger M, Weinmann L, et al. (2008) A human snoRNA with microRNA-like functions. Mol Cell 32: 519-528.

[43] Cole C, Sobala A, Lu C, Thatcher SR, Bowman A, et al. (2009) Filtering of deep sequencing data reveals the existence of abundant Dicer-dependent small RNAs derived from tRNAs. Rna 15: 2147-2160.

[44] Benhamed M, Herbig U, Ye T, Dejean A, Bischof O (2012) Senescence is an endogenous trigger for microRNA-directed transcriptional gene silencing in human cells. Nat Cell Biol 14: 266-275.

[45] Place RF, Li LC, Pookot D, Noonan EJ, Dahiya R (2008) MicroRNA-373 induces expression of genes with complementary promoter sequences. Proc Natl Acad Sci U S A 105: 1608-1613.

[46] Huang V, Place RF, Portnoy V, Wang J, Qi Z, et al. (2012) Upregulation of Cyclin B1 by miRNA and its implications in cancer. Nucleic Acids Res 40: 1695-1707.

[47] Brennecke J, Hipfner DR, Stark A, Russell RB, Cohen SM (2003) bantam encodes a developmentally regulated microRNA that controls cell proliferation and regulates the proapoptotic gene hid in Drosophila. Cell 113: 25-36.

[48] Ambros V (2003) MicroRNA pathways in flies and worms: growth, death, fat, stress, and timing. Cell 113: 673-676.

[49] Chen CZ, Li L, Lodish HF, Bartel DP (2004) MicroRNAs modulate hematopoietic lineage differentiation. Science 303: 83-86.

[50] Dostie J, Mourelatos Z, Yang M, Sharma A, Dreyfuss G (2003) Numerous microRNPs in neuronal cells containing novel microRNAs. Rna 9: 180-186.

[51] Wang Y, Keys DN, Au-Young JK, Chen C (2009) MicroRNAs in embryonic stem cells. J Cell Physiol 218: 251-255.

[52] Xu P, Vernooy SY, Guo M, Hay BA (2003) The Drosophila microRNA Mir-14 suppresses cell death and is required for normal fat metabolism. Curr Biol 13: 790-795.

[53] O'Connell RM, Rao DS, Chaudhuri AA, Baltimore D (2010) Physiological and pathological roles for microRNAs in the immune system. Nat Rev Immunol 10: 111-122.

[54] Lodish HF, Zhou B, Liu G, Chen CZ (2008) Micromanagement of the immune system by microRNAs. Nat Rev Immunol 8: 120-130.

[55] Taganov KD, Boldin MP, Chang KJ, Baltimore D (2006) NF-kappaB-dependent induction of microRNA miR-146, an inhibitor targeted to signaling proteins of innate immune responses. Proc Natl Acad Sci U S A 103: 12481-12486.

[56] O'Connell RM, Chaudhuri AA, Rao DS, Baltimore D (2009) Inositol phosphatase SHIP1 is a primary target of miR-155. Proc Natl Acad Sci U S A 106: 7113-7118.

[57] Thai TH, Calado DP, Casola S, Ansel KM, Xiao C, et al. (2007) Regulation of the germinal center response by microRNA-155. Science 316: 604-608.

[58] Rodriguez A, Vigorito E, Clare S, Warren MV, Couttet P, et al. (2007) Requirement of bic/microRNA-155 for normal immune function. Science 316: 608-611.

[59] Xiao C, Calado DP, Galler G, Thai TH, Patterson HC, et al. (2007) MiR-150 controls B cell differentiation by targeting the transcription factor c-Myb. Cell 131: 146-159.

[60] Li QJ, Chau J, Ebert PJ, Sylvester G, Min H, et al. (2007) miR-181a is an intrinsic modulator of T cell sensitivity and selection. Cell 129: 147-161.

[61] Greco SJ, Rameshwar P (2007) MicroRNAs regulate synthesis of the neurotransmitter substance P in human mesenchymal stem cell-derived neuronal cells. Proc Natl Acad Sci U S A 104: 15484-15489.

[62] Jopling CL, Yi M, Lancaster AM, Lemon SM, Sarnow P (2005) Modulation of hepatitis C virus RNA abundance by a liver-specific MicroRNA. Science 309: 1577-1581.

[63] Poy MN, Eliasson L, Krutzfeldt J, Kuwajima S, Ma X, et al. (2004) A pancreatic islet-specific microRNA regulates insulin secretion. Nature 432: 226-230.

[64] Cheng HY, Papp JW, Varlamova O, Dziema H, Russell B, et al. (2007) microRNA modulation of circadian-clock period and entrainment. Neuron 54: 813-829.

[65] Alvarez-Saavedra E, Horvitz HR (2010) Many families of C. elegans microRNAs are not essential for development or viability. Curr Biol 20: 367-373.

[66] Reinhart BJ, Slack FJ, Basson M, Pasquinelli AE, Bettinger JC, et al. (2000) The 21-nucleotide let-7 RNA regulates developmental timing in Caenorhabditis elegans. Nature 403: 901-906.

[67] Ketting RF, Fischer SE, Bernstein E, Sijen T, Hannon GJ, et al. (2001) Dicer functions in RNA interference and in synthesis of small RNA involved in developmental timing in C. elegans. Genes Dev 15: 2654-2659.

[68] Hatfield SD, Shcherbata HR, Fischer KA, Nakahara K, Carthew RW, et al. (2005) Stem cell division is regulated by the microRNA pathway. Nature 435: 974-978.

[69] Liu J, Carmell MA, Rivas FV, Marsden CG, Thomson JM, et al. (2004) Argonaute2 is the catalytic engine of mammalian RNAi. Science 305: 1437-1441.

[70] Mineno J, Okamoto S, Ando T, Sato M, Chono H, et al. (2006) The expression profile of microRNAs in mouse embryos. Nucleic Acids Res 34: 1765-1771.

[71] Chen CZ, Lodish HF (2005) MicroRNAs as regulators of mammalian hematopoiesis. Semin Immunol 17: 155-165.

[72] Lu J, Qian J, Chen F, Tang X, Li C, et al. (2005) Differential expression of components of the microRNA machinery during mouse organogenesis. Biochem Biophys Res Commun 334: 319-323.

[73] Harris KS, Zhang Z, McManus MT, Harfe BD, Sun X (2006) Dicer function is essential for lung epithelium morphogenesis. Proc Natl Acad Sci U S A 103: 2208-2213.

[74] Liu N, Olson EN (2010) MicroRNA regulatory networks in cardiovascular development. Dev Cell 18: 510-525.

[75] Small EM, Olson EN (2011) Pervasive roles of microRNAs in cardiovascular biology. Nature 469: 336-342.

[76] Zhao Y, Ransom JF, Li A, Vedantham V, von Drehle M, et al. (2007) Dysregulation of cardiogenesis, cardiac conduction, and cell cycle in mice lacking miRNA-1-2. Cell 129: 303-317.

[77] Sokol NS (2012) The role of microRNAs in muscle development. Curr Top Dev Biol 99: 59-78.

[78] Giraldez AJ, Cinalli RM, Glasner ME, Enright AJ, Thomson JM, et al. (2005) MicroRNAs regulate brain morphogenesis in zebrafish. Science 308: 833-838.

[79] Pauli A, Rinn JL, Schier AF (2011) Non-coding RNAs as regulators of embryogenesis. Nat Rev Genet 12: 136-149.

[80] Yoo AS, Staahl BT, Chen L, Crabtree GR (2009) MicroRNA-mediated switching of chromatin-remodelling complexes in neural development. Nature 460: 642-646.

[81] Gao FB (2010) Context-dependent functions of specific microRNAs in neuronal development. Neural Dev 5: 1749-8104.

[82] Krichevsky AM, King KS, Donahue CP, Khrapko K, Kosik KS (2003) A microRNA array reveals extensive regulation of microRNAs during brain development. Rna 9: 1274-1281.

[83] Smirnova L, Grafe A, Seiler A, Schumacher S, Nitsch R, et al. (2005) Regulation of miRNA expression during neural cell specification. Eur J Neurosci 21: 1469-1477.

[84] Schratt GM, Tuebing F, Nigh EA, Kane CG, Sabatini ME, et al. (2006) A brain-specific microRNA regulates dendritic spine development. Nature 439: 283-289.

[85] Lee CT, Risom T, Strauss WM (2006) MicroRNAs in mammalian development. Birth Defects Res C Embryo Today 78: 129-139.

[86] Li C, Feng Y, Coukos G, Zhang L (2009) Therapeutic microRNA strategies in human cancer. Aaps J 11: 747-757.

[87] Tang F, Kaneda M, O'Carroll D, Hajkova P, Barton SC, et al. (2007) Maternal microRNAs are essential for mouse zygotic development. Genes Dev 21: 644-648.

[88] Yu F, Yao H, Zhu P, Zhang X, Pan Q, et al. (2007) let-7 regulates self renewal and tumorigenicity of breast cancer cells. Cell 131: 1109-1123.

[89] Stenvang J, Silahtaroglu AN, Lindow M, Elmen J, Kauppinen S (2008) The utility of LNA in microRNA-based cancer diagnostics and therapeutics. Semin Cancer Biol 18: 89-102.

[90] Ichimura A, Ruike Y, Terasawa K, Tsujimoto G (2011) miRNAs and regulation of cell signaling. Febs J 278: 1610-1618.

[91] Inui M, Martello G, Piccolo S (2010) MicroRNA control of signal transduction. Nat Rev Mol Cell Biol 11: 252-263.

[92] Huang TH, Wu F, Loeb GB, Hsu R, Heidersbach A, et al. (2009) Up-regulation of miR-21 by HER2/neu signaling promotes cell invasion. J Biol Chem 284: 18515-18524.

[93] Christoffersen NR, Silahtaroglu A, Orom UA, Kauppinen S, Lund AH (2007) miR-200b mediates post-transcriptional repression of ZFHX1B. Rna 13: 1172-1178.

[94] Gregory PA, Bert AG, Paterson EL, Barry SC, Tsykin A, et al. (2008) The miR-200 family and miR-205 regulate epithelial to mesenchymal transition by targeting ZEB1 and SIP1. Nat Cell Biol 10: 593-601.

[95] Burk U, Schubert J, Wellner U, Schmalhofer O, Vincan E, et al. (2008) A reciprocal repression between ZEB1 and members of the miR-200 family promotes EMT and invasion in cancer cells. EMBO Rep 9: 582-589.

[96] Stephen AG, Esposito D, Bagni RK, McCormick F (2014) Dragging ras back in the ring. Cancer Cell 25: 272-281.

[97] Yang CH, Yue J, Pfeffer SR, Handorf CR, Pfeffer LM (2011) MicroRNA miR-21 regulates the metastatic behavior of B16 melanoma cells. J Biol Chem 286: 39172-39178.

[98] Lu Z, Li Y, Takwi A, Li B, Zhang J, et al. (2011) miR-301a as an NF-kappaB activator in pancreatic cancer cells. Embo J 30: 57-67.

[99] Ma X, Becker Buscaglia LE, Barker JR, Li Y (2011) MicroRNAs in NF-kappaB signaling. J Mol Cell Biol 3: 159-166.

[100] Permuth-Wey J, Thompson RC, Burton Nabors L, Olson JJ, Browning JE, et al. (2011) A functional polymorphism in the pre-miR-146a gene is associated with risk and prognosis in adult glioma. J Neurooncol 105: 639-646.

[101] Jazdzewski K, Murray EL, Franssila K, Jarzab B, Schoenberg DR, et al. (2008) Common SNP in pre-miR-146a decreases mature miR expression and predisposes to papillary thyroid carcinoma. Proc Natl Acad Sci U S A 105: 7269-7274.

[102] Ryan BM, Robles AI, Harris CC (2010) Genetic variation in microRNA networks: the implications for cancer research. Nat Rev Cancer 10: 389-402.

[103] Shen J, Ambrosone CB, DiCioccio RA, Odunsi K, Lele SB, et al. (2008) A functional polymorphism in the miR-146a gene and age of familial breast/ovarian cancer diagnosis. Carcinogenesis 29: 1963-1966.

[104] Yin JQ, Zhao RC, Morris KV (2008) Profiling microRNA expression with microarrays. Trends Biotechnol 26: 70-76.

[105] Costinean S, Zanesi N, Pekarsky Y, Tili E, Volinia S, et al. (2006) Pre-B cell proliferation and lymphoblastic leukemia/high-grade lymphoma in E(mu)-miR155 transgenic mice. Proc Natl Acad Sci U S A 103: 7024-7029.

[106] Kluiver J, Poppema S, de Jong D, Blokzijl T, Harms G, et al. (2005) BIC and miR-155 are highly expressed in Hodgkin, primary mediastinal and diffuse large B cell lymphomas. J Pathol 207: 243-249.

[107] Kluiver J, Haralambieva E, de Jong D, Blokzijl T, Jacobs S, et al. (2006) Lack of BIC and microRNA miR-155 expression in primary cases of Burkitt lymphoma. Genes Chromosomes Cancer 45: 147-153.

[108] Eis PS, Tam W, Sun L, Chadburn A, Li Z, et al. (2005) Accumulation of miR-155 and BIC RNA in human B cell lymphomas. Proc Natl Acad Sci U S A 102: 3627-3632.

[109] He L, Thomson JM, Hemann MT, Hernando-Monge E, Mu D, et al. (2005) A microRNA polycistron as a potential human oncogene. Nature 435: 828-833.

[110] Hatley ME, Patrick DM, Garcia MR, Richardson JA, Bassel-Duby R, et al. (2010) Modulation of K-Ras-dependent lung tumorigenesis by MicroRNA-21. Cancer Cell 18: 282-293.

[111] He L, He X, Lim LP, de Stanchina E, Xuan Z, et al. (2007) A microRNA component of the p53 tumour suppressor network. Nature 447: 1130-1134.

[112] Tavazoie SF, Alarcon C, Oskarsson T, Padua D, Wang Q, et al. (2008) Endogenous human microRNAs that suppress breast cancer metastasis. Nature 451: 147-152.

[113] Ma L, Teruya-Feldstein J, Weinberg RA (2007) Tumour invasion and metastasis initiated by microRNA-10b in breast cancer. Nature 449: 682-688.

[114] Hoppe R, Achinger-Kawecka J, Winter S, Fritz P, Lo WY, et al. (2013) Increased expression of miR-126 and miR-10a predict prolonged relapse-free time of primary oestrogen receptor-positive breast cancer following tamoxifen treatment. Eur J Cancer 49: 3598-3608.

[115] Roth C, Rack B, Muller V, Janni W, Pantel K, et al. (2010) Circulating microRNAs as blood-based markers for patients with primary and metastatic breast cancer. Breast Cancer Res 12: 3.

[116] van Schooneveld E, Wouters MC, Van der Auwera I, Peeters DJ, Wildiers H, et al. (2012) Expression profiling of cancerous and normal breast tissues identifies microRNAs that are differentially expressed in serum from patients with (metastatic) breast cancer and healthy volunteers. Breast Cancer Res 14.

[117] Heneghan HM, Miller N, Lowery AJ, Sweeney KJ, Newell J, et al. (2010) Circulating microRNAs as novel minimally invasive biomarkers for breast cancer. Ann Surg 251: 499-505.

[118] Tanic M, Andres E, Rodriguez-Pinilla SM, Marquez-Rodas I, Cebollero-Presmanes M, et al. (2013) MicroRNA-based molecular classification of non-BRCA1/2 hereditary breast tumours. Br J Cancer 109: 2724-2734.

[119] Eitan R, Kushnir M, Lithwick-Yanai G, David MB, Hoshen M, et al. (2009) Tumor microRNA expression patterns associated with resistance to platinum based chemotherapy and survival in ovarian cancer patients. Gynecol Oncol 114: 253-259.

[120] Hu Q, Gong JP, Li J, Zhong SL, Chen WX, et al. (2014) Down-regulation of miRNA-452 is Associated with Adriamycin-resistance in Breast Cancer Cells. Asian Pac J Cancer Prev 15: 5137-5142.

[121] Greenburg G, Hay ED (1982) Epithelia suspended in collagen gels can lose polarity and express characteristics of migrating mesenchymal cells. J Cell Biol 95: 333-339.

[122] Tse JC, Kalluri R (2007) Mechanisms of metastasis: epithelial-to-mesenchymal transition and contribution of tumor microenvironment. J Cell Biochem 101: 816-829.

[123] Al Saleh S, Sharaf LH, Luqmani YA (2011) Signalling pathways involved in endocrine resistance in breast cancer and associations with epithelial to mesenchymal transition (Review). Int J Oncol 38: 1197-1217.

[124] Al Saleh S, Al Mulla F, Luqmani YA (2011) Estrogen receptor silencing induces epithelial to mesenchymal transition in human breast cancer cells. PLoS One 6: 21.

[125] Berx G, Raspe E, Christofori G, Thiery JP, Sleeman JP (2007) Pre-EMTing metastasis? Recapitulation of morphogenetic processes in cancer. Clin Exp Metastasis 24: 587-597.

[126] Iorio MV, Ferracin M, Liu CG, Veronese A, Spizzo R, et al. (2005) MicroRNA gene expression deregulation in human breast cancer. Cancer Res 65: 7065-7070.

[127] Sun Y, Wu J, Wu SH, Thakur A, Bollig A, et al. (2009) Expression profile of microRNAs in c-Myc induced mouse mammary tumors. Breast Cancer Res Treat 118: 185-196.

[128] Ma L, Young J, Prabhala H, Pan E, Mestdagh P, et al. (2010) miR-9, a MYC/MYCN-activated microRNA, regulates E-cadherin and cancer metastasis. Nat Cell Biol 12: 247-256.

[129] Gwak JM, Kim HJ, Kim EJ, Chung YR, Yun S, et al. (2014) MicroRNA-9 is associated with epithelial-mesenchymal transition, breast cancer stem cell phenotype, and tumor progression in breast cancer. Breast Cancer Res Treat 147: 39-49.

[130] Derynck R, Akhurst RJ (2007) Differentiation plasticity regulated by TGF-beta family proteins in development and disease. Nat Cell Biol 9: 1000-1004.

[131] Papadimitriou E, Vasilaki E, Vorvis C, Iliopoulos D, Moustakas A, et al. (2012) Differential regulation of the two RhoA-specific GEF isoforms Net1/Net1A by TGF-beta and miR-24: role in epithelial-to-mesenchymal transition. Oncogene 31: 2862-2875.

[132] Schmidt A, Hall A (2002) The Rho exchange factor Net1 is regulated by nuclear sequestration. J Biol Chem 277: 14581-14588.

[133] Bao J, Zervos AS (1996) Isolation and characterization of Nmi, a novel partner of Myc proteins. Oncogene 12: 2171-2176.

[134] Li H, Lee TH, Avraham H (2002) A novel tricomplex of BRCA1, Nmi, and c-Myc inhibits c-Myc-induced human telomerase reverse transcriptase gene (hTERT) promoter activity in breast cancer. J Biol Chem 277: 20965-20973.

[135] Devine DJ, Rostas JW, Metge BJ, Das S, Mulekar MS, et al. (2014) Loss of N-Myc interactor promotes epithelial-mesenchymal transition by activation of TGF-beta/SMAD signaling. Oncogene 33: 2620-2628.

[136] Rostas JW, 3rd, Pruitt HC, Metge BJ, Mitra A, Bailey SK, et al. (2014) microRNA-29 negatively regulates EMT regulator N-myc interactor in breast cancer. Mol Cancer 13: 200.

[137] Gebeshuber CA, Zatloukal K, Martinez J (2009) miR-29a suppresses tristetraprolin, which is a regulator of epithelial polarity and metastasis. EMBO Rep 10: 400-405.

[138] Grelier G, Voirin N, Ay AS, Cox DG, Chabaud S, et al. (2009) Prognostic value of Dicer expression in human breast cancers and association with the mesenchymal phenotype. Br J Cancer 101: 673-683.

[139] Martello G, Rosato A, Ferrari F, Manfrin A, Cordenonsi M, et al. (2010) A MicroRNA targeting dicer for metastasis control. Cell 141: 1195-1207.

[140] Smith AL, Iwanaga R, Drasin DJ, Micalizzi DS, Vartuli RL, et al. (2012) The miR-106b-25 cluster targets Smad7, activates TGF-beta signaling, and induces EMT and tumor initiating cell characteristics downstream of Six1 in human breast cancer. Oncogene 31: 5162-5171.

[141] Johansson J, Berg T, Kurzejamska E, Pang MF, Tabor V, et al. (2013) MiR-155-mediated loss of C/EBPbeta shifts the TGF-beta response from growth inhibition to epithelial-mesenchymal transition, invasion and metastasis in breast cancer. Oncogene 32: 5614-5624.

[142] Hwang MS, Yu N, Stinson SY, Yue P, Newman RJ, et al. (2013) miR-221/222 targets adiponectin receptor 1 to promote the epithelial-to-mesenchymal transition in breast cancer. PLoS One 8: 2013.

[143] Stinson S, Lackner MR, Adai AT, Yu N, Kim HJ, et al. (2011) TRPS1 targeting by miR-221/222 promotes the epithelial-to-mesenchymal transition in breast cancer. Sci Signal 4: 2001538.

[144] Stinson S, Lackner MR, Adai AT, Yu N, Kim HJ, et al. (2011) miR-221/222 targeting of trichorhinophalangeal 1 (TRPS1) promotes epithelial-to-mesenchymal transition in breast cancer. Sci Signal 4: 2002258.

[145] Lambertini E, Lolli A, Vezzali F, Penolazzi L, Gambari R, et al. (2012) Correlation between Slug transcription factor and miR-221 in MDA-MB-231 breast cancer cells. BMC Cancer 12: 1471-2407.

[146] Wei Y, Lai X, Yu S, Chen S, Ma Y, et al. (2014) Exosomal miR-221/222 enhances tamoxifen resistance in recipient ER-positive breast cancer cells. Breast Cancer Res Treat 2014: 10.

[147] Zhang H, Cai K, Wang J, Wang X, Cheng K, et al. (2014) MiR-7, inhibited indirectly by LincRNA HOTAIR, directly inhibits SETDB1 and reverses the EMT of breast cancer stem cells by downregulating the STAT3 pathway. Stem Cells 2014.

[148] Liang YJ, Wang QY, Zhou CX, Yin QQ, He M, et al. (2013) MiR-124 targets Slug to regulate epithelial-mesenchymal transition and metastasis of breast cancer. Carcinogenesis 34: 713-722.

[149] Hu J, Guo H, Li H, Liu Y, Liu J, et al. (2012) MiR-145 regulates epithelial to mesenchymal transition of breast cancer cells by targeting Oct4. PLoS One 7: 26.

[150] Peinado H, Portillo F, Cano A (2004) Transcriptional regulation of cadherins during development and carcinogenesis. Int J Dev Biol 48: 365-375.

[151] Korpal M, Lee ES, Hu G, Kang Y (2008) The miR-200 family inhibits epithelial-mesenchymal transition and cancer cell migration by direct targeting of E-cadherin transcriptional repressors ZEB1 and ZEB2. J Biol Chem 283: 14910-14914.

[152] Park SM, Gaur AB, Lengyel E, Peter ME (2008) The miR-200 family determines the epithelial phenotype of cancer cells by targeting the E-cadherin repressors ZEB1 and ZEB2. Genes Dev 22: 894-907.

[153] Chen Y, Sun Y, Chen L, Xu X, Zhang X, et al. (2013) miRNA-200c increases the sensitivity of breast cancer cells to doxorubicin through the suppression of E-cadherin-mediated PTEN/Akt signaling. Mol Med Rep 7: 1579-1584.

[154] Ward A, Balwierz A, Zhang JD, Kublbeck M, Pawitan Y, et al. (2013) Re-expression of microRNA-375 reverses both tamoxifen resistance and accompanying EMT-like properties in breast cancer. Oncogene 32: 1173-1182.

[155] Li QQ, Chen ZQ, Cao XX, Xu JD, Xu JW, et al. (2011) Involvement of NF-kappaB/miR-448 regulatory feedback loop in chemotherapy-induced epithelial-mesenchymal transition of breast cancer cells. Cell Death Differ 18: 16-25.

[156] Berger C, Qian Y, Chen X (2013) The p53-estrogen receptor loop in cancer. Curr Mol Med 13: 1229-1240.

[157] Turner N, Moretti E, Siclari O, Migliaccio I, Santarpia L, et al. (2013) Targeting triple negative breast cancer: is p53 the answer? Cancer Treat Rev 39: 541-550.

[158] Kim T, Veronese A, Pichiorri F, Lee TJ, Jeon YJ, et al. (2011) p53 regulates epithelial-mesenchymal transition through microRNAs targeting ZEB1 and ZEB2. J Exp Med 208: 875-883.

[159] Piovan C, Palmieri D, Di Leva G, Braccioli L, Casalini P, et al. (2012) Oncosuppressive role of p53-induced miR-205 in triple negative breast cancer. Mol Oncol 6: 458-472.

[160] Sandhu R, Rein J, D'Arcy M, Herschkowitz JI, Hoadley KA, et al. (2014) Over-expression of miR-146a in basal-like breast cancer cells confers enhanced tumorigenic potential in association with altered p53 status. Carcinogenesis 2014.

[161] Adamo V, Iorfida M, Montalto E, Festa V, Garipoli C, et al. (2007) Overview and new strategies in metastatic breast cancer (MBC) for treatment of tamoxifen-resistant patients. Ann Oncol 18: vi53-57.

[162] Peppercorn J, Perou CM, Carey LA (2008) Molecular subtypes in breast cancer evaluation and management: divide and conquer. Cancer Invest 26: 1-10.

[163] Kouros-Mehr H, Kim JW, Bechis SK, Werb Z (2008) GATA-3 and the regulation of the mammary luminal cell fate. Curr Opin Cell Biol 20: 164-170.

[164] Bernardo GM, Lozada KL, Miedler JD, Harburg G, Hewitt SC, et al. (2010) FOXA1 is an essential determinant of ERalpha expression and mammary ductal morphogenesis. Development 137: 2045-2054.

[165] Yan W, Cao QJ, Arenas RB, Bentley B, Shao R (2010) GATA3 inhibits breast cancer metastasis through the reversal of epithelial-mesenchymal transition. J Biol Chem 285: 14042-14051.

[166] Proia TA, Keller PJ, Gupta PB, Klebba I, Jones AD, et al. (2011) Genetic predisposition directs breast cancer phenotype by dictating progenitor cell fate. Cell Stem Cell 8: 149-163.

[167] Dhasarathy A, Kajita M, Wade PA (2007) The transcription factor snail mediates epithelial to mesenchymal transitions by repression of estrogen receptor-alpha. Mol Endocrinol 21: 2907-2918.

[168] Ito I, Hanyu A, Wayama M, Goto N, Katsuno Y, et al. (2010) Estrogen inhibits transforming growth factor beta signaling by promoting Smad2/3 degradation. J Biol Chem 285: 14747-14755.

[169] Wang X, Belguise K, O'Neill CF, Sanchez-Morgan N, Romagnoli M, et al. (2009) RelB NF-kappaB represses estrogen receptor alpha expression via induction of the zinc finger protein Blimp1. Mol Cell Biol 29: 3832-3844.

[170] Wang X, Belguise K, Kersual N, Kirsch KH, Mineva ND, et al. (2007) Oestrogen signalling inhibits invasive phenotype by repressing RelB and its target BCL2. Nat Cell Biol 9: 470-478.

[171] Khajah MA, Al Saleh S, Mathew PM, Luqmani YA (2012) Differential effect of growth factors on invasion and proliferation of endocrine resistant breast cancer cells. PLoS One 7: 30.

[172] Luqmani YA, Al Azmi A, Al Bader M, Abraham G, El Zawahri M (2009) Modification of gene expression induced by siRNA targeting of estrogen receptor alpha in MCF7 human breast cancer cells. Int J Oncol 34: 231-242.

[173] Ye Y, Xiao Y, Wang W, Yearsley K, Gao JX, et al. (2010) ERalpha signaling through slug regulates E-cadherin and EMT. Oncogene 29: 1451-1462.

[174] Volinia S, Calin GA, Liu CG, Ambs S, Cimmino A, et al. (2006) A microRNA expression signature of human solid tumors defines cancer gene targets. Proc Natl Acad Sci U S A 103: 2257-2261.

[175] Bhat-Nakshatri P, Wang G, Collins NR, Thomson MJ, Geistlinger TR, et al. (2009) Estradiol-regulated microRNAs control estradiol response in breast cancer cells. Nucleic Acids Res 37: 4850-4861.

[176] Cochrane DR, Cittelly DM, Howe EN, Spoelstra NS, McKinsey EL, et al. (2010) MicroRNAs link estrogen receptor alpha status and Dicer levels in breast cancer. Horm Cancer 1: 306-319.

[177] Forman JJ, Legesse-Miller A, Coller HA (2008) A search for conserved sequences in coding regions reveals that the let-7 microRNA targets Dicer within its coding sequence. Proc Natl Acad Sci U S A 105: 14879-14884.

[178] Tokumaru S, Suzuki M, Yamada H, Nagino M, Takahashi T (2008) let-7 regulates Dicer expression and constitutes a negative feedback loop. Carcinogenesis 29: 2073-2077.

[179] Cheng C, Fu X, Alves P, Gerstein M (2009) mRNA expression profiles show differential regulatory effects of microRNAs between estrogen receptor-positive and estrogen receptor-negative breast cancer. Genome Biol 10: 2009-2010.

[180] Adams BD, Claffey KP, White BA (2009) Argonaute-2 expression is regulated by epidermal growth factor receptor and mitogen-activated protein kinase signaling and correlates with a transformed phenotype in breast cancer cells. Endocrinology 150: 14-23.

[181] Pandey DP, Picard D (2009) miR-22 inhibits estrogen signaling by directly targeting the estrogen receptor alpha mRNA. Mol Cell Biol 29: 3783-3790.

[182] Xiong J, Yu D, Wei N, Fu H, Cai T, et al. (2010) An estrogen receptor alpha suppressor, microRNA-22, is downregulated in estrogen receptor alpha-positive human breast cancer cell lines and clinical samples. Febs J 277: 1684-1694.

[183] Spizzo R, Nicoloso MS, Lupini L, Lu Y, Fogarty J, et al. (2010) miR-145 participates with TP53 in a death-promoting regulatory loop and targets estrogen receptor-alpha in human breast cancer cells. Cell Death Differ 17: 246-254.

[184] Adams BD, Cowee DM, White BA (2009) The role of miR-206 in the epidermal growth factor (EGF) induced repression of estrogen receptor-alpha (ERalpha) signaling and a luminal phenotype in MCF-7 breast cancer cells. Mol Endocrinol 23: 1215-1230.

[185] Adams BD, Furneaux H, White BA (2007) The micro-ribonucleic acid (miRNA) miR-206 targets the human estrogen receptor-alpha (ERalpha) and represses ERalpha

messenger RNA and protein expression in breast cancer cell lines. Mol Endocrinol 21: 1132-1147.

[186] O'Day E, Lal A (2010) MicroRNAs and their target gene networks in breast cancer. Breast Cancer Res 12: 19.

[187] Yoshimoto N, Toyama T, Takahashi S, Sugiura H, Endo Y, et al. (2011) Distinct expressions of microRNAs that directly target estrogen receptor alpha in human breast cancer. Breast Cancer Res Treat 130: 331-339.

[188] Kondo N, Toyama T, Sugiura H, Fujii Y, Yamashita H (2008) miR-206 Expression is down-regulated in estrogen receptor alpha-positive human breast cancer. Cancer Res 68: 5004-5008.

[189] Iliopoulos D, Hirsch HA, Struhl K (2009) An epigenetic switch involving NF-kappaB, Lin28, Let-7 MicroRNA, and IL6 links inflammation to cell transformation. Cell 139: 693-706.

[190] Iliopoulos D, Hirsch HA, Wang G, Struhl K (2011) Inducible formation of breast cancer stem cells and their dynamic equilibrium with non-stem cancer cells via IL6 secretion. Proc Natl Acad Sci U S A 108: 1397-1402.

[191] Di Leva G, Gasparini P, Piovan C, Ngankeu A, Garofalo M, et al. (2010) MicroRNA cluster 221-222 and estrogen receptor alpha interactions in breast cancer. J Natl Cancer Inst 102: 706-721.

[192] Okuda H, Xing F, Pandey PR, Sharma S, Watabe M, et al. (2013) miR-7 suppresses brain metastasis of breast cancer stem-like cells by modulating KLF4. Cancer Res 73: 1434-1444.

[193] Krutilina R, Sun W, Sethuraman A, Brown M, Seagroves TN, et al. (2014) MicroRNA-18a inhibits hypoxia-inducible factor 1-alpha activity and lung metastasis in basal breast cancers. Breast Cancer Res 16.

[194] Valastyan S, Reinhardt F, Benaich N, Calogrias D, Szasz AM, et al. (2009) A pleiotropically acting microRNA, miR-31, inhibits breast cancer metastasis. Cell 137: 1032-1046.

[195] Li XY, Luo QF, Wei CK, Li DF, Li J, et al. (2014) MiRNA-107 inhibits proliferation and migration by targeting CDK8 in breast cancer. Int J Clin Exp Med 7: 32-40.

[196] Lv XB, Jiao Y, Qing Y, Hu H, Cui X, et al. (2011) miR-124 suppresses multiple steps of breast cancer metastasis by targeting a cohort of pro-metastatic genes in vitro. Chin J Cancer 30: 821-830.

[197] Li L, Luo J, Wang B, Wang D, Xie X, et al. (2013) Microrna-124 targets flotillin-1 to regulate proliferation and migration in breast cancer. Mol Cancer 12: 1476-4598.

[198] Gotte M, Mohr C, Koo CY, Stock C, Vaske AK, et al. (2010) miR-145-dependent targeting of junctional adhesion molecule A and modulation of fascin expression are as-

sociated with reduced breast cancer cell motility and invasiveness. Oncogene 29: 6569-6580.

[199] Sachdeva M, Mo YY (2010) MicroRNA-145 suppresses cell invasion and metastasis by directly targeting mucin 1. Cancer Res 70: 378-387.

[200] Bhaumik D, Scott GK, Schokrpur S, Patil CK, Campisi J, et al. (2008) Expression of microRNA-146 suppresses NF-kappaB activity with reduction of metastatic potential in breast cancer cells. Oncogene 27: 5643-5647.

[201] Bischoff A, Huck B, Keller B, Strotbek M, Schmid S, et al. (2014) miR-149 functions as a tumor suppressor by controlling breast epithelial cell migration and invasion. Cancer Res 2014: 2013.

[202] Luo Q, Wei C, Li X, Li J, Chen L, et al. (2014) MicroRNA-195-5p is a potential diagnostic and therapeutic target for breast cancer. Oncol Rep 31: 1096-1102.

[203] Li D, Zhao Y, Liu C, Chen X, Qi Y, et al. (2011) Analysis of MiR-195 and MiR-497 expression, regulation and role in breast cancer. Clin Cancer Res 17: 1722-1730.

[204] Pinatel EM, Orso F, Penna E, Cimino D, Elia AR, et al. (2014) miR-223 is a coordinator of breast cancer progression as revealed by bioinformatics predictions. PLoS One 9: 2014.

[205] Liang Z, Bian X, Shim H (2014) Inhibition of breast cancer metastasis with microRNA-302a by downregulation of CXCR4 expression. Breast Cancer Res Treat 146: 535-542.

[206] Yang J, Mani SA, Weinberg RA (2006) Exploring a new twist on tumor metastasis. Cancer Res 66: 4549-4552.

[207] Moriarty CH, Pursell B, Mercurio AM (2010) miR-10b targets Tiam1: implications for Rac activation and carcinoma migration. J Biol Chem 285: 20541-20546.

[208] Ahmad A, Sethi S, Chen W, Ali-Fehmi R, Mittal S, et al. (2014) Up-regulation of microRNA-10b is associated with the development of breast cancer brain metastasis. Am J Transl Res 6: 384-390.

[209] Fonseca-Sanchez MA, Perez-Plasencia C, Fernandez-Retana J, Arechaga-Ocampo E, Marchat LA, et al. (2013) microRNA-18b is upregulated in breast cancer and modulates genes involved in cell migration. Oncol Rep 30: 2399-2410.

[210] Zhu S, Wu H, Wu F, Nie D, Sheng S, et al. (2008) MicroRNA-21 targets tumor suppressor genes in invasion and metastasis. Cell Res 18: 350-359.

[211] Frankel LB, Christoffersen NR, Jacobsen A, Lindow M, Krogh A, et al. (2008) Programmed cell death 4 (PDCD4) is an important functional target of the microRNA miR-21 in breast cancer cells. J Biol Chem 283: 1026-1033.

[212] Dobson JR, Taipaleenmaki H, Hu YJ, Hong D, van Wijnen AJ, et al. (2014) hsa-mir-30c promotes the invasive phenotype of metastatic breast cancer cells by targeting NOV/CCN3. Cancer Cell Int 14: 014-0073.

[213] Yan LX, Huang XF, Shao Q, Huang MY, Deng L, et al. (2008) MicroRNA miR-21 overexpression in human breast cancer is associated with advanced clinical stage, lymph node metastasis and patient poor prognosis. Rna 14: 2348-2360.

[214] Foekens JA, Sieuwerts AM, Smid M, Look MP, de Weerd V, et al. (2008) Four miRNAs associated with aggressiveness of lymph node-negative, estrogen receptor-positive human breast cancer. Proc Natl Acad Sci U S A 105: 13021-13026.

[215] Anastasov N, Hofig I, Vasconcellos IG, Rappl K, Braselmann H, et al. (2012) Radiation resistance due to high expression of miR-21 and G2/M checkpoint arrest in breast cancer cells. Radiat Oncol 7: 7-206.

[216] Falkenberg N, Anastasov N, Rappl K, Braselmann H, Auer G, et al. (2013) MiR-221/-222 differentiate prognostic groups in advanced breast cancers and influence cell invasion. Br J Cancer 109: 2714-2723.

[217] Ma F, Zhang J, Zhong L, Wang L, Liu Y, et al. (2014) Upregulated microRNA-301a in breast cancer promotes tumor metastasis by targeting PTEN and activating Wnt/beta-catenin signaling. Gene 535: 191-197.

[218] Bernstein E, Caudy AA, Hammond SM, Hannon GJ (2001) Role for a bidentate ribonuclease in the initiation step of RNA interference. Nature 409: 363-366.

[219] Huang Q, Gumireddy K, Schrier M, le Sage C, Nagel R, et al. (2008) The microRNAs miR-373 and miR-520c promote tumour invasion and metastasis. Nat Cell Biol 10: 202-210.

[220] Cao M, Nie W, Li J, Zhang Y, Yan X, et al. (2014) MicroRNA-495 induces breast cancer cell migration by targeting JAM-A. Protein Cell 2014: 30.

[221] Si ML, Zhu S, Wu H, Lu Z, Wu F, et al. (2007) miR-21-mediated tumor growth. Oncogene 26: 2799-2803.

[222] Tan S, Ding K, Li R, Zhang W, Li G, et al. (2014) Identification of miR-26 as a key mediator of estrogen stimulated cell proliferation by targeting CHD1, GREB1 and KPNA2. Breast Cancer Res 16.

[223] Achari C, Winslow S, Ceder Y, Larsson C (2014) Expression of miR-34c induces G2/M cell cycle arrest in breast cancer cells. BMC Cancer 14: 1471-2407.

[224] Liu S, Patel SH, Ginestier C, Ibarra I, Martin-Trevino R, et al. (2012) MicroRNA93 regulates proliferation and differentiation of normal and malignant breast stem cells. PLoS Genet 8: 7.

[225] Li W, Zang W, Liu P, Wang Y, Du Y, et al. (2014) MicroRNA-124 inhibits cellular proliferation and invasion by targeting Ets-1 in breast cancer. Tumour Biol 2014: 2.

[226] Luthra R, Singh RR, Luthra MG, Li YX, Hannah C, et al. (2008) MicroRNA-196a targets annexin A1: a microRNA-mediated mechanism of annexin A1 downregulation in cancers. Oncogene 27: 6667-6678.

[227] le Sage C, Nagel R, Egan DA, Schrier M, Mesman E, et al. (2007) Regulation of the p27(Kip1) tumor suppressor by miR-221 and miR-222 promotes cancer cell proliferation. Embo J 26: 3699-3708.

[228] Garofalo M, Di Leva G, Romano G, Nuovo G, Suh SS, et al. (2009) miR-221&222 regulate TRAIL resistance and enhance tumorigenicity through PTEN and TIMP3 downregulation. Cancer Cell 16: 498-509.

[229] Miller TE, Ghoshal K, Ramaswamy B, Roy S, Datta J, et al. (2008) MicroRNA-221/222 confers tamoxifen resistance in breast cancer by targeting p27Kip1. J Biol Chem 283: 29897-29903.

[230] Zhang G, Liu Z, Cui G, Wang X, Yang Z (2014) MicroRNA-486-5p targeting PIM-1 suppresses cell proliferation in breast cancer cells. Tumour Biol 2014: 8.

[231] Zhao Z, Li R, Sha S, Wang Q, Mao W, et al. (2014) Targeting HER3 with miR-450b-3p suppresses breast cancer cells proliferation. Cancer Biol Ther 15: 1404-1412.

[232] Camps C, Buffa FM, Colella S, Moore J, Sotiriou C, et al. (2008) hsa-miR-210 Is induced by hypoxia and is an independent prognostic factor in breast cancer. Clin Cancer Res 14: 1340-1348.

[233] Rothe F, Ignatiadis M, Chaboteaux C, Haibe-Kains B, Kheddoumi N, et al. (2011) Global microRNA expression profiling identifies MiR-210 associated with tumor proliferation, invasion and poor clinical outcome in breast cancer. PLoS One 6: 29.

[234] Buffa FM, Camps C, Winchester L, Snell CE, Gee HE, et al. (2011) microRNA-associated progression pathways and potential therapeutic targets identified by integrated mRNA and microRNA expression profiling in breast cancer. Cancer Res 71: 5635-5645.

[235] Radojicic J, Zaravinos A, Vrekoussis T, Kafousi M, Spandidos DA, et al. (2011) MicroRNA expression analysis in triple-negative (ER, PR and Her2/neu) breast cancer. Cell Cycle 10: 507-517.

[236] Sempere LF, Christensen M, Silahtaroglu A, Bak M, Heath CV, et al. (2007) Altered MicroRNA expression confined to specific epithelial cell subpopulations in breast cancer. Cancer Res 67: 11612-11620.

[237] Rodriguez-Gonzalez FG, Sieuwerts AM, Smid M, Look MP, Meijer-van Gelder ME, et al. (2011) MicroRNA-30c expression level is an independent predictor of clinical benefit of endocrine therapy in advanced estrogen receptor positive breast cancer. Breast Cancer Res Treat 127: 43-51.

[238] Gong C, Yao Y, Wang Y, Liu B, Wu W, et al. (2011) Up-regulation of miR-21 mediates resistance to trastuzumab therapy for breast cancer. J Biol Chem 286: 19127-19137.

[239] Qian B, Katsaros D, Lu L, Preti M, Durando A, et al. (2009) High miR-21 expression in breast cancer associated with poor disease-free survival in early stage disease and high TGF-beta1. Breast Cancer Res Treat 117: 131-140.

[240] Kota J, Chivukula RR, O'Donnell KA, Wentzel EA, Montgomery CL, et al. (2009) Therapeutic microRNA delivery suppresses tumorigenesis in a murine liver cancer model. Cell 137: 1005-1017.

[241] Krutzfeldt J, Rajewsky N, Braich R, Rajeev KG, Tuschl T, et al. (2005) Silencing of microRNAs in vivo with 'antagomirs'. Nature 438: 685-689.

[242] Elmen J, Lindow M, Schutz S, Lawrence M, Petri A, et al. (2008) LNA-mediated microRNA silencing in non-human primates. Nature 452: 896-899.

[243] Elmen J, Lindow M, Silahtaroglu A, Bak M, Christensen M, et al. (2008) Antagonism of microRNA-122 in mice by systemically administered LNA-antimiR leads to upregulation of a large set of predicted target mRNAs in the liver. Nucleic Acids Res 36: 1153-1162.

[244] Esau CC (2008) Inhibition of microRNA with antisense oligonucleotides. Methods 44: 55-60.

[245] Lanford RE, Hildebrandt-Eriksen ES, Petri A, Persson R, Lindow M, et al. (2010) Therapeutic silencing of microRNA-122 in primates with chronic hepatitis C virus infection. Science 327: 198-201.

[246] Wang Z (2009) MicroRna Intereference Technologies. DOI: 10.1007/978-3-642-00489-6_2, Springer-Verlag Berlin Heidelberg.

[247] Lewis BP, Shih IH, Jones-Rhoades MW, Bartel DP, Burge CB (2003) Prediction of mammalian microRNA targets. Cell 115: 787– 798.

2

Enantiomerically Pure Substituted Benzo-Fused Heterocycles — A New Class of Anti-Breast Cancer Agents

Joaquín M. Campos, M. Eugenia García-Rubiño, Nawal Mahfoudh and César Lozano-López

1. Introduction

With more than 10 million new cases each year cancer is at present one of the most devastating diseases worldwide with an immense affliction burden not only for affected individuals, their relatives and friends but also representing heavy challenges to health care systems (Steward & Kleihues, 2003). In the year 2000, cancer was responsible for 12% of nearly 56 million deaths worldwide and in many countries this percentage is even higher with more than a quarter of deaths attributable to cancer. Moreover, it is expected that cancer rates further increase by 50% to 15 million new cases in the year 2020, mainly due to steadily ageing populations in both developed and developing countries (Fresco et al., 2010).

In recent years, many studies have shown an association between cell cycle regulation and cancer inasmuch as the cell cycle inhibitors are being considered as a weapon for the management of cancer (Hajduch et al., 1999). Ultimately a great level of interest has arisen in the G_0/G_1 phase regulatory molecules such as cyclin D1, CdkIs, and p53 as potential therapeutic targets in diseases where control of inappropriate cellular proliferation would be a therapeutic benefit (Sherr, 1996).

Apoptosis is an essential physiological process throughout the life of multi-cellular organisms important in the development and in the maintenance of tissue homeostasis. Apoptosis is involved in controlling the cell number and proliferation during embryogenesis, deletion of activated lymphocytes at the end of the immune response, elimination of self-reactive lymphocytes, in controlled destruction of damaged, aged, infected, transformed, and other harmful cells (Nagata, 1997; Testa, 2004). Zivny et al. have recently reviewed the apoptotic pathways, molecules involved in the cross-talk between individual apoptosis pathways, apoptosis regulation as well as mechanisms of action of conventional anticancer drugs and new promising agents, which trigger directly or indirectly apoptosis of hematologic cancer cells (Zivny et al., 2010).

We report herein the synthesis and antiproliferative activities of purine derivatives **1-11** (Chart 2) against the cancerous MCF-7 and MDA-MB-231 human breast cancer cell lines and the corresponding normal one (MCF-10A) to define the *in vitro* therapeutic index (TI) as a measure of the selectivity. From a structural point of view, the compounds studied differ from others previously reported (Díaz-Gavilán et al., 2008b) by the addition of an extra halogen or PhS-groups on the purine ring. Finally the most active racemic compound (**1**) was resolved and the antiproliferative activity of its enantiomers was measured (López-Cara et al., 2011).

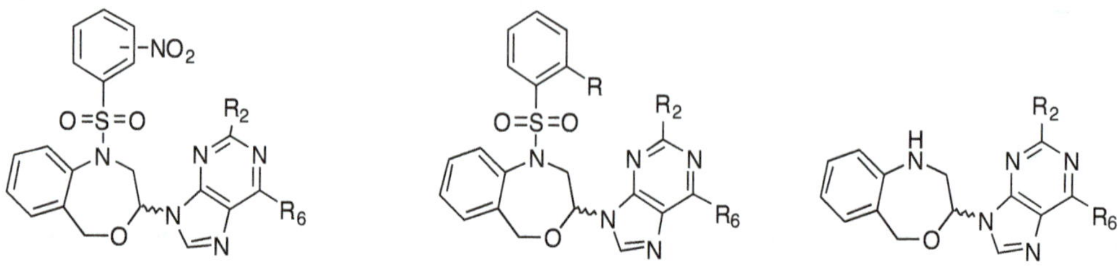

1 Isomer: *p*-NO_2, $R_2 = R_6 = Cl$
2 Isomer: *o*-NO_2, $R_2 = R_6 = Cl$
3 Isomer: *p*-NO_2, $R_2 = H$, $R_6 = Br$
4 Isomer: *o*-NO_2, $R_2 = H$, $R_6 = Br$

5 $R = NO_2$, $R_2 = Cl$, $R_6 = I$
6 $R = NH_2$, $R_2 = R_6 = Cl$
7 $R = NHOH$, $R_2 = R_6 = Cl$

8 $R_2 = R_6 = SPh$
9 $R_2 = Cl$, $R_6 = SPh$

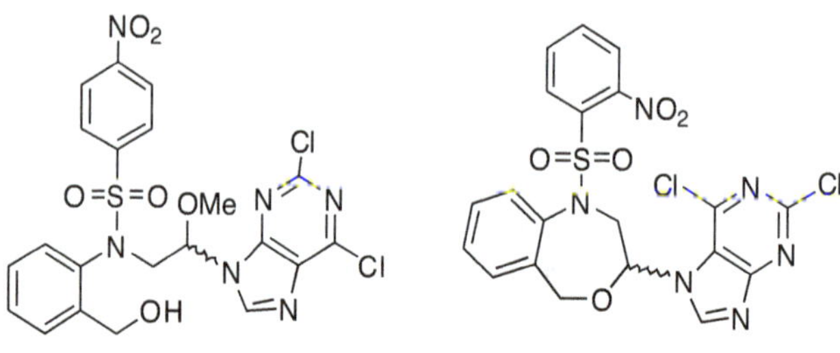

10 **11**

Chart 1. New cyclic (**1-9**) and acyclic (**10, 11**) purinic *O,N*-acetals (López-Cara et al., 2011).

Modern drug discovery relies on high speed organic synthesis. Microwave-assisted organic synthesis is proving to be instrumental for the rapid synthesis of compounds with new and improved biological activities (Al-Obeidi et al., 2003; Kappe & Dallinger, 2006). We previously investigated the Vorbrüggen condensation in microwave-assisted organic synthesis (Conejo-García et al., 2008). Microwave advantage is chiefly the quick access to the target molecules as well as the better yield obtained in the only isomer formed making the purification processes much easier.

2. The chiral switch from the benzo-fused seven-membered *O,N*-acetal (1)

Preparation of the *O,N*-acetals **1-4** was achieved by the microwave-assisted Vorbrüggen one-pot condensation of the cyclic acetals **12** and **13** (Díaz-Gavilán et al., 2004) and the commercially available purine bases 6-chloro-, 6-bromo-and 2,6-dichloro-purines, using chlorotrimethylsilane (TMSCl), 1,1,1,3,3,3-hexamethyldisilazane (HMDS) and tin(IV) chloride as the Lewis acid in anhydrous acetonitrile. The reaction mixture was microwave-irradiated at a temperature of 140 °C or 160 °C for 5 min (Scheme 1).

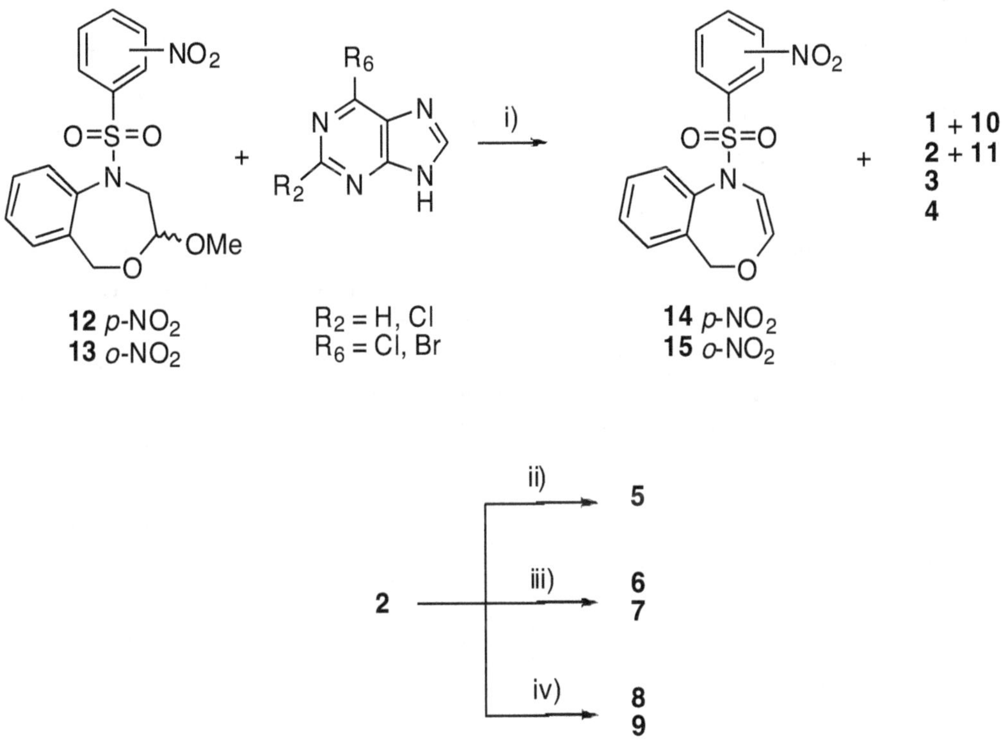

Scheme 1. *Reagents and conditions:* i) purine, TMSCl, HMDS, $SnCl_4$ (1 M solution in CH_2Cl_2), 140 or 160°C, microwave, 5 min; ii) NaI, TFA, butanone, -15°C, 6 hours; iii) $SnCl_2 \cdot 2H_2O$, EtOH, reflux, 2 hours; iv) PhSH, K_2CO_3, DMF, rt, 4 hours.

Compounds **14** and **15** were isolated from the reactions and the acyclic *O,N*-acetal **10** was also obtained in the synthesis of **1**. Traces of the *N*-7′ regioisomer **11** were detected in the synthesis of **2**. The following modifications were carried out on **2**: a) selective nucleophilic substitution of the chorine atom at position 6 of the purine ring using NaI and trifluoroacetic acid (TFA) to yield **5**; b) reduction of the nitro group with $SnCl_2$ to give rise to **6** and **7**; and c) the treatment with the PhSH to produce **8** and **9**.

Compounds **14** and **15** were obtained along with the cyclic and acyclic *O,N*-acetals in the reaction of purines with **12** and **13**, respectively. Their importance lies in the information that they provide of the mechanism of the reaction with purines (López-Cara et al., 2011).

2.1. Resolution of (*RS*)-1 into its eantiomers: Biological activities

The issue of drug chirality is now a major theme in the design and development of new drugs, underpinned by a new understanding of the role of molecular recognition in many pharmacologically relevant events. In general, three methods are utilized for the production of a chiral drug: the chiral pool, separation of racemates, and asymmetric synthesis. Although the use of chiral drugs predates modern medicine, only since the 1980's has there been a significant increase in the development of chiral pharmaceutical drugs. An important commercial reason is that as patents on racemic drugs expire, pharmaceutical companies have the opportunity to extend patent coverage through development of the chiral switch enantiomers with desired bioactivity (Núñez et al., 2009).

(*RS*)-9-[1-(*p*-Nitrobenzenesulfonyl)-1,2,3,5-tetrahydro-4,1-benzoxazepin-3-yl]-2,6-dichloro-9*H*-purine (**1**) is resolved into its two enantiomers: [(*R*)-**1**: $[\alpha]^{25}_{D}$=-43.6 (c=0.22, THF), and (*S*)-**1**: $[\alpha]^{25}_{D}$=+41.0 (c=0.23, THF];] using a semipreparative column CHIRALPAK® IA and a mixture of hexane/*t*-BuOMe/*i*PrOH as eluent (Marchal et al., 2010).

Table 1 shows the antiproliferative activity (IC_{50} values) for **1-11** and 5-fluorouracil (5-FU). All the compounds were first assayed as antiproliferative agents against the human breast adenocarcinoma cell line MCF-7 (p53 wild-type and ras mutated). Compounds (**1**, **2**, **5-7**, and **10**, **11**) were selected to be further assayed on the human breast cancer cell line MDA-MB-231, which has high levels of mutant p53, the most commonly mutated gene in human cancer. Additionally, we used a non-cancerous human mammary epithelial cell line (MCF-10A), in order to study the therapeutic index against breast cancer.

Compound	IC_{50} MCF-7 (μM)	IC_{50} MDA-MB-231 (μM)	IC_{50} MCF-10A(μM)
1	0.355 ± 0.011	0.166 ± 0.063	1.825 ± 0.503
2	0.383 ± 0.027	0.280 ± 0.006	1.530 ± 0.198
3	1.226 ± 0.348	N.D.[b]	N.D.[b]
4	3.618 ± 0.273	N.D.[b]	N.D.[b]
5	0.610 ± 0.043	0.256 ± 0.002	0.351 ± 0.020
6	0.820 ± 0.050	0.467 ± 0.017	1.520 ± 0.498
7	1.530 ± 0.040	0.487 ± 0.006	1.233 ± 0.217
8	9.710 ± 0.380	N.D.[b]	N.D.[b]
9	13.85 ± 1.790	N.D.[b]	N.D.[b]
10	0.355 ± 0.122	0.409 ± 0.074	1.863 ± 0.050
11	0.990 ± 0.090	0.318 ± 0.066	1.265 ± 0.163
5-FU	4.32 ± 0.020	N.D.[b]	N.D.[b]

[a]All experiments were conducted in duplicate and gave similar results. The data are means ± SEM of three independent determinations. The treatment time was 48 h.

[b]N.D.=Not determined.

Table 1. Antiproliferative activities[a] for compounds **1-11** and 5-FU against the cancerous cell lines MCF-7 and MDA-MB-231, and the non-cancerous cell line MCF-10A (López-Cara et al., 2011).

It must be pointed out that from the twenty IC_{50} values against the two cancerous cell lines, the majority of the IC_{50} values were below 1 μM. As shown in Table 1, all the compounds were more active as anti-proliferative agents against MDA-MB-231 than against the MCF-7 human breast cancer cell line, except for the acyclic derivative 10, whose anti-proliferative effect remains the same in both cancer cell lines. The IC_{50}=0.166 μM for compound 1 against the human cancerous cell line MDA-MB-231 stands out over the rest of the values.

A comparison between the cancerous cell lines (MCF-7 and MDA-MB-231) and the corresponding normal one (MCF-10A) was established in an intent to define the *in vitro* therapeutic index as a measure of the selectivity. The *in vitro* TI of a drug is defined as the ratio of the toxic dose to the therapeutic dose (*in vitro* TI=IC_{50} non-tumour cell line/IC_{50} tumour cell line) (Núñez et al., 2007). TI was better for compounds **1**, **2** and **11** against both cancer cell lines with values up to 11.0, 5.50 and 4.55, respectively against MDA-MB-231 cell line. 2,6-Dichloro derivatives **1** and **10** were the most selective compounds against the human breast adenocarcinoma MCF-7 cancer cell line (TIs=5.1 and 5.2, respectively) in relation to the normal one. The iodine derivative **5** showed the most toxic effect against the non-tumour MCF-10A human mammary epithelial cell line (Table 2).

Compound	Therapeutic index (TI)	
	MCF-7	MDA-MB-231
1	5.14	11.0
2	4.00	5.50
5	0.57	1.37
6	1.85	3.25
7	0.80	2.53
10	5.25	4.55
11	1.27	4.00

Table 2. Therapeutic indexes for the most representative compounds.

When the homochiral forms were analyzed we found differences in the IC_{50} values between (*S*)-**1** and (*R*)-**1** enantiomers, although no differences in activity were found between the two enantiomers against the MDA-MB-231 cell line. However both enantiomers present higher anti-proliferative activity than the racemic compound showing the greatest differences against MCF-7 cells. Enantiomer (*S*)-**1** shows higher anti-tumour activity, up to twice that of (*R*)-**1** in the MCF-7 cell line (Table 3). Studies with other compounds showed similar results with more potency in cytotoxicity in an enantiomer in comparison with the racemate. This enantioselective cytotoxicity indicates that the enantiomers of some chiral drugs may differ both quantitatively and qualitatively in their biological activity (Liu et al., 2009; Shelley et al., 1999). Moreover, enantiomers demonstrate minimal *in vitro* but a dramatic *in vivo* chiral dependency in their anti-tumour activities (Lai et al., 2007; Brown et al., 2010).

Compound	MCF-7 (μM)	MDA-MB-231 (μM)
(*RS*)-**1**	0.355 ± 0.011	0.166 ± 0.063
(*R*)-**1**	0.19 ± 0.001	0.11 ± 0.001
(*S*)-**1**	0.10 ± 0.001	0.11 ± 0.001

[a]All experiments were conducted in duplicate and gave similar results. The data are means ± SEM of three independent determinations.

Table 3. Anti-proliferative activities of (*RS*)-**1** and its enantiomers against the cancerous cell lines MCF-7 and MDA-MB-231.

Once the anti-tumour activity of compounds was determined against the different breast cell lines, we carried out a selection between those that showed a great cytotoxic effect against MCF-7, including (*R*)-**1** and (*S*)-**1**, in order to determine their influence on the several cell cycle phases. In this study we have included drugs used in clinic against breast cancer, such 5-FU and paclitaxel, with a known mechanism of action at the level of cell cycle.

In order to analyze if the anti-tumour effects of the drugs involve changes in cell cycle distribution, the non-tumour cell line MCF-10A and the breast cancer cell lines MCF-7 and MDA-MB-231 were treated with the compounds during 48 hours and then analyzed by flow cytometry. The non-accumulation in a specific phase was detected during treatment with the drugs in most of the cell lines analyzed in comparison with control-DMSO-treated cells. Only the (*R*)-**1** enantiomer was able to induce in MDA-MB-231 cells an accumulation in both G_0/G_1 and G_2/M phases with the consequently significant decreased in the S phase. Also an accumulation in the phase G_2/M was detected in MCF-7-**5** treated cells. Treatment with 5-FU and paclitaxel, as has been described previously (Grem et al., 1999), induced accumulation in the S or G_2/M phases depending on the cell line analyzed. Similar data were obtained when cell lines were treated for 24 hours with 0.5 mM mimosine to synchronize the cells in the G_1/S phase (data not shown). These results indicate that compounds inhibited all phases of the cell cycle, probably through the inhibition of protein synthesis as has been proved with other anti-tumour drugs (Duncan et al., 2009).

Finally, to determine if the observed growth inhibition was due to apoptosis, both flow cytometry and confocal microscopy studies were carried out. Cells were treated with the IC_{50} values of compounds and stained using Annexin V and propidium iodide (PI) at 24 and 48 hours post-drug treatment. Apoptosis assays were accomplished in the MCF-7 human breast cancer cell line, where the demonstration of programmed cell death by known apoptosis-inducing agents has proved difficult and only few cytotoxic agents act preferentially through an apoptotic mechanism in human breast cancer cells (Saunders et al., 1997; Chadderton et al., 2000). Paclitaxel (Taxol) induced programmed cell death of up to 43% of the cell population. Simultaneous staining with annexin V-FITC and the PI non-vital dye made it possible to distinguish between early apoptosis (stained positive for annexin V-FITC and negative for PI), and late apoptosis or cell death (stained positive for both annexin V-FITC and PI). In MCF-7 control-DMSO cultures neither early nor late apoptosis were detected after 24 h or 48 h. Similarly, compounds did not induce apoptosis after 24 h of treatment. In contrast, MCF-7 cells treated during 48 h with the novel compounds showed a significant increase of early apoptotic cells in relation to the control culture with percentages varying from 13.93% in cells treated with **11** to 43.30% and 41.99% after treatment with **10** and (*R*)-**1**, respectively. It should be noted that levels of early apoptosis induced by (*R*)-**1** were almost double in comparison with the corresponding racemic **1**, which may explain the enantioselective anti-proliferative activity shown by this enantiomer. These high apoptotic percentages shown by (*R*)-**1** are consistent with the G_1 and G_2/M arrest since cells exposed to specific agents typically enter apoptosis from a given phase of the cell cycle (Saunders et al., 1997; Marchal et al., 2004; Lundberg & Weinberg, 1999). Differences in cytotoxicity, cell cycle analysis or apoptotic levels between (*R*)-**1** and (*S*)-**1** suggest distinct signalling pathways as has been shown with other anti-tumour enantiomers (De Fátima et al., 2008). Moreover, it is possible that the amount of cells undergoing apoptosis in response to the compounds have been higher than these values, because only adherent cells were stained and counted.

The effects of compounds on the pattern of cell death were also confirmed by confocal microscopy after staining with FITC-conjugated annexin V and the nuclear non-vital stain PI. MCF-7 cells treated with compounds showed several staining patterns. Some cells displayed an intense FITC staining located at the plasma membrane and a nucleus with intensely PI-labelled marginated chromatin, suggesting that they were in the course of apoptosis. Other cells showed a peculiar staining pattern, because they exhibited nuclei with the same features observed in true apoptotic cells and, at the same time, cytoplasm homogeneously stained for annexin V. In fact, the FITC staining was located not only at the cell surface, but also within the cytoplasm. Therefore, these cells were considered as aponecrotic cells as has been previously established (Formigli et al., 2002). In addition, patches of localised partially condensed chromatin were found in other cells abutted along the inner part of the nuclear membrane. In the control cultures, most of the cells turned out to be negative for both staining except for some dying cells with the staining features of apoptosis (data not shown). The present data support the effect of the compounds in some of the series of steps of the apoptotic process where a wide range of intermediate morphological and biochemical types of cell death occurs (Marchal et al., 2004; Gooch & Yee, 1999).

Toxicity was determined selecting (*RS*)-**1**, which was the most in vitro cytotoxic compound against MCF-7 cells. We examined the acute-toxicity profile of (*RS*)-**1** in BALB/c mice when it was administered in a single i.p. bolus injection (n=25) at dose levels of 50, 75, 100, 150 and 200 mg/kg or *via* gavage (n=25) in a single p.o. bolus at dose levels of 0.05, 0.5, 5 and 50 mg/kg. Compound (*RS*)-**1** was nontoxic to BALB/c mice even at the highest i.p. bolus dose of 200 mg/kg and p.o. bolus dose of 50 mg/kg after 2 weeks. Control mice (n=10; 5 mice for the i.p. group and 5 mice for the p.o. group) were treated with the vehicle alone. All 50 (*RS*)-**1**-treated mice remained healthy and gained weight throughout the 15-day observation period, with no evidence of morbidity.

3. Purines linked to racemic benzo-fused six-membered heterocycles

Very recently, a series of 2-and 6-substituted (*RS*)-9-(2,3-dihydro-1,4-benzoxathiin-3-ylmethyl)-9*H*-purine derivatives (**16-26**, Chart 2) was obtained by applying a standard Mitsunobu protocol that led to a six-membered ring contraction from (*RS*)-3,4-dihydro-2*H*-1,5-benzoxathiepin-3-ol *via* an episulfonium intermediate (Díaz-Gavilán et al., 2008a). The most active compounds were **17** and **18** with IC_{50}=6.18 ± 1.70 and 8.97 ± 0.83 μM, against MCF-7 cells respectively. These results suggest that the presence of bulky substituents on position 6 of the purine ring reduces the anti-proliferative activity. An approach that has guided the origin of novel drugs is bioisosterism, which we have carried out as suitable structural modifications of the seven-membered building block, such as the modification O-1/S (Núñez et al., 2005; Núñez et al., 2007).

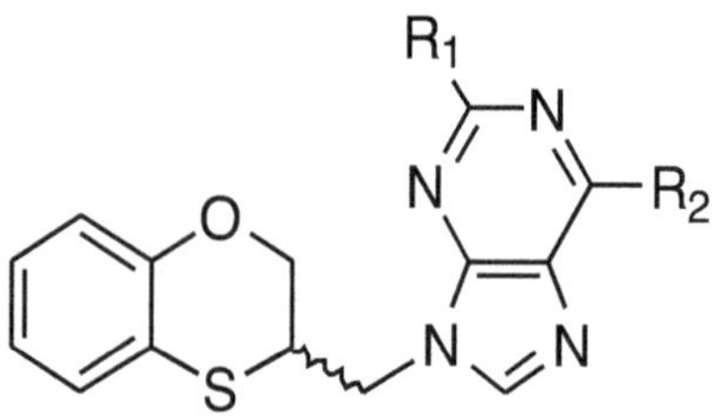

16 R_1 = H, R_2 = Cl
17 R_1 = H; R_2 = Br
18 R_1 = R_2 = Cl
19 R_1 = H; R_2 = SMe
20 R_1 = H; R_2 = OPh
21 R_1 = H; R_2 = SPh
22 R_1 = H; R_2 = NHPh
23 R_1 = H; R_2 = $OCH_2CH{=}CH_2$
24 R_1 = H; R_2 = OCH_2Ph
25 R_1 = H; R_2 = SCH_2Ph
26 R_1 = H; R_2 = $OCH_2C_6H_{11}$

Chart 2. Series of substituted (*RS*)-9-(2,3-dihydro-1,4-benzoxathiin-3-ylmethyl)-9*H*-purine derivatives **16-26** (Díaz-Gavilán et al., 2008a).

The design, synthesis and biological evaluation of two series of substituted (*RS*)-9-(2,3-dihydro-1,4-benzoxathiin-2-ylmethyl)-9*H*-purines **27-30** (Series A, Chart 3), and (*RS*)-9-(2,3-dihydro-1,4-benzodioxin-2-ylmethyl)-9*H*-purines **31-33** (Series B, Chart 3) have been described (Conejo-García et al., 2011). In series A, the methylene linker that connects the six-membered ring and the purine moiety has been changed from position 3 to 2 in relation to derivatives **16-26** (Chart 2). Series B is the isosteric group in which sulfur is replaced by oxygen. We will show the activity of these compounds in the inhibition of MCF-7 breast cancer cell growth to ascertain potential directions for synthetic lead-optimization studies.

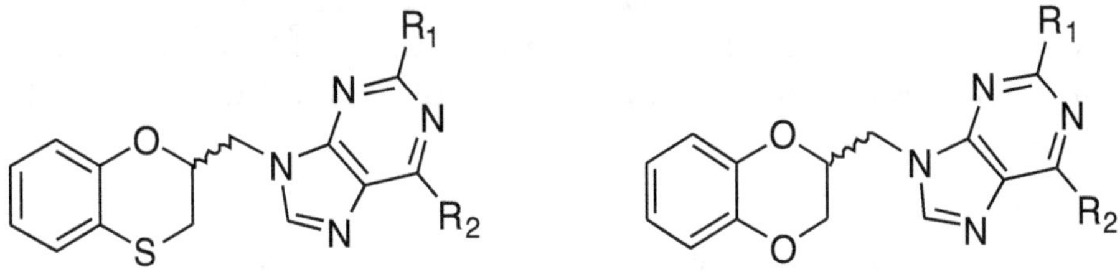

Series A
27 $R_1 = H; R_2 = Cl$
28 $R_1 = H; R_2 = Br$
29 $R_1 = R_2 = Cl$
30 $R_1 = H; R_2 = NH_2$

Series B
31 $R_1 = H; R_2 = Cl$
32 $R_1 = H; R_2 = Br$
33 $R_1 = R_2 = Cl$
34 $R_1 = H; R_2 = NH_2$

Chart 3. Substituted (*RS*)-9-(2,3-dihydro-1,4-benzoxathiin-2-ylmethyl)-9*H*-purines **27-30** (series A) and (*RS*)-9-(2,3-dihydro-1,4-benzodioxin-2-ylmethyl)-9*H*-purines **31-34** (series B).

The starting material (*RS*)-2,3-dihydro-2*H*-1,4-benzoxathiin-2-methanol (**35**) was prepared as previously reported (Díaz-Gavilán et al., 2008a) whilst (*RS*)-(2,3-dihydro-1,4-benzodioxin-2-yl)methanol (**36**) was synthesized by the reaction of cathecol with epichlorohydrin in NaOH and water (Díaz-Gavilán et al., 2007).

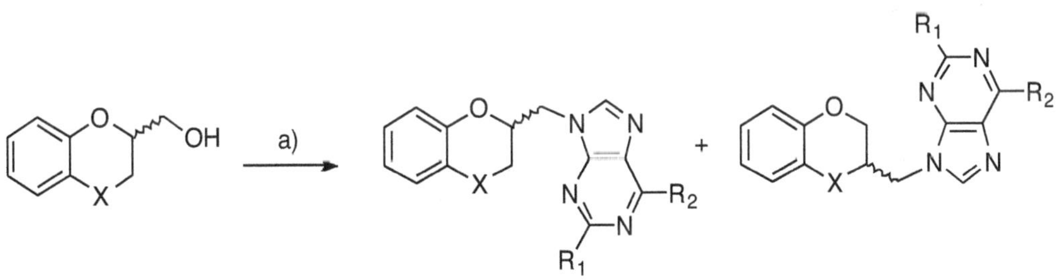

35 X = S
36 X = O

27 X = S, $R_1 = H$, $R_2 = Cl$
28 X = S, $R_1 = H$; $R_2 = Br$
29 X = S, $R_1 = R_2 = Cl$
30 X = S, $R_1 = H$; $R_2 = NH_2$
31 X = O, $R_1 = H$; $R_2 = Cl$
32 X = O, $R_1 = H$; $R_2 = Br$
33 X = O, $R_1 = R_2 = Cl$
34 X = O, $R_1 = H$; $R_2 = NH_2$

16 X = S, $R_1 = H$, $R_2 = Cl$
17 X = S, $R_1 = H$; $R_2 = Br$
18 X = S, $R_1 = R_2 = Cl$

Sheme 2. *Reagents and conditions*: a) Substituted purines, Ph_3P, DIAD, anhydrous THF, microwave irradiation, 140 °C, 5 min, or in the case of 32, 160 °C, 15 min (Conejo-García et al., 2011).

Final compounds **27-34** were synthesized by the Mitsunobu reaction in dry THF between **35** or **36** and the corresponding purines (6-chloropurine, 6-bromopurine, 2,6-dichloropurine and adenine) under microwave-assisted conditions (Scheme 2).

It must be pointed out that when starting from **35** and using 6-chloro-, 6-bromo-, and 2,6-dichloro-purines, apart from the target compounds **27**, **28** and **29**, their corresponding isomers **16**, **17** and **18** (Díaz-Gavilán et al., 2008) previously reported were also obtained as side-products. Therefore we have justified the formation of such "abnormal" products through a neighbouring-group mechanism (Conejo-García et al., 2011).

The anti-carcinogenic potential of the target molecules is reported against the MCF-7 human breast cancer cell line (Table 4). In general, (*RS*)-9-(2,3-dihydro-1,4-benzoxathiin-2-ylmethyl)-9*H*-purines **27-29** (series A) show a better activity than their isosteres (*RS*)-9-(2,3-dihydro-1,4-benzodioxin-2-ylmethyl)-9*H*-purines **31-33** (series B). The anti-cancer activity depends on the substituent of the purine ring. The most active compound **29**, bearing two chlorine atoms at positions 2 and 6 of the purine ring, shows an IC_{50}=2.75 ± 0.02 μM. In general, compounds bearing halogen atoms on the purine ring (**27-29** and **31-33**) present better activity than compounds substituted bearing an amino group (**30** and **34**).

Comp.	IC_{50} (μM)	Comp.	IC_{50} (μM)	Comp.	IC_{50} (μM)
16	10.6 ± 0.66	**28**	4.87 ± 0.02	**32**	7.64 ± 0.03
17	6.18 ± 1.70	**29**	2.75 ± 0.03	**33**	19.58 ± 0.02
18	8.97 ± 0.83	**30**	"/>30	**34**	"/>30
27	9.24 ± 0.01	**31**	18.75 ± 0.02		

Table 4. Anti-proliferative activities against the MCF-7 cell line for the (*RS*)-9-(2,3-dihydro-1,4-benzoxathiin-3-ylmethyl)-9*H*-purines (**16**, **17** and **18**), (*RS*)-9-(2,3-dihydro-1,4-benzoxathiin-2-ylmethyl)-9*H*-purines (**27-30**), and (*RS*)-9-(2,3-dihydro-1,4-benzodioxin-2-ylmethyl)-9*H*-purines (**31-34**).

In recent years, many studies have shown an association between cell cycle regulation and cancer inasmuch as the cell cycle inhibitors are being considered as a weapon for the management of cancer (Hajduch et al., 1999). To study the mechanisms of the anti-tumour activity of the compounds (**27-29** and **32**), the effects on the cell cycle distribution were analysed by flow cytometry (Table 5). DMSO-treated cell cultures contain a 62.79 ± 1.30 % of the cells in the G_0/G_1-phase, and a 19.29 ± 2.98 % of the cells in the S-phase, a 13.26 ± 2.98 % of the cells in the G_2/M-phase. In contrast, MCF-7 cells treated during 48 h with **27-29** and **32** show important differences in the cell cycle progression compared with DMSO-treated control cells. The following can be deduced from the analysis of the cell cycle distribution: compounds **27**, **28**, **29** and **32** accumulate the cancerous cells in the G_2/M-phase (23.35 ± 1.97, 31.37 ± 1.45, 43.89 ± 1.96 and 36.71 ± 7.40, respectively) at the expense of the S-phase cells (13.77 ± 1.13, 17.06 ± 0.75, 10.83 ± 4.70 and 10.27 ± 6.24, respectively) and of the G_0/G_1-phase cells in the case of compounds **28**, **29** and **32** (51.56 ± 1.06, 45.28 ± 2.73 and 53.02 ± 1.16, respectively), except in the case of **27**, which induces a cell cycle arrest in the G_2/M-phase cells (23.35 ± 1.97) at the expense of the S-phase cells (13.77 ± 1.13).

Compound	Cell cycle[a]			Apoptosis[b,c]
	G_0/G_1	S	G_2/M	
Control	62.79 ± 1.30	19.29 ± 1.68	13.26 ± 2.98	0.92 ± 1.29
27	62.87 ± 0.60	13.77 ± 1.13	23.35 ± 1.97	37.99 ± 8.56
28	51.56 ± 1.06	17.06 ± 0.75	31.37 ± 1.45	14.33 ± 1.23
29	45.28 ± 2.73	10.83 ± 4.70	43.89 ± 1.96	70.08 ± 0.33
32	53.02 ± 1.16	10.27 ± 6.24	36.71 ± 7.40	21.66 ± 0.30

[a]Determined by flow cytometry (Marchal et al., 2004).

[b]Apoptosis was determined using an Annexin V-based assay (Marchal et al., 2004). The data indicate the percentage of cells undergoing apoptosis in each sample.

[c]All experiments were conducted in duplicate and gave similar results. The data are means ± SEM of three independent determinations.

Table 5. Cell cycle distribution and apoptosis induction in the MCF-7 human breast cancer cell line after treatment for 48 h with the three most active compounds as anti-proliferative agents.

The protein expression analysis by western blot showed that **27-29** have an important role in the activation and phosphorylation of the initiation factor eIF2α. The initiation factor eIF2α was phosphorylated in MCF-7 human breast cancer cell line after treatment with **27-29**. It is well established that eIF2α phosphorylation correlates with a translational block and consequently produces inhibition of protein synthesis (Holcik & Sonenberg, 2005). These results are in concordance with the delay in the G_2/M cell cycle phase produced by compounds. Furthermore, a prolonged induction of eIF2α finally triggers the cell cycle arrest and/or the apoptosis phenomena (Gil et al., 1999; Dagon et al., 2001).

MCF-7 cells treated for 48 h with compounds **27-29** induced apoptosis, **29** being the compound that showed a significant increase of apoptotic cells in relation to the control culture with a percentage of 70.08 ± 0.33 (Table 5). Apoptosis is a major form of cell death characterized by changes in signalling pathways that lead to the recruitment and activation of caspases, a family of cysteine-containing, aspartate-specific proteases. Caspases exist as inactive proenzymes in cells, and are activated through their processing into two subunits in response to apoptotic stimulation. Activated caspases cleave a variety of important cellular proteins, other caspases, and Bcl-2 family members, leading to a commitment to cell death. Caspase-9 is involved in one of the relatively well-characterized caspase cascades. It is triggered by cytochrome C release from the mitochondria, which promotes the activation of caspase-9 by forming a complex with Apaf-1 in the presence of dATP. Once activated, caspase-9 initiates a caspase cascade that finally induces cell death (Altieri, 2003). Western blot assays showed that compounds **27-29** induced activation of caspase 9 at late times (16 h and 36 h of treatment) similarly to paclitaxel used as control compound. These data confirm that levels of apoptosis showed by annexin V assays that are dependent of intrinsic pathway of cell death. p53 was not activated by the compounds which indicate that apoptosis was induced in a p53 independent manner (Conejo-García et al., 2011).

4. Different apoptosis modulation in breast cancer cells of enantiomers of benzo-fused six-membered heterocycles linked to purines

The intrinsically chiral and non-racemic nature of the living world often results in its different interactions with the enantiomers of a given substance. If this substance is a drug, it might well be that only one of the two isomers is capable of exerting the desired therapeutic effect. The other may be inert, harmful or responsible for possibly undesirable side effects.

García-Rubiño et al. have described the preparation of homochiral **27-29** and **31-33** (García-Rubiño et al., 2013). Compounds (*R*)-**27-29**, (*R*)-**16-18**, (*S*)-**27-29** and (*S*)-**16-18** have been subjected to anti-proliferative, apoptosis (Tables 6 and 7) and cell cycle studies in the MCF-7 and SKBR-3 human breast cancer cell lines.

Comp.	IC_{50} (μM)[a]	Total apoptosis	Comp.	IC_{50} (μM)[a]	Total apoptosis
(*RS*)-**27**	9.24 ± 0.01	67.4 ± 0.90[b] 10.3 ± 0.14[c]	(*RS*)-**16**	10.6 ± 0.66	73.8 ± 0.42b 22.6 ± 0.07c
(*R*)-**27**	4.73 ± 0.02	43.0 ± 0.63[b] 9.70 ± 0.42[c]	(*R*)-**16**	15.2 ± 0.03	72.0 ± 0.21b 20.2 ± 0.21c
(*S*)-**27**	11.4 ± 0.06	89.5 ± 0.70[b] 19.0 ± 0.63[c]	(*S*)-**16**	3.30 ± 0.02	31.6 ± 1.40b 14.0 ± 0.60c
(*RS*)-**28**	4.87 ± 0.02	99.4 ± 0.07[b] 38.4 ± 4.73[c]	(*RS*)-**17**	6.18 ± 1.70	63.4 ± 1.50[b] 30.6 ± 6.78[c]
(*R*)-**28**	4.45 ± 0.07	63.8 ± 6.00[b] 16.0 ± 2.33[c]	(*R*)-**17**	6.17 ± 0.07	55.8 ± 12.0[b] 26.6 ± 0.20[c]
(*S*)-**28**	3.33 ± 0.13	50.2 ± 1.13[b] 25.2 ± 0.49[c]	(*S*)-**17**	6.32 ± 0.04	60.5 ± 9.00[b] 41.8 ± 0.56[c]
(*RS*)-**29**	2.75 ± 0.03	97.7 ± 0.56[b] 29.4 ± 0.30[c]	(*RS*)-**18**	8.97 ± 0.83	51.4 ± 0.21[b] 15.8 ± 0.49[c]
(*R*)-**29**	3.33 ± 0.04	99.1 ± 0.65[b] 77.0 ± 2.80[c]	(*R*)-**18**	10.3 ± 0.01	27.4 ± 0.07[b] 6.25 ± 3.30[c]
(*S*)-**29**	1.85 ± 0.05	89.4 ± 1.50[b] 33.2 ± 0.20[c]	(*S*)-**18**	6.93 ± 0.09	58.8 ± 2.75[b] 60.4 ± 2.40[c]

[a]All experiments were conducted in duplicate and gave similar results. The data are means ± SEM of three independent determinations. IC_{50} was determined after 6 days of treatment. [b]Cells were treated with the 3 × IC_{50} values of compounds. [c]Cells were treated with the IC_{50} values of compounds. Apoptosis was measured after 48 h of treatment.

Table 6. Anti-proliferative effect and apoptosis induction for the target compounds **27-29** and **16-18** in the MCF-7 cell line

Comp.	IC_{50} (μM)[a]	Total apoptosis	Comp.	IC_{50} (μM)[a]	Total apoptosis
(*RS*)-**27**	8.04 ± 0.00	55.2 ± 0.70[b] 23.6 ± 0.10[c]	(*RS*)-**16**	8.17+/-0.00	40.8 ± 0.12b 13.4 ± 0.14c
(*R*)-**27**	6.56 ± 0.11	60.0 ± 1.13[b] 11.7 ± 0.23[c]	(*R*)-**16**	12.1 ± 0.04	29.2 ± 0.11b 9.35 ± 0.12c
(*S*)-**27**	9.46+/-0.00	37.2 ± 0.11[b] 12.4 ± 0.87[c]	(*S*)-**16**	4.50 ± 0.12	42.0 ± 2.31b 18.4 ± 0.44c
(*RS*)-**28**	7.25+/-0.00	95.8 ± 0.21[b] 36.2 ± 1.03[c]	(*RS*)-**17**	8.98+/-0.00	28.6 ± 0.50[b] 7.62 ± 0.70[c]
(*R*)-**28**	5.18+/-0,00	47.5 ± 2.11[b] 8.42 ± 0.41[c]	(*R*)-**17**	9.24+/-0.00	42.7 ± 0.15[b] 7.95 ± 0.02[c]
(*S*)-**28**	7.78+/-0.00	25.7 ± 0.55[b] 10.6 ± 0.09[c]	(*S*)-**17**	9.05 ± 0.14	26.6 ± 1.30[b] 27.2 ± 0.05[c]
(*RS*)-**29**	5+/-0.00	78.2 ± 1.26[b] 27.5 ± 0.33[c]	(*RS*)-**18**	5.73± 0.22	59.8 ± 0.11[b] 20.2 ± 0.04[c]
(*R*)-**29**	4.34+/-0.00	87.4 ± 0.35[b] 37.2 ± 0.30[c]	(*R*)-**18**	7.52+/-0,01	37.5 ± 0.05[b] 10.6 ± 0.32[c]
(*S*)-**29**	7.03+/-0.00	56.1 ± 0.09[b] 4.85 ± 0.19[c]	(*S*)-**18**	4.35+/-0.00	69.0 ± 0.57[b] 27.5 ± 0.60[c]

[a]All experiments were conducted in duplicate and gave similar results. The data are means ± SEM of three independent determinations. IC_{50} was determined after 6 days of treatment. [b]Cells were treated with the 3 × IC_{50} values of compounds. [c]Cells were treated with the IC_{50} values of compounds. Apoptosis was measured after 48 h of treatment.

Table 7. Anti-proliferative effect and apoptosis induction for the target compounds **27-29** and **16-18** in the SKBR3 cell line.

Compounds **27-29**, **16** and **18** show one major bioactive enantiomer against both MCF-7 and SKBR-3 human breast cancer cells whereas compound **17** has presented equally bioactive enantiomers. In general, the IC_{50} values of racemates (*RS*)-**27-29**, **16** and **18** are similar to the average IC_{50} of the corresponding enantiomers (*R*)-**27-29**,**-16**,**-18** and (*S*)-**27-29**,**-16**,**-18**. Structure-activity relationship between the configuration of the enantiomers and the anti-proliferative effect indicates that in general, (*S*)-enantiomers are more active in the MCF-7 cell line. Thus, (*S*)-**28**, (*S*)-**29**, (*S*)-**16** and (*S*)-**18** are more potent than their corresponding enantiomers while (*R*)-**27** is more active than (*RS*)-**27** in the MCF-7 cell line. However, (*R*)-**27-29** and (*S*)-**16** and (*S*)-**18** show more cytotoxicin the SKBR-3 cell line.

In the MCF-7 cell line racemic and homochiral compounds **27**, **28**, and **29**, with the purine moiety at position 2, are more active than their corresponding regioisomers **16**, **17** and **18**, with the purine moiety at position 3, except for (*S*)-**27**. The most active compound (*S*)-**29**, with 2,6-dichloropurine moiety at position 2, shows an IC_{50}=1.85 ± 0.05 μM being 2.5-fold more potent than the clinically used drug 5-FU (IC_{50}=4.32 ± 0.02 μM) (García-Rubiño et al., 2013). In contrast, in the SKBR-3 cell line both racemic and homochiral compounds **27**, **28** and **29** are more active than their corresponding regioisomers **16**, **17** and **18**, except for (*S*)-**16** and (*S*)-**18**. The most active compound in this case is (*R*)-**29** with 2,6-dichloropurine moiety at position 2, shows an IC_{50}=4.34 ± 0.00 μM.

The cell cycle does not show significant differences among the compounds (data not shown). Since it is well established that the eukaryotic initiation factor 2 alpha (eIF2α) phosphorylation correlates with a translational block and consequently leads to the inhibition of protein synthesis and induction of apoptosis (García-Rubiño et al., 2013), we have analyzed the protein activation of this factor by western blot. eIF2α is significantly phosphorylated in MCF-7 cancer cells after treatment with (*S*)-**29**, (*S*)-**17** and (*R*)-**16** at 16 h and 36 h.

Interestingly, (*S*)-**29** induces high eIF2α phosphorylation in the MCF-7 cell line in comparison with its racemate and its enantiomer, where no activation is shown. These results support the highest anti-proliferative activity displayed by (*S*)-**29** and suggest that this activity is in part due to the suppression of protein synthesis provoked by eIF2α phosphorylation (Baltzis et al., 2007). Furthermore, a prolonged induction of eIF2α finally triggers the apoptosis phenomena (Gil et al., 1999; 20, Dagon et al., 2001).

The following can be stated from Tables 6 and 7:

a. In the MCF-7 cell line, compounds are more potent as programmed cell-death inducers than in SKBR-3, and more specifically, (*R*)-**29** and (*S*)-**18** are the more effective apoptotic inducers (77% and 60% at their IC_{50}, respectively) in the MCF-7 cell line.

b. In the SKBR-3 cell line the best apoptotic values are observed at their 3 × IC_{50} concentrations.

c. Compounds (*RS*)-**28**, (*RS*)-**29** and (*R*)-**29** present the best apoptotic percentages in both cancerous cell lines at their 3 × IC_{50} concentrations (99%, 98%, and 99%, respectively in MCF-7, and 96%, 78%, and 87%, respectively, in SKBR-3).

Previous works scarcely reports a different pattern in apoptosis levels between enantiomers. An exception is D-(-)-lentiginosine, the non-natural enantiomer of the iminosugar indolizidine alkaloid that acts as an apoptosis inducer on different tumour cells in contrast to its natural enantiomer (Macchi et al., 2010). All homochiral compounds included in this study show a different apoptosis effect between the two enantiomers. Apoptotic defects in cancer cells are the primary obstacle that limits the therapeutic efficacy of anticancer agents, and hence the development of novel agents targeting novel canonical and non-canonical programmed cell death pathways has become an imperative mission for clinical research (Cummings et al., 2004). Compounds **27-29**, and **16-18** induce strong levels of cell death measured by citotoxicity analysis and by phosphatidylserine externalization (Annexin V binding) (Tables 6 and 7) even in the MCF-7 breast cancer cells that have shown deficiency in the caspase-activation mechanisms (Kagawa et al., 2001).

Whereas compound (*S*)-**27** activates the canonical intrinsic caspase-8/caspase-3 apoptotic pathway on the MCF-7 cell line, compound (*RS*)-**29** induces caspase-2 activation. However, a strong apoptosis induction is also detected in the rest of the compounds analysed. The caspase-independent apoptosis in cells exposed to different drugs with diverse cellular effects has been previously described (Macchi et al., 2010). While caspase-2 activation could induce cell death through cytochrome c/mitochondria damage (Robertson et al., 2002), non-caspase-mediated increase in phosphatidylserine externalization can occur in response to high intracellular Ca^{2+}levels that alters scramblase and translocase (Vanags et al., 1996; 26, Kagan et al., 2000). Additionally, non-caspase proteases may activate and cleave the cytoskeleton proteins attached to phospholipids, including focal adhesion kinase and the actin-capping protein α-adducin (van de Water, 1999). To further confirm the involvement of caspases, including caspase-3, in the apoptosis induced by the most apoptotic compounds in the caspase-3 wild type SKBR-3 cell line, cells were pre-treated with the pan-caspase inhibitor z-VAD-fmk for 2 h, followed by the (*RS*)**-28** and (*RS*)**-29** treatment, and cell viability metabolic-analysis was carried out. Our results show that (*RS*)**-28** and (*RS*)**-29** were sensible to the effect of z-VAD-fmk caspase inhibitor, which could rescue SKBR-3 cells from the cytotoxicity of compounds. These results demonstrate the involvement of caspase activation during cell death induced by the compounds in the SKBR-3 cells as previously described for numerous anti-tumour apoptotic drugs (Yang et al., 2012; Kumar et al., 2013; Lamberto et al., 2013). These and other anti-tumour effects such as autophagy or senescence events could be involved in the caspase-dependent and caspase-independent cell death induced by the compounds included in this study. This fact opens an important line of research that is yet to be explored.

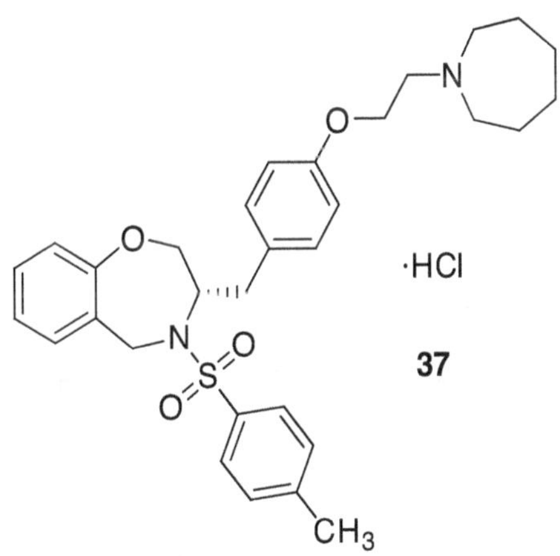

37

Indian researchers have very recently investigated the effect of α tyrosine-based benzoxazepine derivative in MCF-7 and MDA-MB-231 cells (Dwivedi et al., 2013). The anti-proliferative effect of **37** on MCF-7 cells was associated with G_1 cell-cycle arrest. This G_1 growth arrest was followed by apoptosis as **37**-dose dependently increased phosphatidylserine exposure. PARP cleavage and DNA fragmentation that are hallmarks of apoptotic cell death. Compound **37** activated components of both intrinsic and extrinsic pathways of apoptosis characterized by activation of caspase-8 and-9, mitochondrial membrane depolarization and increase in Bax/Bcl2 ratio. However, use of selective caspase inhibitors revealed that the caspase-8-dependent pathway is the major contributor to **37**-induced apoptosis. Compound **37** also significantly reduced the growth of MCF-7 xenograft tumours in athymic nude mice (Dwivedi et al., 2013).

5. Conclusion

Cancer continues to be a major health problem in developing as well as undeveloped countries. Although major advances have been made in the chemotherapeutic management of some patients, the continued commitment to the laborious task of discovering new anticancer agents remains critically important, in the course of identifying various chemical substances, which may serve as leads for designing novel anti-tumour agents.

The ever-increasing use of asymmetric syntheses over many years has been manifested by the biological importance of enantiomerically pure single compound entity factors and further has been strongly guided by drug regulatory bodies because of strict rules and regulations about single isomers. A contributing factor to this effect has been, and continues to be the development of new, novel and efficient methods for accessing single isomers. In general, the binomial enantiomers → different biological activities and in particular, enantiomers → different antiproliferative activities are rarely known, in spite of their great importance. It seems that in the future this topic will receive increasing attention and will help better understanding of the molecular recognition between drugs and biological targets.

Author details

Joaquín M. Campos[1,2*], M. Eugenia García-Rubiño[1,2], Nawal Mahfoudh[1] and César Lozano-López[1]

*Address all correspondence to: jmcampos@ugr.es

1 Departamento de Química Farmacéutica y Orgánica, Facultad de Farmacia, Universidad de Granada, Campus de Cartuja s/n, Granada, Spain

2 Departamento de Química Farmacéutica y Orgánica, Instituto de Investigación Biosanitaria ibs.GRANADA, Universidad de Granada, Granada, Spain

References

[1] Al-Obeidi, F.; Austin, R.E.; Okonya, J.F. & Bond, D.R.S. (2003). Microwave-assisted solid-phase synthesis (MASS): parallel and combinatorial chemical library synthesis. *Mini-Reviews in Medicinal Chemistry*, Vol.3, No.5, (August 2003), pp. 449-460, ISSN 1389-5575.

[2] Altieri, D.C. (2003). Validating survivin as a cancer therapeutic target. *Nature Reviews Cancer*, Vol.3, No.1, (January 2003), pp. 46-54, ISSN 1474-175X.

[3] Baltzis, D.; Pluquet, O.; Papadakis, A.I.; Kazemi, S.; Qu, L.-K & Koromilas, A.E. (2007). The eIF2α Kinases PERK and PKR Activate Glycogen Synthase Kinase 3 to Promote the Proteasomal Degradation of p53. *Journal of Biological Chemistry*, Vol.282, No.43, (October 2007), pp. 31675-31687, ISSN 0021-9258.

[4] Brown, N.M.; Belles, C.A.; Lindley, S.L.; Zimmer-Nechemias, L.D.; Zhao, X.; Witte, D.P.; Kim, M.O. & Setchell, K.D.R. (2010). The chemopreventive action of equol enantiomers in a chemically induced animal model of breast cancer. *Carcinogenesis*, Vol.31, No.5, (May 2010), pp. 886–893, ISSN 0143-3334.

[5] Chadderton, A.; Villeneuve, D.J.; Gluck, S.; Kirwan-Rhude, A.F.; Gannon, B.R.; Blais, D.E. & Parissenti, A.M. (2000). Role of specific apoptotic pathways in the restoration of paclitaxel-induced apoptosis by valspodar in doxorubicin-resistant MCF-7 breast cancer cells. *Breast Cancer Research and Treatment*, Vol.59, No.3, (February 2000), pp. 231-244, ISSN 1573-7217.

[6] Conejo-García, A.; Núñez, M.C.; Marchal, J.A.; Rodríguez-Serrano, F.; Aránega, A.; Gallo, M.A.; Espinosa, A. & Campos, J.M. (2008). Regioespecific Microwave-Assisted Synthesis and Cytotoxic Activity against Human Breast Cancer Cells of (*RS*)-6-Substituted-7-or 9-(2.3-Dihydro-5*H*-1.4-Benzodioxepin-3-yl)-7*H*-or-9*H*-Purines. *European Journal of Medicinal Chemistry*, Vol.43, No.8, (August 2008), pp. 1742-1748, ISSN 0223-5234.

[7] Conejo-García, A.; García-Rubiño, M.E.; Marchal, J.A.; Núñez, M.C.; Ramírez, A.; Cimino, S.; García, M.A.; Aránega, A.; Gallo, M.A. & Campos, J.M. (2011). Synthesis and anticancer activity of (*RS*)-9-(2,3-dihydro-1,4-benzoheteroin-2-ylmethyl)-9*H*-purines. *European Journal of Medicinal Chemistry*, Vol.46, No.9, (September 2011), pp. 3795-3801, ISSN 0223-5234.

[8] Cummings, B.S.; Kinsey, G.R.; Bolchoz, L.J. & Schnellmann, R.G. (2004). Identification of caspase-independent apoptosis in epithelial and cancer cells. *Journal of Pharmacology and Experimental Therapeutics*, Vol.310, No.1, (July 2004), pp. 126-134, ISSN 1521-0103.

[9] Dagon, Y.; Dovrat, S.; Vilchik, S.; Hacohen, D.; Shlomo, G.; Sredni, B.; Salzberg S. & Nir, U. (2001). Double-stranded RNA-dependent protein kinase, PKR, down-regulates CDC2/cyclin B1 and induces apoptosis in non-transformed but not in v-mos transformed cells. *Oncogene*, Vol.20, No.56, (December 2001), pp. 8045-8056, ISSN 0950-9232.

[10] De Fátima, A.; Zambuzzi, W.F.; Modolo, L.V.; Tarsitano, C.A.B.; Gadelha, F.R.; Hyslop, S.; de Carvalho, J.E.; Salgado, I.; Ferreira, C.V. & Pilli, R.A. (2008). Cytotoxicity of goniothalamin enantiomers in renal cancer cells: involvement of nitric oxide, apopto-

sis and autophagy. *Chemico-Biological Interactions*, Vol.176, No.2-3, (November 2008), pp. 143-150, ISSN 0009-2797.

[11] Díaz-Gavilán, M.; Choquesillo-Lazarte, D.; González-Pérez, J.M.; Gallo, M.A.; Espinosa, A. & Campos, J.M. (2007). Synthesis and Reactivity of (*RS*)-6-Chloro-7-or 9-(1,2,3,5-Tetrahydro-4,1-Benzoxazepin-3-yl)-7*H*-or 9*H*-Purines Bearing a Nitrobenzenesulfonyl Group on the Nitrogen Atom. *Tetrahedron*, Vol.63, No.24, (June 2007), pp. 5274-5286, ISSN 0040-4020.

[12] Díaz-Gavilán, M.; Conejo-García, A.; Cruz-López, O.; Núñez, M.C.; Choquesillo-Lazarte, D.; González-Pérez, J.M.; Rodríguez-Serrano, F.; Marchal, J.A.; Aránega, A.; Gallo, M.A.; Espinosa, A. & Campos, J.M. (2008). Synthesis and Anticancer Activity of (*R,S*)-9-(2,3-Dihydro-1,4-Benzoxathiin-3-ylmethyl)-9*H*-Purines. *ChemMedChem*, Vol.3, No.1, (January 2008a), pp. 127-135, ISSN 1860-7187.

[13] Díaz-Gavilán, M.; Gómez-Vidal, J.A.; Rodríguez-Serrano, F.; Marchal, J.A.; Caba, O.; Aránega, A.; Gallo, M.A.; Espinosa, A. & Campos, J.M. (2008). Anticancer Activity of (1.2.3.5-Tetrahydro-4.1-Benzoxazepine-3-yl)-Pyrimidines and-Purines against the MCF-7 Cell Line: Preliminary cDNA Microarray Studies. *Bioorganic & Medicinal Chemistry Letters*, Vol.18, No.4, (February 2008b), pp. 1457-1460, ISSN 0960-894X.

[14] Díaz-Gavilán, M.; Rodríguez-Serrano, F.; Gómez-Vidal, J.A.; Marchal, J.A.; Aránega, A.; Gallo, M.A.; Espinosa, A. & Campos, J.M. (2004). Synthesis of Tetrahydrobenzoxazepine Acetals with Electron-Withdrawing Groups on the Nitrogen Atom. Novel Scaffolds Endowed with Anticancer Activity against Breast Cancer Cells. *Tetrahedron*, Vol.60, No.50, (December 2004), pp. 11547-11557, ISSN 0040-4020.

[15] Duncan, K.J.; Eckert, K.A. & Clawson, G.A. (2009). Mechanisms of growth inhibition in human papillomavirus positive and negative cervical cancer cells by the chloromethyl ketone protease inhibitor, succinyl-alanine-alanine-proline-phenylalanine chloromethyl ketone. *Journal of Pharmacology and Experimental Therapeutics*, Vol.330, No.1, (July 2009), pp. 359-366, ISSN 1521-0103.

[16] Dwivedi, S.K.D.; Samanta, K.; Yadav, M.; Jana, A.K.; Singh, A.K.; Chakravarti, B.; Mondal, S.; Konwar, R,; Trivedi, A.K.; Charttopadhyay, N.; Sanyal, S. & Panda, G. (2013). Amino acids derived benzoxazepines; Design, synthesis and antitumor activity. *Bioorganic & Medicinal Chemistry Letters*, Vol.23, No.24, (December 2013), pp. 6816-6821, ISSN 0960-894X.

[17] Formigli, L.; Zecchi Orlandini, S.; Capaccioli, S.; Poupon, M.F. & Bani, D. (2002). Energy-dependent types of cell death in MCF-7 breast cancer cell tumors implanted into nude mice. *Cells Tissues Organs*, Vol.170, No.2-3, (January 2002), pp. 99-110, ISSN 1422-6405.

[18] Fresco, P.; Borges, F.; Marques, M.P.M. & Diniz, C. (2010). The Anticancer Properties of Dietary Polyphenols and its Relation with Apoptosis. *Current Pharmaceutical Design*, Vol.16, No.1, (January 2010), pp. 114-134, ISSN 1381-6128.

[19] García-Rubiño, M.E.; Conejo-García, A.; Núñez, M.C.; Carrasco, E.; García, M.A.; Choquesillo-Lazarte, D.; García-Ruiz, J.M.; Gallo, M.A.; Marchal, J.A. & Campos, J.M. (2013). Enantiospecific Synthesis of Heterocycles Linked to Purines: Different Apoptosis Modulation of Enantiomers in Breast Cancer Cells. *Current Medicinal Chemistry*, Vol.20, No.38, (December 2013), pp. 4924-4934, ISSN 0929-8673.

[20] Gil, J.; Alcami, J. & Esteban, M. (1999). Induction of apoptosis by double-stranded-RNA-dependent protein kinase (PKR) involves the alpha subunit of eukaryotic translation initiation factor 2 and NF-kappaB. *Molecular and Cellular Biology*, Vol.19, No.7, (July 1999), pp. 4653-4663, ISSN 0270-7306.

[21] Gooch, J.L. & Yee, D. (1999). Strain-specific differences in formation of apoptotic DNA ladders in MCF-7 breast cancer cells. *Cancer Letters*, Vol.144, No.1, (September 1999), pp. 31-37, ISSN 0304-3835.

[22] Grem, J.L.; Nguyen, D.; Monahan, B.P.; Kao, V. & Geoffroy, F.J. (1999). Sequence-dependent antagonism between fluorouracil and paclitaxel in human breast cancer cells. *Biochemical Pharmacology*, Vol.58, No.3, (August 1999), pp. 477-486, ISSN 0006-2952.

[23] Hajduch, M.; Havlieek, L.; Vesely, J.; Novotny, R.; Mihal, V. & Strnad, M. (1999). Synthetic cyclin-dependent kinase inhibitors: new generation of potent anti-cancer drugs. *Advances in Experimental Medicine and Biology*, Vol.457, No.II, (1999), pp. 341-353, ISSN 0065-2598.

[24] Holcik, M. & Sonenberg, N. (2005). Translational control in stress and apoptosis. *Nature Reviews Molecular Cell Biology*, Vol.6, No.4, (April 2005), pp. 318-327, ISSN 1471-0072.

[25] Kagan, V.E.; Fabisiak, J.P.; Shvedova, A.A.; Tyurina, Y.Y.; Tyurin, V.A.; Schor, N.F. & Kawai, K. (2000). Oxidative signaling pathway for externalization of plasma membrane phosphatidylserine during apoptosis. *FEBS Lett*ers, Vol.477, No.1-2, (July 2000), pp. 1-7, ISSN 0014-5793.

[26] Kagawa, S.; Gu, J.; Honda, T.; McDonnell, T.J.; Swisher, S.G.; Roth, J. A. & Fang, B. (2001). Deficiency of caspase-3 in MCF7 cells blocks Bax-mediated nuclear fragmentation but not cell death. *Clinical Cancer Research*, Vol.7, No.5, (May 2001), pp. 1474-1480, ISSN 1078-0432.

[27] Kappe, C. & Dallinger, O.D. (2006). The impact of microwave synthesis on drug discovery. *Nature Reviews Drug Discovery*, Vol.5, No.1, (January 2006), pp. 51-63, ISSN 1474-1776.

[28] Kumar, S.; Kumar, A.; Pathania, A.S.; Guru, S.K.; Jada, S.; Sharma, P.R. Bhushan, S.; Saxena, A.K.; Kumar, H.M. & Malik, F. (2013). Tiron and trolox potentiate the autophagic cell death induced by magnolol analog Ery5 by activation of Bax in HL-60 cells. *Apoptosis*, Vol.18, No.5, (May 2013), pp. 605-617, ISSN 1360-8185.

[29] Lai, J.C.; Brown, B.D.; Voskresenskiy, A.M.; Vonhoff, S.; Klussman, S.; Tan, W.; Colombini, M.; Weeratna, R.; Miller, P.; Benimetskaya, L. & Stein, C.A. (2007). Comparison of D-G3139 and its Enantiomer L-G3139 in melanoma cells demonstrates minimal in vitro but dramatic in vivo chiral dependency. *Molecular Therapy*, Vol.15, No.2 (February 2007), pp. 270-278, ISSN 1525-0016.

[30] Lamberto, I.; Plano, D.; Moreno, E.; Font, M.; Palop, J.; Sanmartín, C. & Encío, I. (2013). Bisacylimidoselenocarbamates cause G2/M arrest associated with the modulation of CDK1 and Chk2 in human breast cancer MCF-7 cells. *Current Medicinal Chemistry*, Vol.20, No.12, (2013), pp. 1609-1619, ISSN 0929-8673.

[31] Liu, H.; Xu, L.; Zhao, M.; Liu, W.; Zhang, C. & Zhou, S. (2009). Enantiomer-specific, bifenthrin-induced apoptosis mediated by MAPK signalling pathway in Hep G2 Cells. *Toxicology*, Vol.261, No.3, (July 2009), pp. 119-125, ISSN 0200-483X.

[32] López-Cara, L.C.; Conejo-García, A.; Marchal, J.A.; Macchione, G.; Cruz-López, O.; Boulaiz, H.; García, M.A.; Rodríguez-Serrano, F.; Ramírez, A.; Cativiela, C.; Jiménez, A.I.; García-Ruiz, J.M.; Choquesillo-Lazarte, D.; Aránega, A. & Campos, J.M. (2011). New (*RS*)-Benzoxazepin-Purines with Antitumour Activity: The Chiral Switch from (*RS*)-2,6-Dichloro-9-[1-(*p*-Nitrobenzenesulfonyl)-1,2,3,5-Tetrahydro-4,1-Benzoxazepin-3-yl]-9*H*-Purine. *European Journal of Medicinal Chemistry*, Vol.46, No.1 (January 2011), pp. 249-258, ISSN 0223-5234.

[33] Lundberg, A.S. & Weinberg, R.A. (1999). Control of the cell cycle and apoptosis. *European Journal of Cancer*, Vol.35, No.4 (April 1999), pp. 531-539, ISSN 0959-8049.

[34] Macchi, B.; Minutolo, A.; Grelli, S.; Cardona, F.; Cordero, F.M.; Mastino, A. & Brandi, A. (2010). The novel proapoptotic activity of nonnatural enantiomer of Lentiginosine. *Glycobiology*, Vol.20, No.5, (May 2010), pp. 500-506, ISSN 0959-6658.

[35] Marchal, J.A.; Aránega, A.; Conejo García, A.; García Chaves, M.A.; Cruz-López, O.; Boulaiz, H.; Rodríguez-Serrano, F.; Cativiela, C.; Perán, M.; Jiménez, A.I.; García-Ruiz, J.M.; Choquesillo-Lazarte, D. & Campos, J.M. Enantiómeros de derivados benzoheteroepínicos y su uso como agentes anticancerígenos. P201030415, 2010, Universidad de Granada.

[36] Marchal, J.A.; Boulaiz, H.; Suárez, I.; Saniger, E.; Campos, J.; Carrillo, E.; Prados, J.; Gallo, M.A.; Espinosa, A. & Aránega, A. (2004). Growth inhibition, G_1-arrest, and apoptosis in MCF-7 human breast cancer cells by novel highly lipophilic 5-fluorouracil derivatives. *Investigational New Drugs*, Vol.22, No.4, (November 2004), pp. 379-389, ISSN 0167-6997.

[37] Nagata, S. (1997). Apoptosis by death factor. *Cell*, Vol.88, No.3, (February 1997), pp. 355-365, ISSN 0092-8674.

[38] Núñez, M.C.; Entrena, A.; Rodríguez-Serrano, F.; Marchal, J.A.; Aránega, A.; Gallo, M.A.; Espinosa, A. & Campos, J.M. (2005). Synthesis of novel 1-(2.3-dihydro-5*H*-4.1-

benzoxathiepin-3-yl)-uracil and –thymine, and their corresponding *S*-oxidized derivatives. *Tetrahedron*, Vol.61, No.43, (October 2005), pp. 10363-10369, ISSN 0040-4020.

[39] Núñez, M.C.; García-Rubiño, M.E.; Conejo-García, A.; Cruz-López, O.; Kimatrai, M.; Gallo, M.A.; Espinosa, A. & Campos, J.M. (2009). Homochiral Drugs: a Demanding Tendency of the Pharmaceutical Industry. *Current Medicinal Chemistry*, Vol.16, No.16, June 2009), pp. 2064-2074, ISSN 0929-8673.

[40] Núñez, M.C.; Rodríguez-Serrano, F.; Marchal, J.A.; Caba, O.; Aránega, A.; Gallo, M.A.; Espinosa, A. & Campos, J.M. (2007). 6′-Chloro-7-or 9-(2,3-dihydro-5*H*-4,1-benzoxathiepin-3-yl)-7*H*-or 9*H*-purines and their corresponding sulfones as a new family of cytotoxic drugs. *Tetrahedron*, Vol.63, No.1, (January 2007), pp. 183-190, ISSN 0040-4020.

[41] Robertson, J.D.; Enoksson, M.; Suomela, M.; Zhivotovsky, B. & Orrenius, S. (2002). Caspase-2 acts upstream of mitochondria to promote cytochrome c release during etoposide-induced apoptosis. *Journal of Biological Chemistry*, Vol.277, No.33, (August 2002), pp. 29803-29809, ISSN 0021-9258.

[42] Saunders, D.E.; Lawrence, W.D.; Christensen, C.; Wappler, N.L.; Ruan, H. & Deppe, G. (1997). Paclitaxel-induced apoptosis in MCF-7 breast cancer cells. *International Journal of Cancer*, Vol.70, No.2, (January 1997), pp. 214-220, ISSN 1097-0215.

[43] Shelley, M.D.; Hartley, L.; Fish, R.G.; Groundwater, P.; Morgan, J.J.G.; Mort, D.; Mason, M. & Evans, A. (1999). Stereo-specific cytotoxic effects of gossypol enantiomers and gossypolone in tumour cell lines. *Cancer Letters*, Vol.135, No.2, (January 1999), pp. 171-180, ISSN 0304-3835.

[44] Sherr, C.J. Cancer cell cycles. *Science*, Vol.274, No.5293, (December 1996), pp. 1672-1677, ISSN 0036-8075.

[45] Stewart, B.W. & Kleihues P. (2003) (Eds.), World Cancer Report, International Agency for Research on Cancer, World Health Organization, 2003.

[46] Testa, U. (2004). Apoptotic mechanisms in the control of erythropoiesis. *Leukemia*, Vol.18, No.7, (July 2004), pp. 1176-1199, ISSN 0887-6924.

[47] van de Water, B.; Nagelkerke, J.F. & Stevens, J.L. (1999). Dephosphorylation of focal adhesion kinase (FAK) and loss of focal contacts precede caspase-mediated cleavage of FAK during apoptosis in renal epithelial cells. *Journal of Biological Chemistry*, Vol. 274, No.19, (May 1999), pp. 13328-13337, ISSN 0021-9258.

[48] Vanags, D.M.; Poern-Ares, M.I.; Coppola, S.; Burgess, D.H. & Orrenius, S. (1996). Protease involvement in fodrin cleavage and phosphatidylserine exposure in apoptosis. *Journal of Biological Chemistry*, Vol.271, No.49, (December 1996), pp. 31075-31085, ISSN 0021-9258.

[49] Yang, F.; Jove, V.; Chang, S.; Hedvat, M.; Liu, L.; Buettner, R.; Tian, Y.; Scuto, A.; Wen, W.; Yip, M.L.; Van Meter, T.; Yen, Y. & Jove, R. (2012). Bortezomib induces

apoptosis and growth suppression in human medulloblastoma cells, associated with inhibition of AKT and NF-κB signaling, and synergizes with an ERK inhibitor. *Cancer Biology Therapy*, Vol.13, No.6, (April 2012), pp. 349-357, ISSN 1538-4047.

[50] Zivny, J.; Klener Jr, P.; Pytlik, R. & Andera, L. (2010). The Role of Apoptosis in Cancer Development and Treatment: Focusing on the Development and Treatment of Hematologic Malignancies. *Current Pharmaceutical Design,* Vol.16, No.1, (January 2010), pp. 11-33, ISSN 1381-6128.

3

Breast Cancer - It's All in the DNA

Somaira Nowsheen, Khaled Aziz, Asef Aziz and
Alexandros G Georgakilas

1. Introduction

Breast cancer is the leading cause of cancer death in women, the second most common cancer worldwide, and the fifth most common cause of cancer-related deaths [1-3]. Not only are the incidence rates of breast cancer increasing, partly due to improved screening and detection techniques, but also the global burden of breast cancer exceeds all other cancers. So it is imperative to improve the quality of life of these patients.

Our knowledge of the process of tumorigenesis has increased significantly over the last decade thanks to continued funding from federal and private organizations, improved technologies enabling affordable sequencing of the entire genome, analysis of large data sets as well as gene expression profiles of human tumor samples, and improved animal models that attempt to resemble tumor formation in humans. The predisposing risk factors, precancerous lesions, and disease progression vary significantly across the tissues of origin. However, common themes have been described that drive a normal cell to undergo transformation and generate a tumor. We plan to lay the groundwork for our discussion utilizing the widely recognized models of colorectal cancer by Bert Vogelstein, the two hit hypothesis by Alfred Knudson, and the common characteristics of cancer cells described by Doug Hanahan and Robert Weinberg.

Furthermore, in this chapter we aim to discuss the early events that cause a normal breast epithelial cell to initiate the process of tumor formation and delineate them from later stage insults to the cell that cause it to progress to advanced metastatic disease. We particularly plan to focus on the role of oxidative stress and one major environmental agent i.e. ionizing radiation inducing DNA damage and chromosomal instability. At the same time we will discuss the cell cycle changes that ensue and the implications of loss of a tumor suppressor gene. Concurrently, there are morphological changes that can be witnessed in experiments performed with cancer cells in vitro which we will tie in with the underlying molecular mechanisms. We will trace the damaged cell along its course to metastasis by focusing on the molecular mechanisms that cause loss of cell-cell adhesion, loss of cellular polarity, ability to migrate through the stroma and gain access to the vascular or lymphatic system, resistance to anoikis and ability to seed a tumor in a new environment. A myriad of hypotheses exists in literature that attempts to explain the process of cancer formation and progression.

Next, we will classify breast tumors as malignant or non-malignant while describing the subtypes of each in a concise manner. Since the therapeutic options available in the clinic are targeted to particular genetic subtypes such as BRCA1 positive, estrogen receptor (ER) positive or triple negative (Her2-/-, ER -/-, PR -/-) etc., we will also discuss these molecular signatures. The clinical diagnosis criteria and imaging modalities will be mentioned concisely. A limited number of clinical trials that have a promising premise behind the study and considered to be ground breaking will be described.

Therapeutic options for breast cancer have expanded in the past 10 years to improve the survival outcomes for the disease. Existing FDA approved pharmacologic agents, small molecule inhibitors in clinical trials and drugs shown to have efficacy in preclinical studies will be methodically described in the final section. In the process, we hope to summarize where we are now with respect to this potent disease that affects millions.

2. How does cancer arise?

As a cell achieves a neoplastic phenotype, its genetic sequence is usually vastly altered and multiple genes are mutated, amplified, or lost. Several models have been proposed regarding what leads to tumorigenesis. One of the models proposed by Dr. Bert Vogelstein proposes the loss of function of tumor suppressors [4-7]. According to his model, loss of function of tumor suppressors such as p53 leads to genomic instability which eventually leads to tumorigenesis via alterations in metabolism, loss of sensitivity to apoptotic signals, and increased invasiveness [8, 9]. Loss of function of the tumor suppressor, p53, is associated with the development of most, if not all, tumor types [10-12]. An inactivating mutation in a tumor suppressor not only leads to hyper-proliferation of epithelial cells, it may also inactivate DNA repair genes. Mutations in proto-oncogene can either create an oncogene or lead to a cascade of inactivation of several more tumor suppressor genes before resulting in cancer. Figure 1 shows this model for colon carcinogenesis.

An alternate theory that accounts for both hereditary and non-hereditary cancer is the two-hit theory of cancer causation proposed by Dr. Alfred Knudson [13, 14]. Normal cells have two undamaged chromosomes, one inherited from each parent. People with a hereditary susceptibility to cancer inherit a damaged gene on one of the chromosomes at conception which is their 'first hit' or mutation. Others receive the 'first hit' in their lifetime. Damage to the same gene on the second chromosome in their lifetime may lead to cancer. An overview of this model is given in Figure 2 and is seen in cancer such as retinoblastoma.

Weinberg and Hanahan have proposed the hallmarks of cancer which helps explain oncogenesis. These are biological capabilities acquired during the complex multistep development of

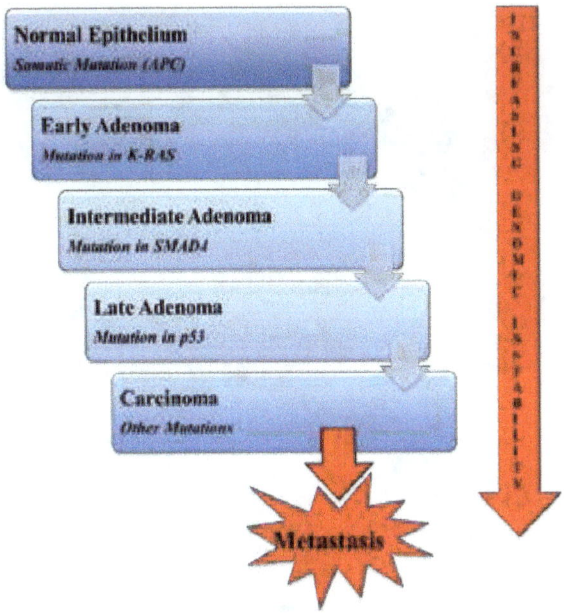

Figure 1. The cascade of events that lead to oncogenesis.

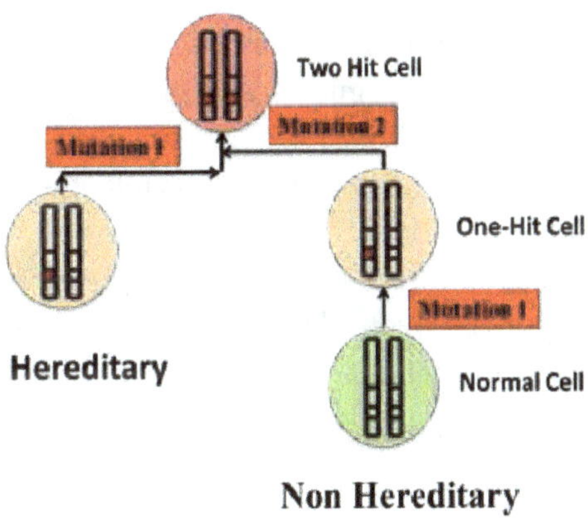

Figure 2. The two-hit model of carcinogenesis.

cancer. Figure 3 summarizes the 8 hallmarks of cancer. They include sustaining proliferative signaling, evading growth suppressors, resisting cell death, enabling replicative immortality, inducing angiogenesis, activating invasion and metastasis, reprogramming of energy metabolism, and evading immune destruction [15]. All these hallmarks lead to genomic instability and persistent inflammation, possibly fueling further genetic diversity, as well as propagation, acquisition and fostering of multiple hallmark functions.

A possible contributing factor that hasn't gained much attention is the role of fragile sites. Common fragile sites (CFSs) are regions of the genome with a predisposition to DNA double-strand breaks in response to intrinsic (oncogenic) or extrinsic replication stress. CFS breakage

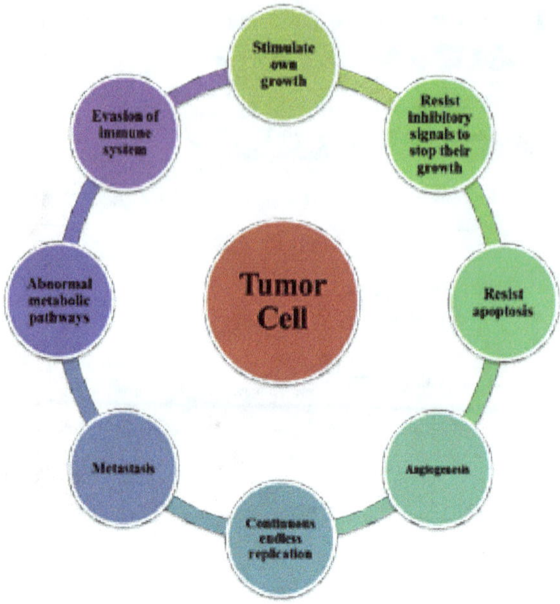

Figure 3. The 8 possible hallmarks of cancer.

is a common feature in carcinogenesis from its earliest stages and through its evolutions. In a recent article the association of several fragile sites stability with key DNA damage response (DDR) and DNA repair proteins like breast cancer type 1 susceptibility protein (BRCA1), Ataxia telangiectasia and Rad3 related (ATR), and Ataxia telangiectasia mutated (ATM) opens another possibility for the induction and/or acceleration of instability in breast tissue [16]. For example *FRA3B*, one of the most frequently expressed fragile sites in the human genome, is located within the tumor suppressor gene *FHIT* region. Deletions within *FHIT* have been associated with various human cancers including breast [17].

3. Events that cause a normal breast epithelial cell to start the process of tumor formation and eventually progress to advanced metastatic disease

A proto-oncogene is a normal gene that can convert to an oncogene due to mutations (generally dominant mutations) or increased expression [18-20]. Proto-oncogenes function in promoting cell division and inhibiting cell differentiation. Oncogenes, however, promote all the markers of a cancer cell such as increased cell division and replication stress, decreased cell differentiation, and inhibition of cell death (usually apoptosis). A proto-oncogene can convert into an oncogene due to various reasons including chromosomal translocation (such as BCR-ABL that is seen in leukemia), gene amplification, point mutations, deletions, alterations in promoter region leading to increased transcription, and insertions that lead to a hyperactive gene product. Human epidermal growth factor receptor 2 (HER2) is a proto-oncogene that is amplified in about 30% of breast cancer [18]. This is discussed in detail in a subsequent section.

To balance the effect of oncogenes, tumor suppressors are present as well to regulate cell growth and cell death but mutations in them can lead to tumor formation. The guardian of the genome, p53, is the most commonly mutated tumor suppressor gene in human cancer [21, 22]. It is involved in multiple pathways including maintenance of genomic stability by causing cell cycle arrest as the cell attempts to repair the damaged DNA, apoptosis, tumor progression, and metastasis [23]. Not surprisingly, a lot of breast cancers harbor mutations in this transcription factor as well. Since p53 has been linked to how BRCA1 dictates DNA repair and cell death, it may have a role in tumor response to treatment as well [24].

Checkpoints are present throughout the cell cycle that halt further progression of DNA replication and cell division, either permanently (senescence) or transiently, when damaged DNA is detected. This activates specific DNA repair pathways (discussed below). ATM and ATR are key proteins in the DNA damage response pathway. ATM is recruited to and activated by DNA double strand breaks while ATR is recruited to and activated by replication protein A-coated double stranded DNA. Two of the best studied ATM/ATR targets are the protein kinases checkpoint kinase 1 (CHK1) and checkpoint kinase 2 (CHK2). Together with ATM and ATR, these proteins reduce cyclin dependent kinase (CDK) activity which slows down or arrests cell-cycle progression at the G1–S, intra-S and G2–M cell cycle checkpoints allowing more time for DNA repair before progression of replication or mitosis. Moreover, ATM/ATR can promote DNA repair by a variety of methods including induction of DNA repair proteins transcriptionally or post-transcriptionally, by recruiting repair factors to the damage-site, and by activating DNA-repair proteins by modulating their post-transcriptional modifications such as phosphorylation, acetylation, ubiquitylation or SUMOylation.

Continuous DNA damage checkpoint activation may lead to selective suppression of the DNA-damage response-induced antitumor barriers. This may be due to inactivating mutations. This process promotes genomic instability and tumor progression [25-28]. Prolonged overexpression of licensing factors such as hCdt1 and hCdc6 prevent cell death and lead to a more aggressive phenotype. Overexpression of the replication licensing factor Cdc6 led to phenotypic changes with mesenchymal features and loss of E cadherin. Analysis in various types of human cancer revealed a strong correlation between increased Cdc6 expression and reduced E-cadherin levels [29]. Cells possessing re-replicated DNA above a critical threshold are typically neutralized by cell death mechanisms but cells with re-replicated elements below a critical threshold are prone to recombination processes leading to genomic instability. As a result these cells are much more resistant to therapy [30].

DNA can be damaged spontaneously during replication stress and cell division as well as due to exogenous/environmental agents. This leads to thousands of DNA lesions/cell per day. In some cases of high oxidative or environmental stresses, repair resistant complex DNA damage can be induced as analytically discussed in a recent review by Kryston et al. 2011 [31]. As little as one unrepaired DNA double strand break can be lethal to the cell. Thus, the DDR and DNA repair pathways are in place to maintain the genomic integrity. This response pathway detects the DNA damage, signals their presence to recruit repair factors and halt cell cycle progression, and promote DNA repair. DNA lesions can block genomic replication and transcription and lead to mutations. Most of the time, cells undergo death in the form of apoptosis or necrosis when there is unrepaired DNA. Cells defective in DNA repair are hypersensitive towards DNA damaging agents. For example, breast cancer cells with defective BRCA proteins are sensitive to poly ADP ribose polymerase (PARP) inhibitors. This is an active area of research with promising results thus far. This is discussed further in a later section. DNA repair pathways include base excision repair (BER), nucleotide excision repair (NER), double strand break repair via homologous recombination (HR) or non-homologous end joining (NHEJ), and mismatch repair (MMR) [32-34]. Frequently, multiple proteins are involved in the repair of the damaged DNA. The repair pathways are briefly described below.

In MMR-mediated repair, nuclease, polymerase and ligase enzymes fix a single-strand cut that is induced upon detection of mismatches and insertion/deletion loops. DNA glycosylase detects a damaged base in BER-mediated repair. This is subsequently removed before nuclease, polymerase and ligase proteins complete the repair. NER-mediated repair recognizes helix-distorting base lesions. The damage is excised as a 22–30-base oligonucleotide, producing single-stranded DNA that is a substrate for DNA polymerases and associated factors. The process ends with ligation. There are 2 major DNA double strand break repair pathways. NHEJ is predominantly used in the repair of radiation induced DNA damage. It is highly efficient but error-prone. The Ku proteins recognize and bind to the damaged site and activate the protein kinase DNA-PKcs, leading to recruitment and activation of end-processing enzymes, polymerases and DNA ligase IV. In contrast, HR uses sister-chromatid sequences as the template to mediate faithful repair. It is used in repair of replicative stress-induced lesions, stalled replication forks, and inter-strand DNA crosslinks. HR starts with single strand DNA generation, which is promoted by various proteins including the MRE11–RAD50–NBS1 (MRN) complex. In events catalyzed by RAD51 and the breast-cancer susceptibility proteins BRCA1 and BRCA2, the single strand DNA then invades the undamaged template and, following the actions of proteins mentioned above such as polymerases, nucleases, helicases, etc., the DNA is repaired.

One of the most famous mutations in cancer is the BRCA family of genes which are critical for HR-mediated repair of DNA double strand breaks [35, 36]. Mutations in the BRCA genes lead to an increased risk for breast cancer as part of the hereditary breast-ovarian cancer syndrome. Women with mutated BRCA1 or BRCA2 gene have up to a 60% risk of developing breast cancer [37, 38]. Hypermethylation of the BRCA1 promoter may be an inactivating mechanism for BRCA1 expression [39, 40]. Many of the mutations in BRCA1 or BRCA2 that predispose to breast cancer cause premature termination of the amino acid coding sequences, resulting in a truncated, dysfunctional protein.

Mutations in ATM, a critical DNA repair protein, lead to Ataxia Telangiectasia (AT). As mentioned above, ATM is a serine/threonine protein kinase that is recruited and activated by DNA double strand breaks and phosphorylates proteins that initiate activation of the DNA damage checkpoint, leading to cell cycle arrest, DNA repair or apoptosis. Several of these targets, including p53, CHK2 and H2AX are tumor suppressors which explains why AT sufferers are predisposed to breast cancer and are hypersensitive to radiation [41, 42]. Another example is the Werner syndrome which is marked by mutations in Werner syndrome ATP-dependent helicase (WRN) and Rad51 genes leading to deficiency in HR- and NHEJ mediated

DNA double strand break repair which, as expected, leads to increased incidence of breast cancer.

Breast cancer often metastasizes to bones, lungs, liver and brain [43-47]. The metastatic cascade is a series of biological steps that tumor cells must complete to exit the primary tumor and develop a new tumor at a distant site. One of the most critical steps involves invasion of the basement membrane and surrounding tissue and enter the bloodstream or lymphatic system. Cells that survive, eventually move into the tissue and establish a new colony that may form a tumor down the line. The host defense system is able to fend off millions of cancer cells that enter the blood stream but a few may escape nonetheless. Invasion involves the loss of cell-cell adhesion which may be mediated by matrix metalloproteinases and urokinases which break down integrins which attach tumor cells to their microenvironment and plasminogen respectively [48-54]. Cadherins are an intricate part of cell-cell adhesion and so downregulation of e-cadherin and upregulation of n-cadherin, involved in epithelial and mesenchymal phenotypes respectively, can promote metastasis [55-60].

Circulating tumor cells (CTCs) which like breast cancer is a heterogeneous population on cells, have a crucial role in the metastatic cascade, tumor dissemination and progression. Epithelial-to-mesenchymal transition (EMT) has an important role in the generation of CTCs and the acquisition of resistance to therapy [61-63]. Fibroblasts and myofibroblasts represent the majority of stromal cells within breast cancer. These cells promote the growth of cells by creating the perfect environment for cell survival and proliferation including enhanced angiogenesis. Tumor cells can express chemokine receptors that not only help direct migrating tumor cells to specific sites, they also determine if the cells will thrive and colonize at those sites. The bloodstream is highly unfavorable to tumor cells owing not only to the presence of immune cells, but also physical forces and anoikis, which combats metastasis. Interestingly, binding of tumor cells to coagulation factors, including tissue factor, fibrinogen, fibrin and thrombin, creates an embolus and facilitates arrest in capillary beds followed by the establishment of metastasis [64].

EMT is an important process in metastasis. Here, epithelial cells lose cell-to-cell contacts and cell polarity, downregulate epithelial-associated genes, upregulate mesenchymal-genes, and undergo major changes in their cytoskeleton. This confers greater motility and invasiveness. Expression of stem-cell markers and acquisition of stem-cell characteristics are important processes in this pathway as well. Once the tumor cells seed at the secondary site, they undergo redifferentiation to an epithelial phenotype [65]. One of the factors involved in EMT is epithelial derived growth factor (EGFR) which induces tissue factor which in turn promotes tumor seeding via the process described above. The transcription factor Twist-related protein 1 (TWIST1), the receptor ligand tumor derived growth factor β (TGFβ), Hypoxia-inducible factor 1 (HIF1), HER2, and Phosphatidylinositol-4,5-bisphosphate 3-kinase (PI3K)/ Protein kinase B (AKT) signaling pathways have also been implicated in metastases. In preclinical models, expression of TWIST reduces metastasis and number of CTCs. CTCs often express NOTCH1 which confers self-renewal abilities. Some cells also express Aldehyde dehydrogenase 1 (ALDH1), another gene associated with stem cell like properties. Interleukin 6 (IL6) and Interleukin 8 (IL8) attract CTCs while Matrix metalloproteinase-1 (MMP1)–collagenase 1 and the actin cytoskeleton component fascin 1 help CTCs infiltrate into tumors. Overexpression of the chemokine receptor C-X-C chemokine receptor type 1 (CXCR1) in CTCs is associated with decreased metastases and may be a therapeutic target.

4. Risk factors for breast cancer

Risk factors for malignant breast tumors include increased estrogen exposure which can be due to a number of reasons. For example, a woman can be exposed to increased estrogen due to increased total number of menstrual cycles, older age at 1st live birth, and obesity (increased estrogen exposure as adipose tissue converts androstenedione to estrone). BRCA1 and BRCA2 gene mutations also increase the risk of breast cancer and much research has been done in this avenue. Interestingly, increased incidence of triple negative breast cancer is seen in the African American population. Breast cancer risk is also increased with increased alcohol intake. Research suggests alcohol stimulates tumor growth by fuelling the production of growth factors that promote angiogenesis and by suppressing the immune system [66].

5. Classification of breast tumors as malignant or non-malignant

The breast is an organized organ and diseases may arise at any of its structural subunits. The stroma provides a supporting environment and this is where fibroadenoma and phyllodes tumor can arise. The smallest subunit is the lobule where we can see lobular carcinoma. Lobules give rise to terminal ducts where we can see tubular carcinoma. Next are major ducts where fibrocystic changes, DCIS, and invasive ductal carcinoma are often seen. These join to form the lactiferous sinus where intraductal papilloma may arise. Finally, Paget disease can be seen at the nipple. Figure 4 summarizes the different breast pathologies.

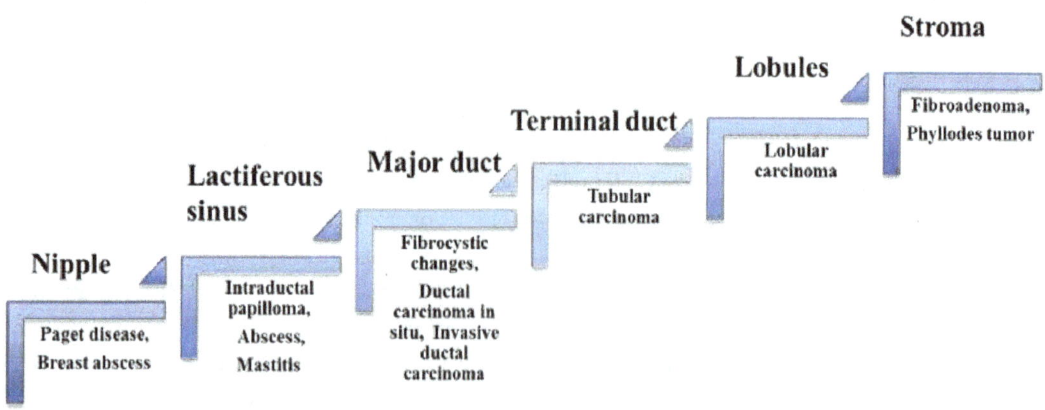

Figure 4. Pathologies that can affect the different breast tissues.

Not all breast tumors are malignant. Fibroadenoma are small, mobile, firm mass with sharp edges. They are most common in those <35 years old and increase in size and tenderness in response to estrogen as is seen in pregnancy and prior to menstruation. As mentioned, it does not lead to breast cancer. Similarly, intraductal papillomas are small benign tumors that grow in lactiferous ducts, typically beneath the areola. They can cause serous (faintly yellow and thin) or bloody nipple discharge. Of note, they do increase the risk for carcinoma be approximately 2-fold [67]. Phyllodes tumor are large bulky mass of connective tissue and cysts with leaf-like projections. They are most common in the 6th decade of life and similar to intraductal papilloma, can become malignant.

Malignant breast tumors are more common in postmenopausal women. They usually arise from terminal duct lobular unit. Overexpression of different proteins such as HER2 and EGFR are often seen. As discussed in a later section, receptor status can affect the therapy and prognosis. Since approximately 70% of the breast is drained by the axillary lymph node, involvement of this node indicating metastasis is the single most important prognostic factor. Since there is more tissue in the upper outer quadrant of the breast, tumors often arise here.

Malignant breast tumors can be subdivided into noninvasive and invasive tumors. Noninvasive tumors include ductal carcinoma in situ (DCIS), Paget disease, and comedocarcinoma. Comedocarcinoma is a subtype of DCIS where ductal caseous necrosis is seen. DCIS fills the ductal lumen and arises from ductal atypia. They are often seen as microcalcification on mammography due to necrosis. Paget disease results from underlying DCIS and results in eczematous patches on the nipple. Invasive breast tumors include invasive ductal and lobular cancer. A firm, fibrous mass with sharp margins and small, glandular, duct-like cells are seen in invasive ductal tumors. They are the worst and most invasive of the tumors as well as the most common, comprising of over 70% of all breast cancer. Invasive lobular cancer often presents bilaterally with multiple lesions in the same location. Pathologically, they present as an orderly row of cells. Fleshy, cellular lymphocytic infiltrate is seen with medullary breast carcinoma and it has a good prognosis. Finally, inflammatory breast tumor presents with dermal lymphatic invasion and has approximately 50% survival at 5 years. Due to blockage of the lymphatic drainage, Peau d'orange is often seen with this condition.

The classification is important because treatment varies based on the type of cancer. When a tumor is diagnosed as benign, it is often left alone. With malignant tumors, biopsy is performed to determine the severity and aggressiveness of the tumor.

5.1. Subtypes of breast cancer

Molecular subtypes of breast cancer may be useful in planning treatment and developing new therapies and so a lot of research is being conducted in this field. Figure 5 depicts some of the more common subtypes. Most studies divide breast cancer into six major molecular subtypes:

i. Luminal A

ii. Luminal B

iii. Triple negative/basal-like

iv. HER2 positive

v. Claudin low

vi. Normal-like

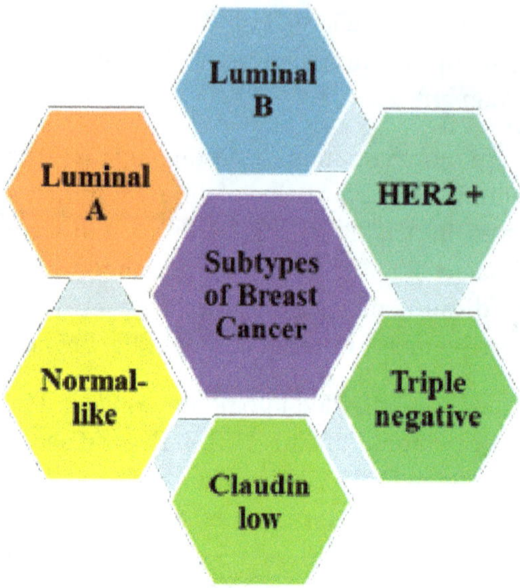

Figure 5. Subtypes of breast cancer.

Some of the less common subtypes include apocrine molecular type. Molecular apocrine breast cancers are aggressive estrogen receptor negative tumors overexpressing either HER2 or gross cystic disease fluid protein-15 (GCDFP15) [68]. Breast cancers that do not fall into any of these subtypes are often listed as unclassified.

i. Luminal A

Most breast cancers are luminal tumors. Luminal tumor cells look the most like the cells of breast cancers that start in the inner (luminal) cells lining the mammary ducts. Luminal A tumors tend to be ER+ and/or PR+, HER2-, and tumor grade 1 or 2. Less than 15% of luminal A tumors have p53 mutations. Hence, luminal A tumors tend to have the best prognosis, with fairly high survival rates and fairly low recurrence rates. Since luminal A tumors tend to be ER+, treatment often includes hormonal therapy which is discussed in a subsequent section.

ii. Luminal B

As mentioned above, luminal tumors have cells that look like those of breast cancers that start in the inner (luminal) cells lining the mammary ducts. Luminal B tumors tend to be ER+ and/ or PR+. Since they have highly mitotically active cells, they are positive for Ki67. They are often HER2+ as well. Interestingly, women with luminal B tumors are often diagnosed at a younger age than those with luminal A tumors and have a poorer prognosis due to poorer tumor grade, larger tumor size and lymph node involvement. About 30% of the tumors also have mutations in p53.

iii. Triple negative/basal-like

Triple negative breast cancers are: ER-, PR-, and HER2-; hence the name triple negative. There are several subsets of triple negative breast cancer. One subset is referred to as basal-like because the tumors have cells with features similar to those of the outer (basal) cells surrounding the mammary ducts. Most basal-like tumors have mutations in p53. About 15 to 20% of breast cancers are triple negative or basal-like. These tumors tend to occur more often in younger and African American women. Of note, most BRCA1 breast cancers are both triple negative and basal-like. Triple negative/basal-like tumors are often aggressive and have a poorer prognosis. These tumors are usually treated with some combination of surgery, radiation therapy and chemotherapy.

iv. HER2 type

The molecular subtype HER2 type is not the same as HER2+ and is not used to guide treatment. Although most HER2 type tumors are HER2+ (and named for this reason), about 30 percent are HER2-. HER2 type tumors tend to be ER-, PR-, with lymph node involvement and poor tumor grade. About 10% to 15% of breast cancers fall under this category and about 75% of HER2 type tumors contain p53 mutations. HER2 type tumors have a fairly poor prognosis and are prone to early and frequent recurrence and metastases. Women with HER2 type tumors appear to be diagnosed at a younger age than those with luminal A and luminal B tumors. HER2/neu-positive tumors can be treated with the drug trastuzumab (Herceptin) and this is discussed in further detail in a subsequent section.

v. Claudin-low

Claudin low is often triple-negative, but distinct in that there is low expression of cell-cell junction proteins including E-cadherin and frequently there is infiltration of lymphocytes. It is also enriched in mesenchymal and stem cell features [69].

vi. Normal-like

About 6 to 10% of all breast cancers are classified as normal-like. These tumors are usually small and tend to have a good prognosis.

6. Clinical diagnosis criteria and imaging modalities for breast cancer

Breast cancer is divided into different stages. Table 1 summarizes these stages.

The extent of cancer can be used to stratify patients. Patients with clinical stage I, IIA, or a subset of stage IIB disease (T2N1 where T= tumor, N= node) are classified as having early-stage breast cancer. Patients with a T3 tumor without nodal involvement or stage IIIA to IIIC disease are classified as having locally advanced breast cancer. Stage IV is when there are distant metastases present and is seen in about 5% of newly diagnosed patients.

Stage	Description
0	Restricted to membrane of the milk duct (DCIS, LCIS)
1	<2cm tumor restricted to the breast
2	2-5 cm tumor +/- metastasis to draining lymph node
3	Metastasis to the lymph nodes +/- superficial skin and surrounding muscles
4	Metastasis to other parts of the body

Table 1. Stages of breast cancer

i. Early-stage breast cancer

The surgical approach to the primary tumor depends on the size of the tumor, whether or not multifocal disease is present, and the size of the breast. Options include breast-conserving therapy or mastectomy and both have similar outcomes.

The risk for metastatic disease in the regional nodes is related to tumor size, histologic grade, and the presence of lymphatic invasion within the primary tumor. As mentioned above, the axillary nodes drain most of the breast tissue. Tumor characteristics are used to select adjuvant treatment for patients with breast cancer. Patients with hormone receptor-positive breast cancer should receive adjuvant endocrine therapy. For patients with triple-negative breast cancer, treatment option includes adjuvant chemotherapy if the tumor size is >0.5 cm. Patients with HER2-positive breast cancer >1 cm in size typically receive a combination of chemotherapy plus HER2-directed therapy. Following chemotherapy, patients with ER-positive disease generally receive adjuvant endocrine therapy.

ii. Locally advanced breast cancer

Most patients with locally advanced, inoperable breast cancer should receive neoadjuvant systemic therapy rather than proceeding with primary surgery in an attempt to shrink the tumor. Typically, these patients are usually not candidates for breast conservation. Neoadjuvant treatment improves the rate of breast conservation without compromising survival outcomes and so most patients get chemotherapy in the neoadjuvant setting rather than endocrine therapy. Due to its greater toxicity to cancer cells, chemotherapy is associated with higher response rates in a faster time frame. As mentioned earlier, HER2-directed agent (ie, trastuzumab) should be added to the chemotherapy regimen for tumors that are HER2-positive. Following surgery, all patients who undergo breast-conserving surgery generally undergo adjuvant radiation therapy (RT) to maximize locoregional control. Some patients treated by a mastectomy should receive postmastectomy RT in order to kill any cancer cells that may have escaped during the procedure.

Patients with hormone receptor-positive breast cancer should receive adjuvant endocrine therapy. The selection of endocrine therapy is made according to menopausal status. In patients with ER-positive breast cancer, in whom surgery is not an option or life expectancy is limited, primary hormonal treatment with either tamoxifen or an aromatase inhibitor without surgery is generally used.

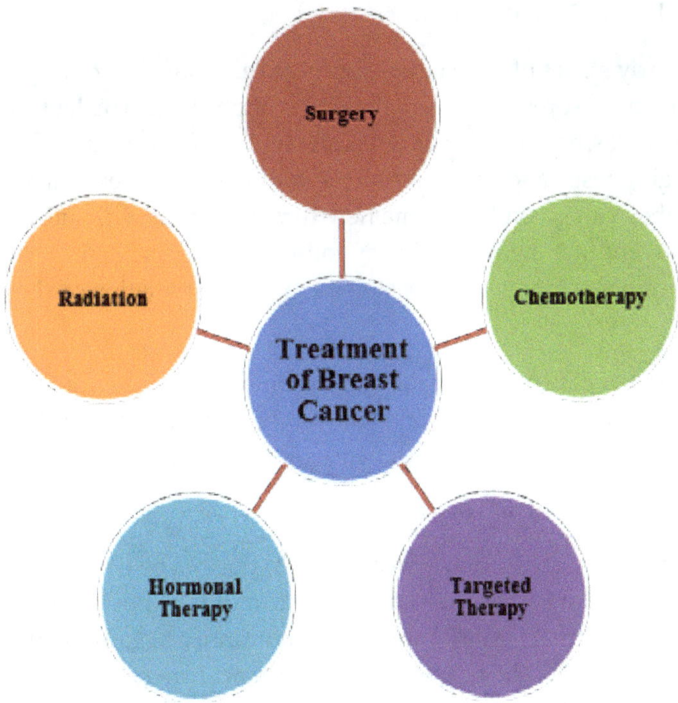

Figure 6. Different treatments available for breast cancer.

7. Therapeutic options for breast cancer

The heterogeneity of breast cancers makes it a challenge to diagnose and treat this solid tumor.

The main types of treatment for breast cancer are:

i. Surgery

ii. Radiation therapy

iii. Chemotherapy

iv. Hormone therapy

v. Targeted therapy

Treatments can be classified into broad groups (Figure 6), based on how they work and when they are used.

a. Local and systemic therapy

As the name implies, local therapy is intended to treat a tumor at the site without affecting the rest of the body. Examples include surgery and radiation therapy. Systemic therapy refers to drugs which can be given by mouth or directly into the bloodstream to reach cancer cells anywhere in the body. Chemotherapy, hormone therapy, and targeted therapy are systemic therapies that are widely used.

b. Adjuvant and neoadjuvant therapy

Since even in the early stages of breast cancer, cancer cells may break away from the primary breast tumor and begin to spread, adjuvant therapy is often given to patients with no detectable cancer after surgery. A small number of cells can't be 'felt' on a physical exam or seen on X-rays or other imaging tests, and they cause no symptoms until they reach a certain number but, menacingly, they can go on to become new tumors in nearby tissues, other organs, and bones. Hence, adjuvant therapy is a mainstay following surgery. Both systemic therapy like chemotherapy, hormone therapy, and targeted therapy, and radiation can be used as adjuvant therapy.

In neoadjuvant therapy, patients are treated with chemotherapy or hormonal therapy prior to surgery. The goal of this treatment is to shrink the tumor in the hope it will allow a less extensive operation to be done. This also lowers the chance of the cancer coming back later.

i. Surgery

For both DCIS and early-stage invasive breast cancer, doctors generally recommend surgery to remove the tumor. To make sure that the entire tumor is removed, the surgeon will also remove a small area of normal tissue around the tumor until a negative margin is achieved. A lumpectomy is the removal of the tumor and a small cancer-free margin while a mastectomy is the removal of the entire breast. It is important to lower the risk of recurrence and to get rid of any remaining cancer cells that can lead to both local and distant recurrence of cancer. Adjuvant therapies include radiation therapy, chemotherapy, targeted therapy, and/or hormonal therapy which are described below. Surgical treatment for breast cancer involves removal of the lymph nodes and can also include resection of the surrounding axillary nodes.

ii. Radiation therapy

This involves killing the cancer cells by inducing clustered DNA damage using ionizing radiation. By overwhelming the cell with DNA damage, the cell undergoes apoptosis. As little as one DNA double strand break can be lethal to the cell. By giving multiple doses of radiation broken up into fractions, the hope is to prolong survival. Some of the side effects include dermatologic issues, fibrosis, nausea etc. due to the radiation. Although most side effects usually go away after radiation therapy has been concluded, some long-term side effects may occur months or even years after treatment ends. These late effects which usually associate with persistent inflammation and oxidative stress may include developing a secondary primary cancer. However, we must mention that the risk of developing a second cancer because of radiation therapy is relatively low, and this risk is generally outweighed by the benefit of treating the primary, existing cancer and offering survival to the patient.

iii. Chemotherapy

This involves using drugs and small molecules to selectively kill the cancer cells. Examples include: carboplatin, cisplatin, cyclophosphamide, docetaxel, doxorubicin, fluorouracil (5-FU), gemcitabine, methotrexate, paclitaxel, etc. A patient may receive one drug at a time or combinations of different drugs at the same time. Research has shown that combinations of certain drugs are sometimes more effective than single drugs for adjuvant treatment and so combinations are often used. Carboplatin and cisplatin are alkylating agents and belong to the group of platinum-based antineoplastic agents. They interact with DNA to interfere with DNA repair. These drugs cross-link with the DNA strands, mostly to guanine groups. This causes intra- and inter-strand DNA cross-links, resulting in inhibition of DNA, RNA and protein synthesis. Antimetabolites, such as methotrexate, are more active against S-phase cells where they block DNA synthesis whereas vinca alkaloids are more active in the M-phase where they inhibit spindle formation and alignment of chromosomes. Antimetabolites are compounds that bear a structural similarity to naturally occurring substances such as vitamins, nucleosides or amino acids. They compete with the natural substrate for the active site on an essential enzyme or receptor. Methotrexate competitively inhibits dihydrofolate reductase, which is responsible for the formation of tetrahydrofolate from dihydrofolate. This plays an important role in the synthesis of, among others, purines and methionine. Anthracyclines such as doxorubicin intercalate with DNA and affect the topoisomerase II enzyme. This DNA gyrase splits the DNA helix and reconnects it to overcome the torsional forces that would interfere with replication. The anthracyclines stabilize the DNA topoisomerase II complex and thus prevent reconnection of the strands. Paclitaxel promotes assembly of microtubules and inhibits their disassembly which interferes with cell division.

One of the more recent treatment options for breast are PARP inhibitors which showed initial promise in patients with tumors that have BRCA1 or BRCA2 mutations and therefore deficient double strand break repair. PARP inhibitors achieve an enhanced or synthetic lethality for tumor cells by blocking DNA repair pathways. PARP, which has multiple family members, detects single strand DNA breaks and participates in BER. It forms poly (ADP-ribose) polymers on itself and a number of substrates which can alter a number of pathways including DNA repair. Inhibition of PARP leads to persistent single strand break which converts to a double strand break as the cell attempts to replicate the DNA. Normal cells have an intact HR-mediated repair pathway and so are able to repair the DNA double strand break. However, in the absence of intact HR-mediated repair pathway which can happen with loss of or mutation in BRCA proteins, the cell is unable to repair the double strand break. As a result, typically, the cell undergoes apoptosis. A phase II study of the PARP inhibitor olaparib in patients with advanced breast cancer with BRCA1 or BRCA2 mutations has shown promising results with a response rate of 11/27, a progression-free survival of 5.7 months, and a median objective response duration of 144 days [70]. Phase III trials are currently in progress to evaluate olaparib in breast cancer [71]. TNBC also demonstrates BRCAness and so PARP inhibitors may be useful in this setting as well. Data from clinical trials have not been conclusive in this regard thus far.

Phosphatase and tensin homolog (PTEN) regulates RAD51 mediated DNA repair to maintain genomic stability. PTEN mutations, which occur in 30–50% of breast cancers, cause genomic instability similar to that seen in BRCA-deficient cells and so may be targets of PARP inhibitors as well [72].

iv. Hormonal therapy

Hormonal therapy is widely used in breast cancer treatment. These are used in the setting of ER+ and PR+ tumors. Since these tumors use hormones to fuel their growth, blocking the hormones can help prevent or at least slow down the growth of the tumor.

Selective estrogen receptor modulators (SERMs) are a class of compounds that act on the estrogen receptor. Tamoxifen blocks estrogen from binding to breast cancer cells. It is effective for not only lowering the risk of recurrence in the breast that had cancer, it also reduces the risk of developing cancer in the other breast, and the risk of distant recurrence. It is also approved to reduce the risk of breast cancer in women at high risk for developing breast cancer and for lowering the risk of a local recurrence for women with DCIS who have had a lumpectomy. Tamoxifen is also an effective treatment for metastatic hormone receptor-positive breast cancer. However, chronic Tamoxifen use has been linked with some toxicity and adverse effects like persistent oxidative stress and others as reviewed in [73].

Aromatase inhibitors (AIs) decrease the amount of estrogen made by tissues other than the ovaries in postmenopausal women by blocking the aromatase enzyme, which converts androgens into estrogen. These drugs include anastrozole and exemestane. Similar to Tamoxifen, AIs are also an effective treatment for metastatic hormone receptor positive breast cancer.

Fulvestrant, a SERM, is an additional hormonal therapy approved for patients with metastatic breast cancer. Fulvestrant is an estrogen-receptor targeting therapy that is used for the treatment of advanced-stage breast cancer in postmenopausal women with endocrine-sensitive cancer [74-77].

v. Targeted therapy

Targeted therapy is a treatment that targets specific genes or proteins. One of the advantages of this is that it limits damage to healthy cells. Trastuzumab, a monoclonal antibody, is approved for both the treatment of advanced breast cancer and as an adjuvant therapy for early-stage HER2+ breast cancer. Trastuzumab does have cardio toxic effects. Pertuzumab is a monoclonal antibody marketed by Genentech for the treatment of HER2+ breast cancer, in combination with trastuzumab and docetaxel. It inhibits the dimerization of HER2 with other HER receptors, which reduces tumor growth. Lapatinib, a dual tyrosine kinase inhibitor which interrupts the HER2/neu and epidermal growth factor receptor (EGFR) pathways, is commonly used for women with HER2-positive metastatic breast cancer when trastuzumab and pertuzumab in combination with docetaxel are no longer effective at controlling the cancer's growth. Lapatinib decreases tumor-causing breast cancer stem cells and inhibits receptor signal processes by binding to the ATP-binding pocket of the EGFR/HER2 protein kinase domain, preventing auto-phosphorylation and subsequent activation of the signal mechanism.

Table 2 lists some of the current trials evaluating different therapies for breast cancer.

ClinicalTrials.gov Identifier	Description
NCT00065325	Compare the efficacy of Faslodex (fulvestrant) to Aromasin (exemestane) in hormone receptor positive postmenopausal women with advanced breast cancer.
NCT00103181	Compare whole breast radiation therapy to partial breast radiation therapy in treating women who have undergone surgery for ductal carcinoma in situ or stage I or stage II breast cancer.
NCT00176488	Evaluate epirubicin (an anthracycline) together with vinorelbine (an anti-mitotic drug) in treating patients with stage II, stage III, or stage IV breast cancer.
NCT00281697	Evaluate the efficacy and safety of bevacizumab when combined with standard chemotherapy compared with chemotherapy alone in subjects with previously treated metastatic breast cancer.
NCT00372710	Evaluate the safety and efficacy of zoledronic acid (a bisphosphonate) when added to standard therapies in breast cancer patients with metastatic bone lesions.
NCT00399529	Examine combination therapy with Trastuzumab, Cyclophosphamide, and an allogeneic Granulocyte-macrophage colony-stimulating factor (GM-CSF)-secreting whole cell breast cancer vaccine in patients with stage IV HER2/neu-overexpressing breast cancer.
NCT00454532	Assess the toxicity, maximum tolerated dose, safety and preliminary efficacy of BZL101, an aqueous extract from herba Scutellaria Barbata D. Don of the Lamiaceae family, for the treatment of advanced metastatic breast cancer.
NCT00466102	Determine whether RAD001 can inhibit growth of tumor cells and/or stop the formation and activity of bone degrading osteoclasts.
NCT00494234	To see if the drug KU 0059436 (olaparib) is effective and well tolerated in treating patients with measurable BRCA1- or BRCA2-positive advanced breast cancer and for whom no curative therapeutic option exists.
NCT00503841	How well does erlotinib work in treating women undergoing surgery for stage I, stage II, or stage III breast cancer?
NCT00629616	Efficacy of Anastrozole with fulvestrant in treating postmenopausal women with stage II or stage III breast cancer that can be removed by surgery.
NCT00817362	Efficacy and safety of IPI-504 (heat shock protein 90 inhibitor) with Trastuzumab in pretreated, locally advanced or metastatic HER2+ breast cancer
NCT00817531	Efficacy of Dasatinib in locally advanced triple negative breast cancer patients
NCT01031446	Evaluate cisplatin and paclitaxel together with everolimus and to see how well it works in treating patients with metastatic breast cancer
NCT01132664	Assess the safety and efficacy of BKM120 (PI3K inhibitor) in combination with trastuzumab in patients with relapsing HER2 overexpressing breast cancer who have previously failed trastuzumab.

ClinicalTrials.gov Identifier	Description
NCT01351597	Evaluate the efficacy and safety of combination chemotherapy with DoceTaxel (Detaxel) and Oxaliplatin (Oxalitin) in recurrent or metastatic breast cancer
NCT01509625	Assess the response to treatment with fulvestrant at a dose of 500 mg/month with a loading dose of 500 mg, in terms of progression free survival, overall survival, and clinical benefit rate, in post-menopausal women with advanced breast cancer and estrogen receptor positive, who were treated with this medicinal product and at said dose after having progressed with a previous anti-estrogen therapy.
NCT01534455	Compare the efficacy and tolerability of two dose-schedules of eribulin (a ketone analog) plus lapatinib in HER2-positive breast cancer, pre-treated with trastuzumab in the adjuvant and/or metastatic setting.
NCT01880385	Evaluating the treatment of bevacizumab in association with pre-operative chemotherapy, followed by surgery, adjuvant chemotherapy and radiotherapy in patients with inflammatory breast cancer.
NCT01881230	Compare the safety and efficacy of nab-paclitaxel in combination with either gemcitabine or carboplatin to the combination of gemcitabine and carboplatin as first line treatment in female subjects with triple negative metastatic breast cancer or metastatic triple negative breast cancer.
NCT02000622	Assess the efficacy and safety of single agent olaparib, a PARP inhibitor, vs standard of care based on physician's choice of capecitabine (that is converted to 5-FU during metabolism), vinorelbine (anti-mitotic drug) or eribulin (a ketone analog) in metastatic breast cancer patients with germline BRCA 1/2 mutations.
NCT02202746	Determine whether lucitanib, a potent tyrosine kinase inhibitor, is safe and effective in the treatment of patients with fibroblast growth factor aberrant metastatic breast cancer.

Table 2. Current clinical trials evaluating therapies for breast cancer

8. Conclusion

Breast cancer continues to be a threat and a challenge to treat. While a lot has been accomplished in the past decade, there is more that can be done. Further understanding of tumor evolution will lead to the eradication and effective prevention of this disease. At the same time delineating the breast oncogenic mechanisms like DNA damage response, conversion of DNA lesions to mutations, etc. will help us target initiating events and further optimize personalized therapies and possibly develop new ones. Therefore we believe that it is the 'DNA' which plays the dominant role and holds the key for effective treatment of the whole phenomenon of breast carcinogenesis.

Abbreviations

5-FU: Fluorouracil

AI: Aromatase inhibitor

AKT: Protein kinase B

ALDH1: Aldehyde dehydrogenase 1

AT: Ataxia telangiectasia

ATM: Ataxia telangiectasia mutated

ATR: Ataxia telangiectasia and Rad3 related

BER: Base excision repair

BRCA1: Breast cancer type 1 susceptibility protein

CDK: Cyclin dependent kinase

CFS: Common fragile sites

Chk1: Checkpoint kinase 1

Chk2: Checkpoint kinase 2

CTC: Circulating tumor cells

CXCR1: C-X-C chemokine receptor type 1

DCIS: Ductal carcinoma in situ

DDR: DNA damage response

EGFR: Epidermal derived growth factor

EMT: Epithelial-to-mesenchymal transition

GCDFP15: Gross cystic disease fluid protein-15

GM-CSF: Granulocyte-macrophage colony-stimulating factor

HER2: Human epidermal growth factor receptor 2

HIF1: Hypoxia-inducible factor 1

HR: Homologous recombination

IL6: Interleukin 6

IL8: Interleukin 8

MMP1: Matrix metalloproteinase-1

MMR: Mismatch repair

MRN: MRE11–RAD50–NBS1

NER: Nucleotide excision repair

NHEJ: Non-homologous end joining

PARP: Poly ADP ribose polymerase

PI3K: Phosphatidylinositol-4,5-bisphosphate 3-kinase

PTEN: Phosphatase and tensin homolog

RT: Radiation therapy

SERM: Selective estrogen receptor modulator

TGFβ: Tumor derived growth factor β

TWIST: Twist-related protein

WRN: Werner syndrome ATP-dependent helicase

Acknowledgements

Somaira Nowsheen and Khaled Aziz thank the Mayo Clinic Medical Scientist Training Program for fostering an outstanding environment for physician-scientist training. Somaira Nowsheen was supported by the Laura J. Siegel Breast Cancer Fellowship Award from the Foundation for Women's Wellness. Dr. Georgakilas was supported by an EU Marie Curie Reintegration Grant MC-CIG-303514, Greek National funds through the Operational Program Educational and Lifelong Learning of the National Strategic Reference Framework (NSRF)-Research Funding Program: THALES (Grant number MIS 379346) and COST Action CM1201 Biomimetic Radical Chemistry.

Author details

Somaira Nowsheen[1], Khaled Aziz[1], Asef Aziz[2] and Alexandros G Georgakilas[3*]

*Address all correspondence to: alexg@mail.ntua.gr

1 Medical Scientist Training Program, Mayo Graduate School, Mayo Medical School, Mayo Clinic, Rochester, MN, USA

2 Baylor University, Waco, TX, USA

3 Department of Physics, School of Applied Mathematical and Physical Sciences, National Technical University of Athens, Zografou Campus, GR, Athens, Greece

References

[1] Siegel R, Ma J, Zou Z, Jemal A. Cancer statistics, 2014. CA: A Cancer Journal for Clinicians. 2014;64(1):9-29.

[2] Ma J, Jemal A. Breast cancer statistics. Breast Cancer Metastasis and Drug Resistance: Springer; 2013. p. 1-18.

[3] DeSantis C, Ma J, Bryan L, Jemal A. Breast cancer statistics, 2013. CA: A Cancer Journal for Clinicians. 2014;64(1):52-62.

[4] Vogelstein B, Lane D, Levine AJ. Surfing the p53 network. Nature. 2000;408(6810): 307-10.

[5] Toshiyuki M, Reed JC. Tumor suppressor p53 is a direct transcriptional activator of the human bax gene. Cell. 1995;80(2):293-9.

[6] Greenblatt M, Bennett W, Hollstein M, Harris C. Mutations in the p53 tumor suppressor gene: clues to cancer etiology and molecular pathogenesis. Cancer Research. 1994;54(18):4855-78.

[7] Latif F, Tory K, Gnarra J, Yao M, Duh F-M, Orcutt ML, et al. Identification of the von Hippel-Lindau disease tumor suppressor gene. Science. 1993;260(5112):1317-20.

[8] El-Deiry WS, Tokino T, Velculescu VE, Levy DB, Parsons R, Trent JM, et al. WAF1, a potential mediator of p53 tumor suppression. Cell. 1993;75(4):817-25.

[9] Fearon ER, Vogelstein B. A genetic model for colorectal tumorigenesis. Cell. 1990;61(5):759-67.

[10] Selivanova G. p53: fighting cancer. Current cancer drug targets. 2004;4(5):385-402.

[11] Whibley C, Pharoah PD, Hollstein M. p53 polymorphisms: cancer implications. Nature Reviews Cancer. 2009;9(2):95-107.

[12] Muller PA, Vousden KH. Mutant p53 in Cancer: New Functions and Therapeutic Opportunities. Cancer Cell. 2014;25(3):304-17.

[13] Knudson AG. Two genetic hits (more or less) to cancer. Nature Reviews Cancer. 2001;1(2):157-62.

[14] Michor F, Iwasa Y, Nowak MA. Dynamics of cancer progression. Nature Reviews Cancer. 2004;4(3):197-205.

[15] Hanahan D, Weinberg Robert A. Hallmarks of Cancer: The Next Generation. Cell. 2011;144(5):646-74.

[16] Georgakilas AG, Tsantoulis P, Kotsinas A, Michalopoulos I, Townsend P, Gorgoulis VG. Are common fragile sites merely structural domains or highly organized "functional" units susceptible to oncogenic stress? Cellular and Molecular Life Sciences. 2014:1-26.

[17] Dillon LW, Burrow AA, Wang Y-H. DNA instability at chromosomal fragile sites in cancer. Current genomics. 2010;11(5):326.

[18] Slamon DJ, Godolphin W, Jones LA, Holt JA, Wong SG, Keith DE, et al. Studies of the HER2/neu proto-oncogene in human breast and ovarian cancer. Science. 1989;244(4905):707-12.

[19] Finlay CA, Hinds PW, Levine AJ. The p53 proto-oncogene can act as a suppressor of transformation. Cell. 1989;57(7):1083-93.

[20] Franke TF, Yang S-I, Chan TO, Datta K, Kazlauskas A, Morrison DK, et al. The protein kinase encoded by the Akt proto-oncogene is a target of the PDGF-activated phosphatidylinositol 3-kinase. Cell. 1995;81(5):727-36.

[21] Malkin D, Li FP, Strong LC, Fraumeni J, Nelson CE, Kim DH, et al. Germ line p53 mutations in a familial syndrome of breast cancer, sarcomas, and other neoplasms. Science. 1990;250(4985):1233-8.

[22] Hollstein M, Sidransky D, Vogelstein B, Harris CC. p53 mutations in human cancers. Science. 1991;253(5015):49-53.

[23] Brosh R, Rotter V. When mutants gain new powers: news from the mutant p53 field. Nature Reviews Cancer. 2009;9(10):701-13.

[24] Yang ES, Nowsheen S, Rahman MA, Cook RS, Xia F. Targeting BRCA1 localization to augment breast tumor sensitivity to poly(ADP-ribose) polymerase inhibition. Cancer Res. 2012; 72(21): 5547-5555.

[25] Bartkova J, Horejsi Z, Koed K, Kramer A, Tort F, Zieger K, et al. DNA damage response as a candidate anti-cancer barrier in early human tumorigenesis. Nature. 2005;434(7035):864-70.

[26] Bartkova J, Rezaei N, Liontos M, Karakaidos P, Kletsas D, Issaeva N, et al. Oncogene-induced senescence is part of the tumorigenesis barrier imposed by DNA damage checkpoints. Nature. 2006;444(7119):633-7.

[27] Gorgoulis VG, Vassiliou LV, Karakaidos P, Zacharatos P, Kotsinas A, Liloglou T, et al. Activation of the DNA damage checkpoint and genomic instability in human precancerous lesions. Nature. 2005;434(7035):907-13.

[28] Halazonetis TD, Gorgoulis VG, Bartek J. An oncogene-induced DNA damage model for cancer development. Science. 2008;319(5868):1352-5.

[29] Sideridou M, Zakopoulou R, Evangelou K, Liontos M, Kotsinas A, Rampakakis E, et al. Cdc6 expression represses E-cadherin transcription and activates adjacent replication origins. The Journal of cell biology. 2011;195(7):1123-40.

[30] Liontos M, Koutsami M, Sideridou M, Evangelou K, Kletsas D, Levy B, et al. Deregulated Overexpression of hCdt1 and hCdc6 Promotes Malignant Behavior. Cancer Research. 2007;67(22):10899-909.

[31] Kryston TB, Georgiev AB, Pissis P, Georgakilas AG. Role of oxidative stress and DNA damage in human carcinogenesis. Mutation Research/Fundamental and Molecular Mechanisms of Mutagenesis. 2011;711(1):193-201.

[32] Polo SE, Jackson SP. Dynamics of DNA damage response proteins at DNA breaks: a focus on protein modifications. Genes Dev. 2011;25(5):409-33.

[33] Stratton MR. Exploring the genomes of cancer cells: progress and promise. Science. 2011;331(6024):1553-8.

[34] Stricker T, Catenacci DV, Seiwert TY. Molecular profiling of cancer--the future of personalized cancer medicine: a primer on cancer biology and the tools necessary to bring molecular testing to the clinic. Semin Oncol. 2011;38(2):173-85.

[35] Bartek J, Lukas C, Lukas J. Checking on DNA damage in S phase. Nat Rev Mol Cell Biol. 2004;5(10):792-804.

[36] Jackson SP, Bartek J. The DNA-damage response in human biology and disease. Nature. 2009;461(7267):1071-8.

[37] Graeser MK, Engel C, Rhiem K, Gadzicki D, Bick U, Kast K, et al. Contralateral Breast Cancer Risk in BRCA1 and BRCA2 Mutation Carriers. Journal of Clinical Oncology. 2009;27(35):5887-92.

[38] King M-C, Marks JH, Mandell JB, The New York Breast Cancer Study G. Breast and Ovarian Cancer Risks Due to Inherited Mutations in BRCA1 and BRCA2. Science. 2003;302(5645):643-6.

[39] Esteller M, Silva JM, Dominguez G, Bonilla F, Matias-Guiu X, Lerma E, et al. Promoter Hypermethylation and BRCA1 Inactivation in Sporadic Breast and Ovarian Tumors. Journal of the National Cancer Institute. 2000;92(7):564-9.

[40] Marsit CJ, Liu M, Nelson HH, Posner M, Suzuki M, Kelsey KT. Inactivation of the Fanconi anemia//BRCA pathway in lung and oral cancers: implications for treatment and survival. Oncogene. 2003;23(4):1000-4.

[41] Alderton G. Radiation sensitivity: Tolerance is not a virtue. Nat Rev Cancer. 2007;7(4):230-1.

[42] Shiloh Y. ATM and related protein kinases: safeguarding genome integrity. Nat Rev Cancer. 2003;3(3):155-68.

[43] Minn AJ, Gupta GP, Siegel PM, Bos PD, Shu W, Giri DD, et al. Genes that mediate breast cancer metastasis to lung. Nature. 2005;436(7050):518-24.

[44] Coleman R, Rubens R. The clinical course of bone metastases from breast cancer. British journal of cancer. 1987;55(1):61.

[45] Weigelt B, Peterse JL, Van't Veer LJ. Breast cancer metastasis: markers and models. Nature Reviews Cancer. 2005;5(8):591-602.

[46] Mehrotra J, Vali M, McVeigh M, Kominsky SL, Fackler MJ, Lahti-Domenici J, et al. Very high frequency of hypermethylated genes in breast cancer metastasis to the bone, brain, and lung. Clinical Cancer Research. 2004;10(9):3104-9.

[47] Bos PD, Zhang XH-F, Nadal C, Shu W, Gomis RR, Nguyen DX, et al. Genes that mediate breast cancer metastasis to the brain. Nature. 2009;459(7249):1005-9.

[48] Gomez D, Alonso D, Yoshiji H, Thorgeirsson U. Tissue inhibitors of metalloproteinases: structure, regulation and biological functions. European journal of cell biology. 1997;74(2):111-22.

[49] Nagase H, Woessner JF. Matrix metalloproteinases. Journal of Biological Chemistry. 1999;274(31):21491-4.

[50] Gialeli C, Theocharis AD, Karamanos NK. Roles of matrix metalloproteinases in cancer progression and their pharmacological targeting. FeBS Journal. 2011;278(1):16-27.

[51] Kessenbrock K, Plaks V, Werb Z. Matrix metalloproteinases: regulators of the tumor microenvironment. Cell. 2010;141(1):52-67.

[52] Bourboulia D, Stetler-Stevenson WG, editors. Matrix metalloproteinases (MMPs) and tissue inhibitors of metalloproteinases (TIMPs): Positive and negative regulators in tumor cell adhesion. Seminars in cancer biology; 2010: Elsevier.

[53] Leblanc R, Lee S, David M, Bordet J, Norman D, Patil R, et al. Interaction of platelet-derived autotaxin with tumor integrin $\alpha V\beta 3$ controls metastasis of breast cancer cells to bone. Blood. 2014.

[54] Lorger M, Felding-Habermann B. Integrin Signaling in Angiogenesis and Metastatic Cancer Progression in the Brain. Signaling Pathways and Molecular Mediators in Metastasis: Springer; 2012. p. 311-29.

[55] Oka H, Shiozaki H, Kobayashi K, Inoue M, Tahara H, Kobayashi T, et al. Expression of E-cadherin cell adhesion molecules in human breast cancer tissues and its relationship to metastasis. Cancer Research. 1993;53(7):1696-701.

[56] Graff JR, Herman JG, Lapidus RG, Chopra H, Xu R, Jarrard DF, et al. E-cadherin expression is silenced by DNA hypermethylation in human breast and prostate carcinomas. Cancer Research. 1995;55(22):5195-9.

[57] Yoshida R, Kimura N, Harada Y, Ohuchi N. The loss of E-cadherin, α-and β-catenin expression is associated with metastasis and poor prognosis in invasive breast cancer. International journal of oncology. 2001;18(3):513-20.

[58] Hazan RB, Phillips GR, Qiao RF, Norton L, Aaronson SA. Exogenous expression of N-cadherin in breast cancer cells induces cell migration, invasion, and metastasis. The Journal of cell biology. 2000;148(4):779-90.

[59] Nass SJ, Herman JG, Gabrielson E, Iversen PW, Parl FF, Davidson NE, et al. Aberrant methylation of the estrogen receptor and E-cadherin 5′ CpG islands increases with malignant progression in human breast cancer. Cancer Research. 2000;60(16):4346-8.

[60] Nieman MT, Prudoff RS, Johnson KR, Wheelock MJ. N-cadherin promotes motility in human breast cancer cells regardless of their E-cadherin expression. The Journal of cell biology. 1999;147(3):631-44.

[61] Chaffer CL, Weinberg RA. A perspective on cancer cell metastasis. Science. 2011;331(6024):1559-64.

[62] Creighton CJ, Chang JC, Rosen JM. Epithelial-mesenchymal transition (EMT) in tumor-initiating cells and its clinical implications in breast cancer. Journal of mammary gland biology and neoplasia. 2010;15(2):253-60.

[63] Yu M, Bardia A, Wittner BS, Stott SL, Smas ME, Ting DT, et al. Circulating breast tumor cells exhibit dynamic changes in epithelial and mesenchymal composition. Science. 2013;339(6119):580-4.

[64] Palumbo JS, Kombrinck KW, Drew AF, Grimes TS, Kiser JH, Degen JL, et al. Fibrinogen is an important determinant of the metastatic potential of circulating tumor cells. Blood. 2000;96(10):3302-9.

[65] Burgess DJ. Breast cancer: Circulating and dynamic EMT. Nature Reviews Cancer. 2013;13(3):148-9.

[66] Pelucchi C, Tramacere I, Boffetta P, Negri E, Vecchia CL. Alcohol Consumption and Cancer Risk. Nutrition and Cancer. 2011;63(7):983-90.

[67] Ban KA, Godellas CV. Epidemiology of Breast Cancer. Surgical oncology clinics of North America. 2014;23(3):409-22.

[68] Lehmann-Che J, Hamy A-S, Porcher R, Barritault M, Bouhidel F, Habuellelah H, et al. Molecular apocrine breast cancers are aggressive estrogen receptor negative tu-

mors overexpressing either HER2 or GCDFP15. Breast Cancer Research. 2013;15(3):R37.

[69] Prat A, Parker J, Karginova O, Fan C, Livasy C, Herschkowitz J, et al. Phenotypic and molecular characterization of the claudin-low intrinsic subtype of breast cancer. Breast Cancer Research. 2010;12(5):R68.

[70] Tutt A, Robson M, Garber JE, Domchek SM, Audeh MW, Weitzel JN, et al. Oral poly(ADP-ribose) polymerase inhibitor olaparib in patients with BRCA1 or BRCA2 mutations and advanced breast cancer: a proof-of-concept trial. The Lancet. 2010;376(9737):235-44.

[71] Tutt A, Balmana J, Robson M, Garber J, Kaufman B, Geyer C, et al. 331TiPOlympia, Neo-Olympia and Olympiad: Randomized phase III trials of Olaparib in patients with breast cancer and a germline BRCA1/2 mutation. Annals of Oncology. 2014;25(suppl 4):iv109.

[72] Zhang HY, Liang F, Jia ZL, Song ST, Jiang ZF. PTEN mutation, methylation and expression in breast cancer patients. Oncology letters. 2013;6(1):161-8.

[73] Yang G, Nowsheen S, Aziz K, Georgakilas AG. Toxicity and adverse effects of Tamoxifen and other anti-estrogen drugs. Pharmacology & therapeutics. 2013;139(3): 392-404.

[74] Clemons MJ, Cochrane B, Pond GR, Califaretti N, Chia SK, Dent RA, et al. Randomised, phase II, placebo-controlled, trial of fulvestrant plus vandetanib in postmenopausal women with bone only or bone predominant, hormone-receptor-positive metastatic breast cancer (MBC): the OCOG ZAMBONEY study. Breast Cancer Research and Treatment. 2014;146(1):153-62.

[75] Massarweh S, Romond E, Black EP, Van Meter E, Shelton B, Kadamyan-Melkumian V, et al. A phase II study of combined fulvestrant and everolimus in patients with metastatic estrogen receptor (ER)-positive breast cancer after aromatase inhibitor (AI) failure. Breast Cancer Research and Treatment. 2014;143(2):325-32.

[76] Schwartzberg LS, Wang G, Somer BG, Blakely LJ, Wheeler BM, Walker MS, et al. Phase II Trial of Fulvestrant With Metronomic Capecitabine for Postmenopausal Women With Hormone Receptor-Positive, HER2-Negative Metastatic Breast Cancer. Clinical breast cancer. 2014;14(1):13-9.

[77] Bachelot T, McCool R, Duffy S, Glanville J, Varley D, Fleetwood K, et al. Comparative efficacy of everolimus plus exemestane versus fulvestrant for hormone-receptor-positive advanced breast cancer following progression/recurrence after endocrine therapy: a network meta-analysis. Breast Cancer Research and Treatment. 2014;143(1):125-33.

4

MicroRNAs as Therapeutic Targets in Human Breast Cancer

Hacer Esra Gurses, Omer Faruk Hatipoğlu,
Mehmet Gunduz and Esra Gunduz

1. Introduction

Cancer, which has unrestricted cell growth with the potential to invade or metastasize to other parts of the body is a complex group of diseases with many possible causes. The American Cancer Society reported that the most common type of cancer and the leading cause of cancer-related mortality among females in the world is breast cancer (BC), with about 235,000 new cases expected in the United States in 2014. One in eight women has a chance of developing BC in her lifetime.

Technological improvements in the last decade have helped researchers to understand this complex disease more thoroughly. In spite of the presence of promising tools for breast cancer therapy, the mortality rate of metastatic breast cancer cases is still high. Thus it is necessary to identify significant therapeutic targets by investigating the molecular basis of the disease. In recent years, studies aimed at determining the possible molecular mechanisms of breast cancer have increased in number. Many treatment strategies have been developed. Nevertheless, these methods induce a range of therapeutic responses and therapeutic resistance can develop in breast cancer patients, therefore new methods must be developed.

MicroRNAs (miRNAs) have been reported as playing important roles in cancer development. miRNAs are potential alternative therapeutic targets for cancer. They are also candidate diagnostic and prognostic indicators of breast cancer. miRNAs are small non-coding RNAs that bind to the 3' untranslated region of target mRNAs and down-regulate their translation to protein or degrade the mRNAs. miRNAs play critical roles in many different cellular processes including metabolism, apoptosis, differentiation, and development. They are also linked to human diseases, including cancer. Since their initial discovery in 1993, during a study of the gene lin-4 in *Caenorhabditis elegans*, more than 2000 molecules have been identified in humans, regulating the expression of almost 30% of genes.

miRNAs role as mainly in a tumor suppressive or oncogenic manner. Significantly increased miRNA expression can cause differences in cancer initiation, progression, migration, invasion and metastasis. If circulating extracellular miRNAs are detectable in plasma of BC patients, they can supply novel, non-invasive biomarkers for BC diagnosis and prognosis. Furthermore, new discoveries about miRNAs indicate that they may be involved in the response to chemotherapy or radiotherapy. For instance, MiR-21 is a significant BC-related intracellular and extra-cellular biomarker and a therapeutic target with upregulated expression detected in human BC tissues and cell lines, and plays a key role in all phases of BC pathogenesis. Today, investigation of the association of miRNAs with breast cancer has advanced. miRNAs are being utilized as diagnostic and prognostic biomarkers for patient stratification and also as therapeutic targets and agents in clinical laboratories.

Consequently, the aim of this chapter is to present the current knowledge and concepts concerning the involvement of microRNAs in breast cancer. The oncogenic role of miRNAs in BC etiopathogenesis and as treatment response predictors and therapeutic targets in BC management will be described.

2. The regulation of MicroRNAs

MicroRNAs (miRNAs) are a class of endogenous small RNAs displaying a role in gene regulation at the post transcriptional level in the cell. They have roles in the central dogma and exist extensively in the genome of high level eukaryotic cells in which miRNA genes constitute 1–2% of introns or genes [1]. miRNAs control gene expression via transcription and translation of genes, including mRNA deterioration and translation suppression. The removal of an adenylate group is followed by loss of poly(A)-binding protein initiation 5' decapping, hence promoting exonucleolytic digestion from the 5' end [2]. miRNA interferes with gene expression through inhibition of translation. miRNAs can thereby independently stop translation, beginning by a cap-dependent mechanism. For translationally active polysomes of lower mass initiation is impaired [3]. Furthermore, recent studies indicate that miRNAs cause an m^7 G cap-dependent impediment to the recruitment of 80S ribosomes to mRNA [4]. As a result, the basis of the cap binding affinity of the miRNA-binding protein Ago was identified, in which the cap is inaccessible and thus unable to be bound to the initiation factor eIF4E [5]. Although, several proteins interfere with mRNA degradation and translational repression, some of them are necessary components of the RNA induced silencing complex (RISC) that transports those small RNAs to complementary sites within mRNA [6]. miRNAs assert their silencing role generally by interactions with the 3'-untranslated related RISC complex and can affect miRNA targeting specificity. The result of these miRNA interactions is that they regulate a huge number of protein coding genes. These targets include several signalling pathways, and their effects trigger amplification of certain genes. miRNAs have characteristic roles in changing cellular and signalling pathways which can induce cancer developmnet and progression [7] (Figure 1).

miRNAs are transcribed by RNA polymerase II by using large RNA precursors known as pri-miRNAs [8]. The variation of transcription factors just as of protein-coding genes regulate transcription of miRNA genes [9]. The regulatory network of miRNAs and their targets is complicated. A single miRNA can regulate various mRNAs, and conversely a single mRNA can be targeted by a number of distinct miRNAs. Based on computational estimations, it has been determined that miRNAs regulate one third of all human protein-coding genes [10].

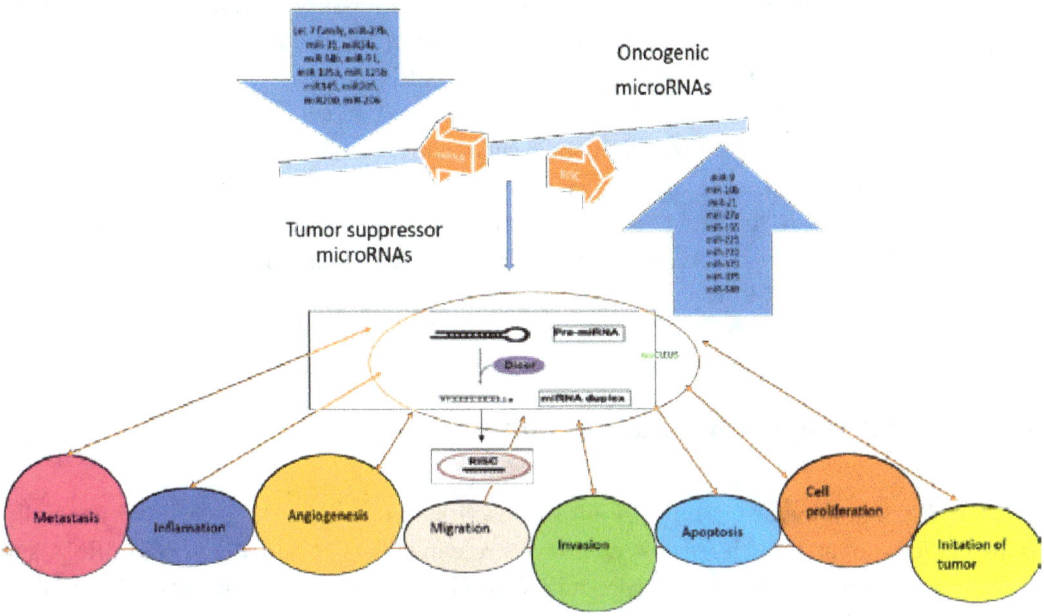

Figure 1. The changes induced by miRNAs in breast cancer pathogenesis. The decreased of suppressive miRNA control inhibition on oncogenes in breast cancer. The upregulation of miRNA inhibits tumor suppressors. Both mechanisms control gene expression and play specific roles in BC predisposition, initiation, cell proliferation, resistance to apoptosis, invasion, angiogenesis, inflammation and metastasis in BC cells. (RISC: RNA-induced silencing complex)

3. Types of microRNAs

miRNAs are 20-21 nucleotides in length and regulate the expression of almost 30% of genes. Approximately 706 miRNAs have been identified in humans. In the miRBase database there are more than 5000 miRNAs that have been identified in various organisms, each with a different genomic organization and different biogenetic mechanisms [11]. Since their initial discovery in 1993, in a study of the gene lin-4 in *Caenorhabditis elegans*, more than 2000 molecules have been identified in humans so far, and these are involved in regulating the expression of almost 30% of genes identified. The first microRNA gene to be discovered was lin-4 in *C. Elegans*, a gene associated with development [12]. miRNAs have different roles in gene regulation, and thereby control complex networks in eukaryotic organisms, including hematopoietic cell differentiation, cell proliferation, apoptosis and organ development [13].

While clustering miRNA genes, they were stratified as hosted and non-hosted. miRNA clusters generally contain between two to three miRNA genes, however there are also larger clusters. For example, the human hsa-miR-17 cluster has six members [14].

Lately, the expression of an enormous cluster of 40 miRNA genes located in the ~1 Mb human imprinted 14q32 domain was identified [15]. miRNA genes are clustered according sequence similarities. However, some of them can differ [16].

These miRNAs have different roles in oncogenesis, tumor-suppression, cancer initiation, progression and metastasis. Recent studies have shown that the miR-17-92 family contain miRNAs which play a role in carcinogenesis. These miRNAs are miR-17, miR-18a, miR-19a, miR-20a, miR-19b, and miR- 92a. The same polycistronic cluster are all transcribed from chromosome 13. In mammals, the miR-106b-25 cluster on chromosome 7, and the miR-106a-363 cluster on the X chromosome are also two paralogs, miRNAs which have the same seed sequence and can share the same targets. According to the homology of the seed sequences, miRNAs in these paralogous clusters can be grouped into four different families, miR-17, miR-18, miR-19 and miR-92 [1].

4. MicroRNA biogenesis and function

By using RNA polymerase II, miRNA joins transcription of pri-miRNA precursor generally. In the nucleus, an endonuclease enzyme plays a role in the processing of the pri-miRNA and conversion into precursor miRNA (pre-miRNA). The pri-miRNAs are processed to mature miRNAs by the RNaseIII family enzymes, Drosha and Dicer. Drosha and Dicer, the RNaseIII family enzymes, process the pri-miRNAs to mature miRNAs. The Drosha and pasha cleaves pri-miRNA to pre-miRNA in the nucleus a nd subsequently Dicer processes it to a miRNA/ miRNA* duplex of ~20 bp in the cytoplasm. This constitutes the miRNA-induced silencing complex, miRISC. miRNA (pre-miRNA) contain a stem loop secondary structure and have 80-100nt long sequences. Transportation of pre-miRNA from the nucleus to cytoplasm happens thanks to Exportin-5. Translation of a complement messenger RNA is controlled by the RNA induced silencing complex. Mature miRNA can detect and attach the 3` untranslated regions of an mRNA from the core region, that is generally position 2-7 in the miRNA. High complementarity is not required for regulation and a single miRNA can target multiple genes. miRNAs have a variety of roles including the development of heart and skeletal muscle, cell cycle control, different cell signalling pathways, neurogenesis, insulin secretion, cholesterol metabolism, aging, immune responses and viral replication [17]. Furthermore, miRNAs regulate histone modification and DNA methylation of promoter sites for expression of target genes [18].

Some miRNAs, such as the miR-17/20 cluster, the miR-221/222 cluster, and the let-7 and miR-34 families, play important roles in cell cycle control by targeting cell cycle regulators. These regulators include myc, E2Fs, and cyclin D1 which regulate miR-17/20 during transcription which triggers regulation of translation levels of E2F, pRb, and cyclin D1. miR-15/16 inhibits cyclin D1, cyclin E, CDK4/6 and the miR-34 family suppresses E2F, cyclin D1, and cyclin E expression and they, in turn, control cell cycle [11] (Figure 2).

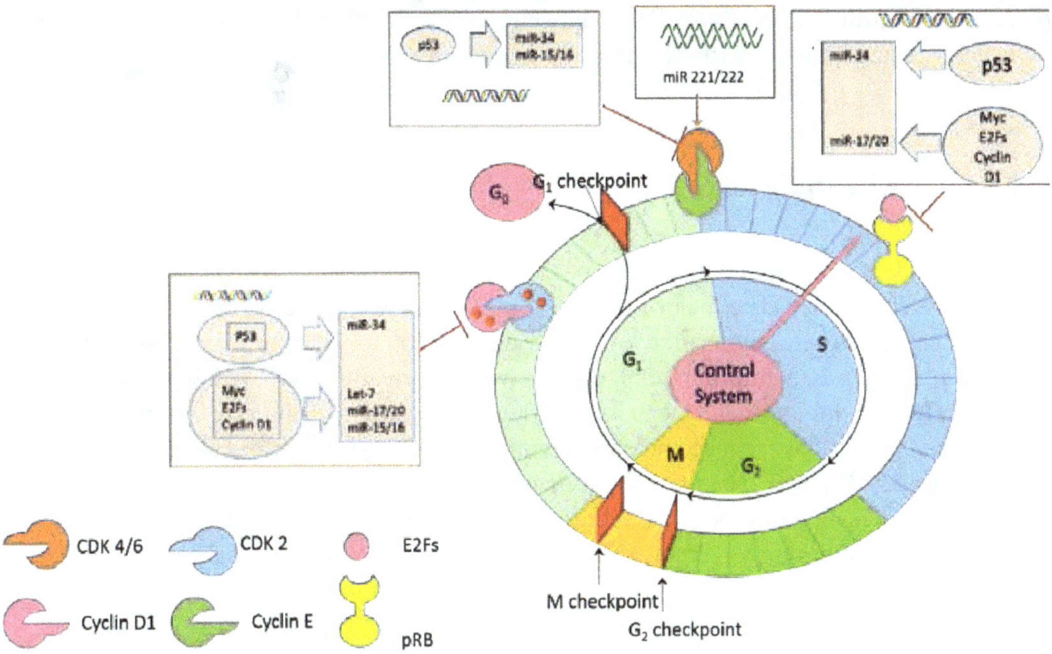

Figure 2. miRNAs in cell cycle regulation

miRNAs detect the specificity and sensitivity of post-transcriptional gene silencing. In order to find out mechanisms of miRNA, provide a chance to get knowledge about biological processes of organisms and covered reasons of diseases [19].

5. MicroRNAs and diseases

In eukaryotic organisms, altered expression of miRNAs can trigger disease development [20]. The association between human disease and miRNA dysregulation can be seen in miR2Disease, a publicly available database [21]. miRNAs play various roles in cell proliferation, metabolism, apoptosis, development, neuronal gene expression, brain morphogenesis [22] cell differentiation, muscle differentiation [23], cell growth and stem cell division [24, 25].

In addition, miRNAs have significant roles in cancer development. miRNAs make decisions as to the fate of the cell [26]. miRNAs are regulated differently in each human cancer, with some of them upregulated and others down-regulated [27].

miRNAs have been determined to play a role in most biological processes and different human diseases including: cardiovascular disease [28], acute and chronic disease [29], neurodevelopmental diseases [30], autoimmune disease [31], liver disease [32], skeletal muscle disease [33] and skin disease [34].

Scientists foresee that miRNA present an immense prospect in diagnosis as well as therapy of diseases in thefuture. Recently, miRNA, antisense blocking and miRNA alteration techniques have been considered as alternative treatments for different cancers [35].

6. MicroRNAs and cancer

Thanks to advancing technology, the genetic study of disease at the molecular level has increased precipitously. The majority of these molecular studies are concerned with understanding cancer. At the molecular level, the etiology of cancer lies in various signalling pathways. Cancer is a multifactorial disease with many different varieties which differ significantly from one another. Due to its complexity and variety, common occurence and high death rate, scientists have focused heavily on cancer research. In Singh and Mo's reserach, they indicated that miRNAs can be used to predict response to therapy as well as in prognosis in clinical cases. To illustrate, a variety of anticancer agents, when combined with miRNA reagents, such as anti-miR-21, result in more effective therapeutic approaches [7].

7. MicroRNAs and breast cancer

7.1. The role of MicroRNAs in breast cancer

Recently, the importance of microRNAs (miRNA/miRs) in cellular regulation has been shown. Some miRNAs are oncogenic and are related to breast cancer. They cause metastasis and then deregulation in cancer [36] (Figure 3). Circulating miRNAs can potentially be used to detect and prognose cancer early [37]. While in this field there are no studies about treatment with circulating miRNA, they can be used as a marker of chemoresistance in BC [38]. In the blood plasma of patients with BC, let-7, miR-10b, miR-34, miR-155 and miR-200c are low, while miR-21, miR-195 and miR-221 are abundant.. Plasma levels of these miRNAs were measured and used to characterize treatment response [39].

In each breast cancer subtype, the expression and regulation of miRNAs in disease initiation is different. In a comparison of 10 normal breast samples and 76 breast cancer samples, the most significantly dysregulated miRNAs were identified as miR-125b, miR-145, miR-21 and miR-155 [40]. These miRNAs play different roles in BC. In order to prove the miRNAs capability of regulation of transition from ductal carcinoma in situ to invasive ductal carcinoma, 94 biopsies were analysed. Then, a nine-miRNA signature was identifiedin invasion, and five miRNAs were identified in metastasis. The downregulation of let-7d, miR-210 and miR-221 in ductal carcinoma in situ, and upregulation of them in the invasive transition is indicated [41]. There are a number of studies about miRNA in BC. In one of these, the peripheral blood samples of 189 patients and89 healthy individuals were collected to determine characteristic miRNA genotyping and expression. miR-499, miR-146a and miR-196a-2 were detected in postmenopausal patients and miR- 196a-2 was determined in premenopausal breast cancer patients. This differs from healthy individuals [42]. In another study that included 23 BC patients and10 controls, next-generation sequencing was used for analysis. Specific miRNAs were found to be co-expressed in the serum and tissue of BC patients. miR-103, miR-23a, miR-29a, miR-222, miR-23b, miR-24 and miR-25 are all upregulated. miR-222 has an especially high level in the serum of BC patients and serves as a specific biomarker [43].

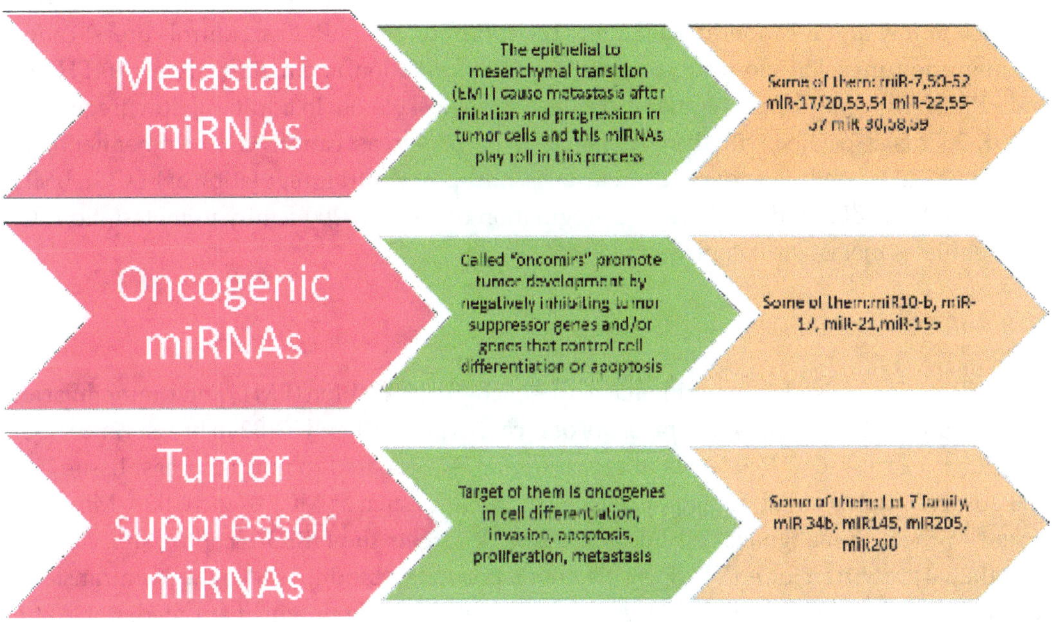

Figure 3. Classes of miRNAs in breast cancer

7.2. Tumor Suppressor MicroRNAs in Breast Cancer

7.2.1. let-7 family

The Let-7 family is crucial for cell type determination during embryogenesis. This family was first discovered in *Caenorhabditis elegans* and was one of the first two microRNAs to be identified [44]. The subtypes of the let-7 family are: let-7a, let-7b, let-7c, let-7d, let-7e, let-7f, let-7g, let-7i, miR-98 and miR-202. They have functions in cell regulation, gene expression and development. Lin28 regulates biogenesis of let-7 at the post- transcriptional stage [45]. Downregulation of let-7 causes different cancers. The role of let-7 was determined in stem cells.

Let-7 was found to play role in self-renewal, differentiation and tumorigenicity in both breast tumor initiating cells (BT-IC) and non-BT-IC, all of which were isolated from primary breast cancer, Overexpression of let-7 family miRNAs decreases proliferation, leads to formation of mammospheres by BT-ICs *in vitro* and tumor formation and metastasis in NOD/SCID mice. Let-7 also targets H-RAS and HMGA2 and regulates BT-IC stem cell-like properties [46].

7.2.2. miR-200 family

The miR-200 family includes five subgroups: miR-200a, miR-200b, miR-200c, miR-141 and miR-429. The miR-200 family suppresses EMT which is mediated via the regulation of E-cadherin. The miR-200 family is not present in invasive breast cancer cell lines of mesenchymal phenotype; also, these cell lines did not express e-cadherin. [47]. There is a correlation between miR-200 family and E-cadherin, so it alters cell morphology. miR-200c controls breast cancer cell migration, invasion, elongatioon and stress fiber formation, and metastasis targets FHOD1 and PPM1F which are direct regulators of the actin cytoskeleton. In addition, downregulation of miR-200c is associated with drug resistance in human breast cancer. On the other hand, the role of miR-200c family is not clear in metastasis. miR-200c controls regulation of PLCG1, BMI1, TGF-β2, FAP-1, ZEB and Suz12 [48]. Upregulation of the miR-200 family in metastatic 4TO7 cells regulates metastatic colonization [49].

7.2.3. miR-205

This miRNA is involved in the epithelial to mesenchymal transition (EMT) and tumor invasion by targeting the transcriptional repressors of E-cadherin, ZEB1 and ZEB2 in breast cancer [50]. miR-205 is expressed at low levels in breast tumor as compared to normal breast tissue [51]. The observed down-regulation in breast cancer cell lines such as MCF-7 and MDA-MB-231 is absent in the non-malignant cell line MCF-10A. It targets the HER3 receptor and vascular endothelial growth factor A (VEGF-A) via interaction with a binding site in the 3'-untranslated region (3'-UTR) of ErbB3 and VEGF-A. Also, activation of the downstream mediator Akt is inhibited by miR-205 which has a role in the proliferation pathway mediated by the HER receptor family [51, 52].

7.2.4. miR-145

When Iorio et al. compared normal breast tissue and breast cancer by microarray and northern blot analyses, they found that miR-145 in downregulated in breast cancer. miRNAs can be a novel biomarker for early cancer detection, because of its early appearance [53]. Spizzo et al. also reported the relation of TP53 activation and miR-145 as pro-apoptotic. The target of miR-145 may be estrogen receptor-α (ER-α) protein expression and cause apoptosis in both ER-α positive and wild type TP53-expressing breast cancer cells [54]. The oncogene c-Myc, which plays a role in cell proliferation and development in vitro and in vivo, is a target of miR-145 [7]. The transcription factor p53 is mutated in breast cancer. Several miRNAs such as miR-145 play a role in the trancriptional control of p53. There are different mechanisms in response to DNA damage, cell cycle arrest, apoptosis associated with p53 [55] (Figure 4).

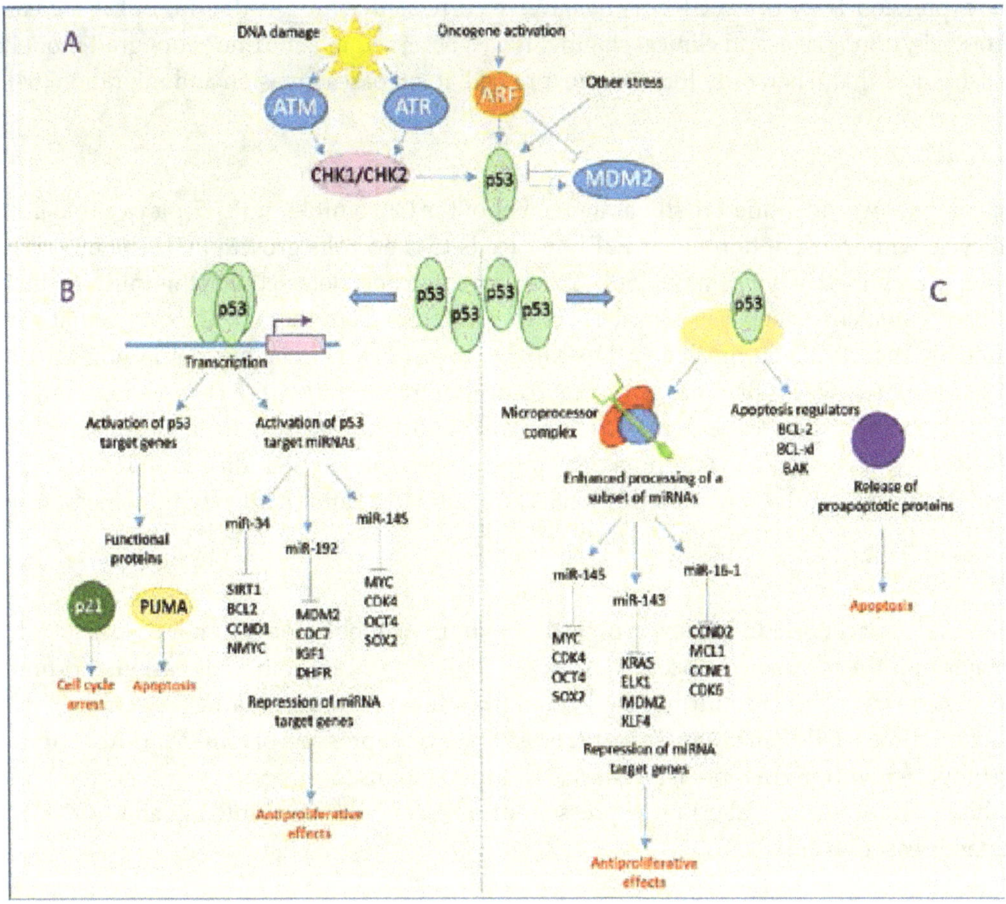

Figure 4. The effect of miRNAs in the p53 pathway. A. The main genes involved in the posttranscriptional control of p53. B. The mission of transcription factor p53 and activation of it by proteins and miRNAs. C. Post-transcription stage of p53. An association between miRNAs, p53, and apoptotic genes was demonstrated [55].

7.3. Oncogenic MicroRNAs in breast cancer

Some miRNAs, which suppress the expression of antioncogenes in apoptosis, metastasis, invasion and cell proliferation play roles as oncomirs and their expression is increased in breast cancer [56]. The oncogenic miRNAs and their families have been identfied as miR-10, miR-15, miR-16, miR-17~92 cluster, miR-18, miR-19, miR-20, miR-21 family, miR-92 miR-155, miR-569.

7.3.1. miR-10

miR-10a and miR-10b are subtypes of the miR-10 family and play a role in metastasis and development [57]. The miR-10 family regulate Hox transcripts, and thus function in development [58]. The dysregulation of this miRNA family was identified not only in breast cancer, but also in colon cancer [59], melanoma [57], acute myeloid leukemia [60], glioblastoma [61], hepatocellular carcinoma [62] and pancreatic cancer [63].

The expression level of miR-10b is negatively correlated with E-cadherin, but it increases metastasis, tumor size, and clinical staging. It was observed in a murine xeno- graft model of breast cancer that when miR-10b is overexpressed, it increases invasion and migration [64].

7.3.2. miR-17

This miRNA was identified firstly as a member of the OncomiR-1. miR-17 plays a role in the cell cycle with transcription factor E2F1 and leads to cancerous growth [65]. The miR-17~92 cluster is amplified in lymphomas [66]. Although researchers detected that this miRNA cluster is downregulated in metastasis, miR-17-5p was different from them. It is expressed at very/ extremely high levels in invasive MDA-MB-231 breast cancer cells but not in non-invasive MCF-7 breast cancer cells. This group can cause migration in MCF-7 cells by targeting the HBP1/β-catenin pathway and reduction of miR-17-5p suppresses the invasion of MDA-MB-231 cells in vitro [67]. In addition, this miRNAs has subtypes including miR-18b, miR-19b, miR-20a, miR-92, miR-93 and miR-106 which are found to be amplified in lymphomas [66, 68].

7.3.3. miR-21

Chan et al. first reported high levels of miR-21 in human glioblastoma tumor tissues [69]. It is a major miRNA for breast cancer, because of it roles in cell migration, invasion and tumor progression [70]. This is confirmed by studies from several groups. For instance, Singh et al., using real time RT-PCR array analysis, reported that overexpression of miR-21 in breast tumors as compared with normal breast tissues [71]. Iorio et al. used microarray and northern blot analyses, and found the aberrant expression of miR-21, miR-125b, miR-145 and miR-155 in human breast cancer [40].

Clinicopathologic features of miR-21 and the association of PTEN were determined in a study by Huang et al. using real-time RT-PCR and immunohistochemistry (IHC) analyses. They researched miR-21 expression in non-tumor and tumor tissues of 40 human invasive ductal carcinoma of the breast and reported that the association of PTEN (phosphatase and tensin homolog deleted on chromosome 10) and miR-21 expression inversely correlated in breast cancer and that miR-21 causes metastasis [72].

7.3.4. miR-155

This oncomir is highly expressed in human cancers. Suppressor of cytokine signaling 1 (SOCS1) is a target gene of miR-155 in human breast cancer. Research indicates that SOCS1 is negatively regulated by miR-155, and may be a potential target in breast cancer therapy [73].

7.4. Metastatic MicroRNAs in breast cancer

Metastasis is the primary cause of mortality in breast cancer. In metastasis, cancer migrates from a primary solid tumor to distant parts of the body [74]. Mesenchymal to epithelial transition (MET) and epithelial to mesenchymal transition (EMT) are causes of metastasis [75]. Recent research shows that some miRNAs levels decrease, but others accumulated during metastasis of breast cancer [76]. The miR-9,36 miR-10b,37,38 miR-21,39-45 miR-29a,46 miR-15547 and miR-373/520 families promote metastasis in BC [77]. For instance, miR-9 plays a role cell motility focusing on E-cadherin and raises the level of vascular endothelial growth factor (VEGF) [78]. Tristetraprolin, the target of miR-29a, regulates EMT and metastasis in BC [79]. miR-373/520 can increase invasion and migration by CD44. The connection of miR-373 and CD44 expression was displayed thanks to clinical metastasis samples [77]. Subgroups of miRNA that prevent metastasis in BC are: miR-7,50-52 miR-17/20, 53, 54 miR-22,55- 57 miR-30, 58, 59 miR-31,60-62 miR-126,63-68 miR-145,69-72 miR- 146, 73, 74 miR-193b,75 miR-205,76,77 miR-206,78-80 miR-335,32,81 miR-448,82 miR-66183,84 and let-7 [46].

Some miRNAs were selected to determine their roles in metastasis. Epidermal growth factor receptor (EGFR), a regulator of cellular processes and overexpressed in breast cancer, is associatede with miR-7 and causes metastatis [80]. Several cancer types are inhibited by miR-7 include p21-activated kinase 1 expression which is a signaling kinase. If overexpression of miR-7 is present in BC cells, it causes migration to other tissues in BC [81].

miR-17 is known as an oncogenic miRNA in other cancers. When miR-17/20 is overexpressed in breast cancer cell lineage, it stops cell proliferation and causes G1 cell cycle arrest. This miRNA's target is cyclin D1 rolled in G1-S phase transition. In ~50% of human breast cancers cyclin D1 expression is increased. It has an inverese correlation with miR-17/20 [82].

When analyzed non-invasive breast cancer cell MCF-7 and invasive MDA-MB-231 cell line, miRNAs' role in inhibition of invasion was determined. While miRNA is inhibiting invasion, it connects IL-8 and cytokeratin 8 through cyclin D1 [83]. In vivo and in vitro investigation about breast cancer shows that overexpression of miRNA causes a reduction in cell motility through targetting CDK6, SIRT1 and Sp1. Furthermore, miR-22 targets estrogen receptor α (Erα) and supresses cell proliferation on ERα-dependent breast cancer [84]. miR-145 and miR-146 are very important tumor suppressors miRNAs in breast cancer. miR-145 prevents metastasis by targeting IRS-1, mucin-1, c-myc, JAM-A and fascin [54]. In an MDA-MB-231 mouse model experiment, miR-146 induces EGFR, which plays a role in inhibition of metastasis [85]. It also downregulates interleukin receptor associated kinase and TNF associated factor 6 and controls NFκB [86]. Mo's research displayed that the overexpession of miR-30 suppresses cell growth by targetting Ubc9, and plays a role in cell growth and cancer development. This pathway was also seen in breast cancer [87].

8. Conclusion

Recently, breast cancer has been thoroughly studied, because approximately 13 million women will be diagnosed with breast cancer globally and about 465,000 will die from the disease [10]. Researchers have conducted a variety of experiments concerning breast cancer and its pathways. Although there are many breast cancer therapies, alternative methods are being developed. In particular, research focused on molecular mechanisms are currently popular. miRNAs are an alternative methodology as a potential therapeutic target for breast cancer. The association of miRNAs and breast cancer is discussed, including miRNAs as candidate diagnostic and prognostic indicators in breast cancer. Combinations of different anticancer agents with miRNA can be more effective as therapeutic approaches. Hence, some of miRNAs can be utilized as breast cancer biomarkers. Briefly, the main subtypes of miRNAs are discussed in this chapter, and several lines reseache focus on other types of miRNAs.

Author details

Hacer Esra Gurses, Omer Faruk Hatipoğlu, Mehmet Gunduz and Esra Gunduz

*Address all correspondence to: esragunduz@outlook.com

Department of Medical Genetics, Faculty of Medicine, Turgut Ozal University, Ankara, Turkey

References

[1] Walker, K.E.C.a.A.M., *Potential Roles of miR-106a in Breast Cancer* in *intech*, m. gündüz, Editor. 2011. p. 523-540.

[2] Eulalio, A., et al., *Target-specific requirements for enhancers of decapping in miRNA-mediated gene silencing.* Genes Dev, 2007. 21(20): p. 2558-70.

[3] Pillai, R.S., et al., *Inhibition of translational initiation by Let-7 MicroRNA in human cells.* Science, 2005. 309(5740): p. 1573-6.

[4] Mathonnet, G., et al., *MicroRNA inhibition of translation initiation in vitro by targeting the cap-binding complex eIF4F.* Science, 2007. 317(5845): p. 1764-7.

[5] Kiriakidou, M., et al., *An mRNA m7G cap binding-like motif within human Ago2 represses translation.* Cell, 2007. 129(6): p. 1141-51.

[6] Hock, J., et al., *Proteomic and functional analysis of Argonaute-containing mRNA-protein complexes in human cells.* EMBO Rep, 2007. 8(11): p. 1052-60.

[7] Singh, R. and Y.Y. Mo, *Role of microRNAs in breast cancer.* Cancer Biol Ther, 2013. 14(3): p. 201-12.

[8] Ding, X.C., J. Weiler, and H. Grosshans, *Regulating the regulators: mechanisms controlling the maturation of microRNAs.* Trends Biotechnol, 2009. 27(1): p. 27-36.

[9] O'Donnell, K.A., et al., *c-Myc-regulated microRNAs modulate E2F1 expression.* Nature, 2005. 435(7043): p. 839-43.

[10] Fu, S.W., L. Chen, and Y.G. Man, *miRNA Biomarkers in Breast Cancer Detection and Management.* J Cancer, 2011. 2: p. 116-22.

[11] Yu, Z., et al., *microRNA, cell cycle, and human breast cancer.* Am J Pathol, 2010. 176(3): p. 1058-64.

[12] Lee, R.C., R.L. Feinbaum, and V. Ambros, *The C. elegans heterochronic gene lin-4 encodes small RNAs with antisense complementarity to lin-14.* Cell, 1993. 75(5): p. 843-54.

[13] Bartel, D.P., *MicroRNAs: genomics, biogenesis, mechanism, and function.* Cell, 2004. 116(2): p. 281-97.

[14] Mourelatos, Z., et al., *miRNPs: a novel class of ribonucleoproteins containing numerous microRNAs.* Genes Dev, 2002. 16(6): p. 720-8.

[15] Seitz, H., et al., *A large imprinted microRNA gene cluster at the mouse Dlk1-Gtl2 domain.* Genome Res, 2004. 14(9): p. 1741-8.

[16] Aravin, A.A., et al., *The small RNA profile during Drosophila melanogaster development.* Dev Cell, 2003. 5(2): p. 337-50.

[17] Kayani, M., et al., *Role of miRNAs in breast cancer.* Asian Pac J Cancer Prev, 2011. 12(12): p. 3175-80.

[18] Tan, Y., et al., *Transcriptional inhibiton of Hoxd4 expression by miRNA-10a in human breast cancer cells.* BMC Mol Biol, 2009. 10: p. 12.

[19] Liu, B., J. Li, and M.J. Cairns, *Identifying miRNAs, targets and functions.* Brief Bioinform, 2014. 15(1): p. 1-19.

[20] Mraz, M. and S. Pospisilova, *MicroRNAs in chronic lymphocytic leukemia: from causality to associations and back.* Expert Rev Hematol, 2012. 5(6): p. 579-81.

[21] Jiang, Q., et al., *miR2Disease: a manually curated database for microRNA deregulation in human disease.* Nucleic Acids Res, 2009. 37(Database issue): p. D98-104.

[22] Giraldez, A.J., et al., *MicroRNAs regulate brain morphogenesis in zebrafish.* Science, 2005. 308(5723): p. 833-8.

[23] Naguibneva, I., et al., *The microRNA miR-181 targets the homeobox protein Hox-A11 during mammalian myoblast differentiation.* Nat Cell Biol, 2006. 8(3): p. 278-84.

[24] Hatfield, S.D., et al., *Stem cell division is regulated by the microRNA pathway.* Nature, 2005. 435(7044): p. 974-8.

[25] Mattick, J.S. and I.V. Makunin, *Small regulatory RNAs in mammals.* Hum Mol Genet, 2005. 14 Spec No 1: p. R121-32.

[26] McManus, M.T., *MicroRNAs and cancer.* Semin Cancer Biol, 2003. 13(4): p. 253-8.

[27] Naeini, M.M. and A.M. Ardekani, *Noncoding RNAs and Cancer.* Avicenna J Med Biotechnol, 2009. 1(2): p. 55-70.

[28] Zhao, Y., E. Samal, and D. Srivastava, *Serum response factor regulates a muscle-specific microRNA that targets Hand2 during cardiogenesis.* Nature, 2005. 436(7048): p. 214-20.

[29] Silvestre, J.S., et al., *Post-ischaemic neovascularization and inflammation.* Cardiovasc Res, 2008. 78(2): p. 242-9.

[30] Nelson, P.T., W.X. Wang, and B.W. Rajeev, *MicroRNAs (miRNAs) in neurodegenerative diseases.* Brain Pathol, 2008. 18(1): p. 130-8.

[31] Pauley, K.M., S. Cha, and E.K. Chan, *MicroRNA in autoimmunity and autoimmune diseases.* J Autoimmun, 2009. 32(3-4): p. 189-94.

[32] Chen, X.M., *MicroRNA signatures in liver diseases.* World J Gastroenterol, 2009. 15(14): p. 1665-72.

[33] McCarthy, J.J. and K.A. Esser, *MicroRNA-1 and microRNA-133a expression are decreased during skeletal muscle hypertrophy.* J Appl Physiol (1985), 2007. 102(1): p. 306-13.

[34] Yi, R., et al., *Morphogenesis in skin is governed by discrete sets of differentially expressed microRNAs.* Nat Genet, 2006. 38(3): p. 356-62.

[35] Ardekani, A.M. and M.M. Naeini, *The Role of MicroRNAs in Human Diseases.* Avicenna J Med Biotechnol, 2010. 2(4): p. 161-79.

[36] Braicu, C., G.A. Calin, and I. Berindan-Neagoe, *MicroRNAs and cancer therapy - from bystanders to major players.* Curr Med Chem, 2013. 20(29): p. 3561-73.

[37] Humphreys, D.T., et al., *MicroRNAs control translation initiation by inhibiting eukaryotic initiation factor 4E/cap and poly(A) tail function.* Proc Natl Acad Sci U S A, 2005. 102(47): p. 16961-6.

[38] Thermann, R. and M.W. Hentze, *Drosophila miR2 induces pseudo-polysomes and inhibits translation initiation.* Nature, 2007. 447(7146): p. 875-8.

[39] Gezer, U., et al., *Abundant circulating microRNAs in breast cancer patients fluctuate considerably during neoadjuvant chemotherapy.* Oncol Lett, 2014. 8(2): p. 845-848.

[40] Iorio, M.V., et al., *MicroRNA gene expression deregulation in human breast cancer.* Cancer Res, 2005. 65(16): p. 7065-70.

[41] Volinia, S., et al., *Breast cancer signatures for invasiveness and prognosis defined by deep sequencing of microRNA.* Proc Natl Acad Sci U S A, 2012. 109(8): p. 3024-9.

[42] Alshatwi, A.A., et al., *Differential expression profile and genetic variants of microRNAs sequences in breast cancer patients.* PLoS One, 2012. 7(2): p. e30049.

[43] Wu, Q., et al., *Analysis of serum genome-wide microRNAs for breast cancer detection.* Clin Chim Acta, 2012. 413(13-14): p. 1058-65.

[44] Reinhart, B.J., et al., *The 21-nucleotide let-7 RNA regulates developmental timing in Caenorhabditis elegans.* Nature, 2000. 403(6772): p. 901-6.

[45] Wang, X., et al., *Regulation of let-7 and its target oncogenes (Review).* Oncol Lett, 2012. 3(5): p. 955-960.

[46] Yu, F., et al., *let-7 regulates self renewal and tumorigenicity of breast cancer cells.* Cell, 2007. 131(6): p. 1109-23.

[47] Korpal, M., et al., *The miR-200 family inhibits epithelial-mesenchymal transition and cancer cell migration by direct targeting of E-cadherin transcriptional repressors ZEB1 and ZEB2.* J Biol Chem, 2008. 283(22): p. 14910-4.

[48] Park, S.M., et al., *The miR-200 family determines the epithelial phenotype of cancer cells by targeting the E-cadherin repressors ZEB1 and ZEB2.* Genes Dev, 2008. 22(7): p. 894-907.

[49] Korpal, M., et al., *Direct targeting of Sec23a by miR-200s influences cancer cell secretome and promotes metastatic colonization.* Nat Med, 2011. 17(9): p. 1101-8.

[50] Gregory, P.A., et al., *The miR-200 family and miR-205 regulate epithelial to mesenchymal transition by targeting ZEB1 and SIP1.* Nat Cell Biol, 2008. 10(5): p. 593-601.

[51] Wu, H., S. Zhu, and Y.Y. Mo, *Suppression of cell growth and invasion by miR-205 in breast cancer.* Cell Res, 2009. 19(4): p. 439-48.

[52] !!! INVALID CITATION !!!

[53] Sempere, L.F., et al., *Altered MicroRNA expression confined to specific epithelial cell subpopulations in breast cancer.* Cancer Res, 2007. 67(24): p. 11612-20.

[54] Spizzo, R., et al., *miR-145 participates with TP53 in a death-promoting regulatory loop and targets estrogen receptor-alpha in human breast cancer cells.* Cell Death Differ, 2010. 17(2): p. 246-54.

[55] Jansson, M.D. and A.H. Lund, *MicroRNA and cancer.* Mol Oncol, 2012. 6(6): p. 590-610.

[56] Zhang, B., et al., *microRNAs as oncogenes and tumor suppressors.* Dev Biol, 2007. 302(1): p. 1-12.

[57] Zhang, L., et al., *microRNAs exhibit high frequency genomic alterations in human cancer.* Proc Natl Acad Sci U S A, 2006. 103(24): p. 9136-41.

[58] Lund, A.H., *miR-10 in development and cancer.* Cell Death Differ, 2010. 17(2): p. 209-14.

[59] Volinia, S., et al., *A microRNA expression signature of human solid tumors defines cancer gene targets.* Proc Natl Acad Sci U S A, 2006. 103(7): p. 2257-61.

[60] Jongen-Lavrencic, M., et al., *MicroRNA expression profiling in relation to the genetic heterogeneity of acute myeloid leukemia.* Blood, 2008. 111(10): p. 5078-85.

[61] Gaur, A., et al., *Characterization of microRNA expression levels and their biological correlates in human cancer cell lines.* Cancer Res, 2007. 67(6): p. 2456-68.

[62] Varnholt, H., et al., *MicroRNA gene expression profile of hepatitis C virus-associated hepatocellular carcinoma.* Hepatology, 2008. 47(4): p. 1223-32.

[63] Bloomston, M., et al., *MicroRNA expression patterns to differentiate pancreatic adenocarcinoma from normal pancreas and chronic pancreatitis.* Jama, 2007. 297(17): p. 1901-8.

[64] Ma, L., J. Teruya-Feldstein, and R.A. Weinberg, *Tumour invasion and metastasis initiated by microRNA-10b in breast cancer.* Nature, 2007. 449(7163): p. 682-8.

[65] Hammond, S.M., *MicroRNAs as oncogenes.* Curr Opin Genet Dev, 2006. 16(1): p. 4-9.

[66] Ota, A., et al., *Identification and characterization of a novel gene, C13orf25, as a target for 13q31-q32 amplification in malignant lymphoma.* Cancer Res, 2004. 64(9): p. 3087-95.

[67] Li, H., et al., *miR-17-5p promotes human breast cancer cell migration and invasion through suppression of HBP1.* Breast Cancer Res Treat, 2011. 126(3): p. 565-75.

[68] Fassina, A., et al., *The miR-17-92 microRNA cluster: a novel diagnostic tool in large B-cell malignancies.* Lab Invest, 2012. 92(11): p. 1574-82.

[69] Chan, J.A., A.M. Krichevsky, and K.S. Kosik, *MicroRNA-21 is an antiapoptotic factor in human glioblastoma cells.* Cancer Res, 2005. 65(14): p. 6029-33.

[70] Han, M., et al., *Re-expression of miR-21 contributes to migration and invasion by inducing epithelial-mesenchymal transition consistent with cancer stem cell characteristics in MCF-7 cells.* Mol Cell Biochem, 2012. 363(1-2): p. 427-36.

[71] Si, M.L., et al., *miR-21-mediated tumor growth.* Oncogene, 2007. 26(19): p. 2799-803.

[72] Huang, G.L., et al., *Clinical significance of miR-21 expression in breast cancer: SYBR-Green I-based real-time RT-PCR study of invasive ductal carcinoma.* Oncol Rep, 2009. 21(3): p. 673-9.

[73] Jiang, S., et al., *MicroRNA-155 functions as an OncomiR in breast cancer by targeting the suppressor of cytokine signaling 1 gene.* Cancer Res, 2010. 70(8): p. 3119-27.

[74] Jemal, A., et al., *Cancer statistics, 2010.* CA Cancer J Clin, 2010. 60(5): p. 277-300.

[75] Yang, J. and R.A. Weinberg, *Epithelial-mesenchymal transition: at the crossroads of development and tumor metastasis.* Dev Cell, 2008. 14(6): p. 818-29.

[76] Wang, L. and J. Wang, *MicroRNA-mediated breast cancer metastasis: from primary site to distant organs.* Oncogene, 2012. 31(20): p. 2499-511.

[77] Huang, Q., et al., *The microRNAs miR-373 and miR-520c promote tumour invasion and metastasis.* Nat Cell Biol, 2008. 10(2): p. 202-10.

[78] Ma, L., et al., *miR-9, a MYC/MYCN-activated microRNA, regulates E-cadherin and cancer metastasis.* Nat Cell Biol, 2010. 12(3): p. 247-56.

[79] Gebeshuber, C.A., K. Zatloukal, and J. Martinez, *miR-29a suppresses tristetraprolin, which is a regulator of epithelial polarity and metastasis.* EMBO Rep, 2009. 10(4): p. 400-5.

[80] Webster, R.J., et al., *Regulation of epidermal growth factor receptor signaling in human cancer cells by microRNA-7.* J Biol Chem, 2009. 284(9): p. 5731-41.

[81] Reddy, S.D., et al., *MicroRNA-7, a homeobox D10 target, inhibits p21-activated kinase 1 and regulates its functions.* Cancer Res, 2008. 68(20): p. 8195-200.

[82] Fu, M., et al., *Minireview: Cyclin D1: normal and abnormal functions.* Endocrinology, 2004. 145(12): p. 5439-47.

[83] Yu, Z., et al., *microRNA 17/20 inhibits cellular invasion and tumor metastasis in breast cancer by heterotypic signaling.* Proc Natl Acad Sci U S A, 2010. 107(18): p. 8231-6.

[84] Pandey, D.P. and D. Picard, *miR-22 inhibits estrogen signaling by directly targeting the estrogen receptor alpha mRNA.* Mol Cell Biol, 2009. 29(13): p. 3783-90.

[85] Hurst, D.R., et al., *Breast cancer metastasis suppressor 1 up-regulates miR-146, which suppresses breast cancer metastasis.* Cancer Res, 2009. 69(4): p. 1279-83.

[86] Bhaumik, D., et al., *Expression of microRNA-146 suppresses NF-kappaB activity with reduction of metastatic potential in breast cancer* cells. Oncogene, 2008. 27(42): p. 5643-7.

[87] Wu, F., et al., MicroRNA-mediated regulation of Ubc9 expression in cancer cells. Clin Cancer Res, 2009. 15(5): p. 1550-7.

5

DNA Methylation

Majed S. Alokail and Amal M. Alenad

1. Introduction

DNA methylation is a major epigenetic modification that is strongly involved in the physiological control of genome expression. Developmental processes and proper biological functions are tightly dependent on hierarchical and regulated gene expression patterns. Numerous molecular processes control gene expression. DNA methylation is a physiological epigenetic process that leads to long term-repression of gene expression. DNA methylation is a common epigenetic modification involving the methylation of 5'-cytosine residues and is often detected in the dinucleotides of CpG sequences. Methylation is often localized in promoter regions and occasionally in transcriptional regulatory regions in mammals, plants and even prokaryotes. DNA methylation may be classified as hyper-and hypomethylation, according to increased and decreased levels of genomic modification, respectively. Hypermethylation is an epigenetic alteration often leading to gene-inactivating deletions and translocations. Hypermethylated cells may exhibit a phenotype of drug-resistance or malignant proliferation. Aberrant methylation in eukaryotic cells may lead to silencing of important genes, such as tumour suppressor genes, affecting their related transcriptional pathways and ultimately leading to the development of disease such as cancer. Therefore, it is considered to be a hallmark of cancer, it is detected in several types of cancer cells, including colon, breast, ovarian and cervical cancer cells and is associated with alterations in specific gene expression.

Hypermethylation of tumour suppressor gene promoters and global disruption of many histone modifications are characteristic features of cancer. Deregulation of the epigenetic profile alters the transcription profile of many genes. In the case of tumour suppressors DNA methylation reduces gene expression and subsequently removes regulatory proteins required for normal cell growth and development. Therefore, DNA methylation in cancer would be predicted to influence multiple gene networks rather than single genes. Because of heterogeneity of breast cancer at both histological and molecular levels staging breast cancer fails to predict prognosis or therapeutic response of the disease, therefore, DNA methylation targeted therapies, in recent years, play an increased role in the treatment of breast cancer. DNA methylation targeted therapies, in recent years, play an increased role in the treatment of breast cancer. Two groups of agents targeting epigenetic modifications have been studied previously, namely histone deacetylase inhibitors and DNA methyl transferase inhibitors. The associations between DNA methylation mechanism and breast cancer classification and prognosis will be reviewed in this chapter in detail by describing the DNA methylation mechanism and gene expression in breast cancer, as well as functional genomics and genome wide DNA methylation in breast cancer.

2. What is epigenetics?

The term epigenetic was introduced by Conard Waddington in 1942 as a concept of environmental influence in inducing phenotype modification. His work on developmental plasticity states that the environmental influences during development could induce alternative phenotypes from one genotype, one of the clearest examples is polyphenisms in insects. He showed that exposing the pupae of wild type Drosophila melanogaster to heat shock treatment, results in altered wing vein patterns [1,2]. Breeding individuals who have been exposed to these environmentally induced changes led to a stable population exhibiting the phenotype without the environmental stimulus. The concept of epigenetics was not clarified until the late 1990s when Wolffe and Matzkeset the modern definition, which was 'the study of heritable changes in gene expression that occur without a change in DNA sequence'[4]. Bird came with a wider definition of epigenetic which is 'the structural adaptation of chromosomal regions so as to register, signal or perpetuate activity states' [5]. The term epigenome has emerged to describe the epigenetic modifications all over the epigenome, thus, the epigenome controls the genome in both normal and abnormal cellular processes and events [6]. Epigenetic mechanisms include; DNA methylation, histone modification and non-coding RNAs, which work cooperatively to control gene expression.

3. DNA methylation

DNA methylation is a well conserved process that occurs in eukaryotes and prokaryotes [7]. DNA methylation refers to the covalent addition of a methyl group to carbon number five in the nitrogenous base cytosine at the DNA strand. Only cytosine residues where adjacent to guanine are targets for the methylation by the methyltransferases enzymes and the distribution of methylated and unmethylated CpGs is tissue-specific which leads to cell-specific pattern of DNA methylation [8]. The CpG may occur in multiple repeats which are known as CpG islands [9]. These regions are often associated with the promoter regions of genes. Almost half of the genes in our genome have CpG rich promoter regions. In the whole genome, about 80% of the CpG dinucleotides not associated with CpG islands are heavily methylated [10]. In contrast, the CpG islands associated with gene promoters are usually unmethylated [11].

There are a number of factors that may maintain the undermethylated state of CpG islands, such as sequence feature, SP1 binding sites, specific acting enhancer elements, as well as specific histone methylation mark H3K4me3, which prevents the binding of de novo methylation complexes [12]. Methylation of the CpG islands in the promoter region silences gene expression, and the absence of methylation is associated with active transcription. Thus unmethylated CpG islands are associated with the promoters of transcriptionally active genes, such as housekeeping genes and many regulated genes, such as genes showing tissue specific expression [13]. DNA methylation information at every cytosine can be determined, but it was targeted at few candidate genes using methylation-sensitive restriction enzymes or gene-specific DNA methylation mapping by sequencing bisulfite-converted DNA. In contrast, development of advance technology in DNA methylation mapping, including high-density oligonucleotide arrays, illumina bead arrays and next-generation high-throughput sequencing, together with advances in bioinformatics, have enable examination of broad regions of the genome and provide high-content profiles of DNA methylation.

3.1. DNA Methyltransferases (DNMTs)

The methylation process is catalysed by the DNA methyltransferases enzymes (DNMTs) which are known as DNMTs; DNMT1, DNMT3A, DNMT3B, and DNMT3L [14]. DNMT3A and DNMT3B are the de novo methyltransferases while DNMT1 maintains the methylation patterns during DNA replication (mitosis) [15]. However, the actual function of DNMT2 is not clear, bur several forms of DNMT1 have been detected which differ in their translation start sites and prefer hemimethylated DNA. Overexpression of DNMT1 has been reported in human tumours and may contribute to the global methylation abnormalities seen in cancer cells although increased expression of the DNMTs is likely to be only partially responsible for the observed methylation abnormalities since not all tumours overexpress these enzymes [10]. Cytosine (C^5)-DNA methyltransferases catalyze the transfer of a methyl group from S-adenosyl-methionine onto cytosine residues in specific sequences of duplex DNA, with production of 5-methyl cytosine and S-adenosyl-homocystein (SAMe) (Figure1). For most proteins, cytosine (C^5)-DNA methyltransferases have up to 10 conservative regions arranged in a strictly defined sequence [16]. Comparison of the primary structures of cytosine (C^5)-DNA methyltransferases reveals the association of their major functions with their conservative motifs, whereas the site-specific recognition belongs to a variable region of the target-recognizing domain (TRD) [17]. Among ten conservative blocks of amino acids in cytosine (C^5)-DNA methyltransferases, the N-terminal domain of DNMT1 contains varied specific functional sequences, such as the nuclear localization signal (NLS), the cysteine–enriched zinc-binding motif, and a special sequence directing the methylase into the area of DNA replication. In addition, DNMT1 interact with the proliferating cell nuclear antigen (PCNA) which is required for DNA replication, and the DNMT1-PCNA interaction allow rapid remethylation of the newly synthesised daughter strands before packed into chromatin [18]. A null mutation of the mouse methylase DNMT1 gene resulted in a significant (up to 70%) decrease in the genome methylation and death of developing embryos [19]. The remaining 30% level of DNA methylation and the ability of embryonic stem cells deprived of the DNMT1 methylase for de novo methylation of DNA suggest that these functions were performed by other DNA methylases

[19]. Such methylases were searched for in animals, and new enzymes of the DNMT2 and DNMT3 families were found [20]. Cell-cycle regulators p21 and retinoblastoma gene product Rb can bind to DNMT1 and inhibit its methyltransferase activity during DNA replication in the cell cycle [18]. This observations show complex interaction between DNMT1 and cellular proteins involved in gene regulation and epigenetic signalling during cell replication [21].

The DNMT3 family consists of two genes, DNMT3a and DNMT3b, which are highly expressed in undifferentiated ES cells but downregulated after differentiation and expressed at low levels in adult somatic tissues and are overexpressed in tumour cells [22]. Both DNMT3a and DNMT3b are required for genome-wide de novo methylation and are essential for mammalian development [22]. Both DNMT3a and DNMT3b had been mapped by the unigene consortium via polymorphisms in 3' –untranslated region sequences. DNMT3b mapped to the region of chromosome 20q that contains the trait for ICFNS (immunodeficiency centromeric instability, facial ubnormalities) syndrome. This syndrome presents with variable combined immunodeficiency, mild facial anomalies and extravagant cytogenetic abnormalities which largely affect the pericentric region of chromosomes 1, 9 and 16. These pericentric regions contain a type of satellite DNA termed classical satellite, or satellites 2 and 3. It is normally heavily methylated, but is nearly completely unmethylated in the DNA of ICF patients. It was found that immunodeficiency centromeric instability (ICF) patients had mutations in the C-terminal DNA methyltransferase domain of DNMT3b. DNMT3b remains the only DNA methyltransferase shown to be mutated in a human disease [15]. DNMT3b has been shown to play a crucial role in hypermethylation of promoter CpG-rich regions of tumour suppressor genes and thus its inactivation within human cancer cells [22].

3.2. How does demethylation occur?

The key question is how the enzymes know where to methylate? Two theories have been suggested. Firstly, it has been suggested that all genes are methylated by default except for active genes [23]. Actively transcribed genes have a preponderance of attached transcriptional factors, giving no physical access to the methyltransferses to reach their targets. On the other hand, inactive DNA is susceptible to the methyltransferases and subsequently become methylated. This model was confirmed by the study of the transcription factor SP1. It has been shown that as long as SP1 is attached to its site, no methylation could occur in the adjacent CpG sites, and removal of the SP1 leads to de novo methylation at this site [24]. The second theory is that methylation is directed by sequence specific binding proteins so the methyltransferases bind with certain proteins such as a histone deacetylases (HDACs) and other transcription repressors, and form a complex would bind to specific sequence on the DNA [23].

Methylated genes may need to be activated in response to environmental signals and thus demethylation is an important dynamic epigenetic mechanism and it was originally thought that demethylation only occured through passive demethylation (Figure 2). However, the rapid demethylation of the paternal genomes upon fertilization and examples of rapid demethylation of genes in post-mitotic neurons suggest that an active demethylase must exist [23,25]. A number of enzymes have been suggested to have demethylase activity these include MBD2b, MBD4, the DNA repair endonucleases XPG (Gadd45a) and a G/T mismatch repair

DNA glycosylase which is glycosidase dependent. In this mechanism, the methylated cytosine is recognized by glycosidase which cleaves the bond between the DNA back bone and base. The base is subsequently removed and replaced with unmethylated cytosine by the DNA repair system.

4. Histone Deacetylases (HDACs)

Histones are five basic nuclear proteins that form the core of the nucleosome and the histone octamer contains two molecules each of histones H2A, H2B, H3 and H4. Histone H1 the linker histone is located outside the core and involve in the packing of DNA [26]. Histone modifications play a major role in regulating gene expression and extend the information potential of the DNA which explains the growing interest of the 'Histone Code' [27]. Modifications to amino acids on the N-terminal tails of histones protruding from the nucleosome core can induce both an open or closed chromatin structure and these affect the ability of transcription factors to access promoter regions to activate transcription. The covalent modification can be acetylation, methylation, phosphorylation and ubiquitination. Methylation of some residues is associated with both transcriptional repression, such as methylation of histone 3 lysine 9 (H3 K9) and others with transcriptional activation, such as methylation of histone 3 lysine 4 (H3 K4) [28,29].

Histone methylation is performed by histone methltransferase (HMTs) which can transfer up to three methyl groups to lysine residues within the tails of the histones with different effects on gene activity. Acetylation which occurs at lysine residue is associated with transcriptional activation [30]. This modification is performed by histone acetylases (HATs) and removed by the HDACs [31]. The HDACs are critical in the regulation of expression of genes important for cell survival, proliferation, differentiation, and apoptosis [32]. HDACs also act as members of a protein complex responsible for recruitment of transcription factors to the promoter region of genes, including those of tumour suppressors, and regulation of acetylation status of specific cell cycle regulatory proteins [33]. High HDAC expression and histone hypoacetylation have been observed in cancer with associated transcriptional repression of genes, providing a rationale for the investigation of HDAC inhibitors in cancer therapeutics [34].

Additionally, acetylation of histones has been extensively studied as one of the key regulatory mechanisms of gene expression [35]. Histone acetylation was found to affect RNA transcription as early as the 1960s [36]. The highly conserved lysine residue at the N-terminal of H3 at position 9, 14, 18 and 23, and H4 lysine 5,8,12 and 16, are frequently targeted for modification [37]. Acetylations of the lysine residues neutralize the positive charge of the histone tails. Therefore, decrease their affinity for DNA which results in open chromatin conformation allowing the transcriptional machinery to reach its target [38]. The acetyltransferases added the acetyl groups from acetyl coenzyme A (acetyl-CoA) to the epsilon-amino group of specific lysine residues [39]. There are eighteen HDAC enzymes in mammalian cells which are divided into two families: a) zinc metalloenzymes that catalyses the hydrolysis of acetylated specific residues on histone tails and include class I, II and 1V HDACs, and b) NAD-dependent Sir2 deactylases which are considered as class III HDACs [40,41].

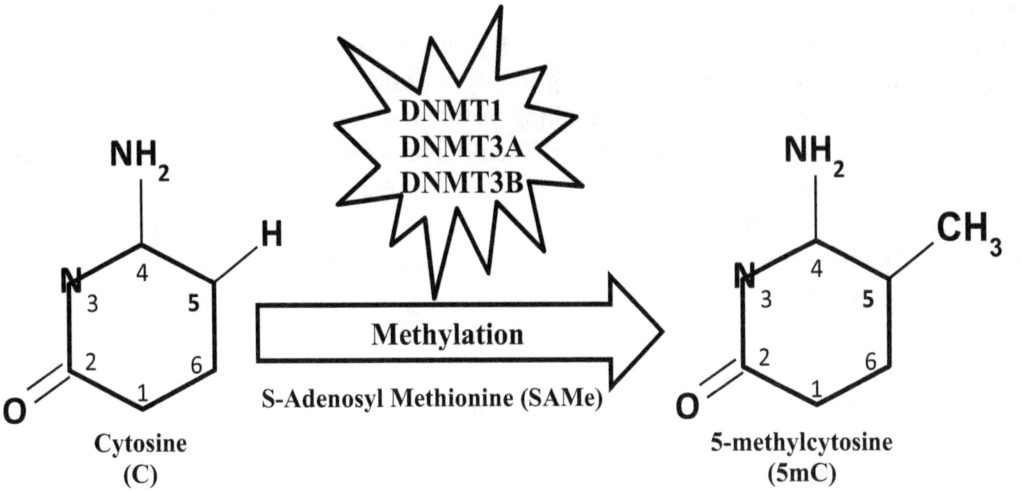

Figure 1. Methylation of DNA by DNA methyltransferases enzymes (DNMTs) DNMT1, DNMT3A, DNMT3B. A methyl group transfer from S-adenosyl-methionine onto cytosine residues leading to production of 5-methyl cytosine and S-adenosyl-homocystein (SAMe).

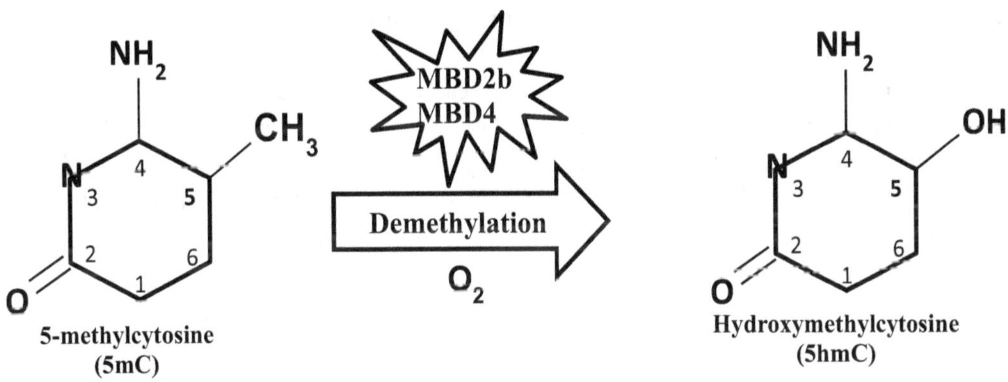

Figure 2. DNA demethylation appears to be a shared attribute of reprogramming events, and understanding DNA methylation dynamics is thus of considerable interest. Some enzymes such as MBD2b and MBD4 convert 5-methylcytosine (5mC) to 5-hydroxymethylcytosine (5hmC).

Class I is a group of four enzymes known as HDAC1, 2, 3 and 8 and this class is associated with gene regulation. They are expressed ubiquitously and they function exclusively in the nucleus [40]. Class II is subdivided into class IIA, which includes HDAC 4, 5, 7 and 9 and class IIB that includes HDAC 6 and 10. Class II enzymes shuttle between cytoplasm and nucleus, and they involve mainly in cell differentiation and are highly expressed in certain tissues [40]. Class III includes the NAD-dependent deacetylases which is a group of seven enzymes that are involved in maintaining the chromatin stability. They can remove the acetyl groups from histones besides other proteins [42]. Class IV contains one member which is HDAC11 which is closely related to class I thus some reviewers consider it as a member of that class. The function of HDAC11 has not been characterized yet [43], however, there is increasing evidence showing that changes in chromatin structure would alter DNA methylation patterns. The targeting of DNA methylation enzymes to gene promoters is guided by chromatin modifying enzymes. The fact is that chromatin configuration is dynamic and that chromatin modifying enzymes are activated by cellular signalling pathways. This provides a link between the extracellular environment and the state of DNA methylation [44]. Evidence of the link between chromatin modelling and DNA methylation in humans and mice arises from mutations of the SWI-SNF proteins which are involved in chromatin remodelling. These mutations result in defects in DNA methylation [44]. A number of histone methyltransferases, such as G9a, SUV39H1 and EZH2, a member of the multi-protein polycomb complex PRC2 can regulate DNA methylation by either recruiting or regulating the stability of DNMTs. DNMTs in turn can recruit HDACs and MBPs to achieve chromatin condensation and gene silencing [45]. This relationship between the epigenetic machinery makes the epigenetic mechanisms of genome expression a tightly regulated process.

5. DNA methylation and breast cancer

During the last decade, the study of epigenetic mechanisms in cancer, such as DNA methylation, histone modification, nucleosome positioning, and micro RNA expression, has provided extensive information about the mechanisms that contribute to the neoplastic phenotype through the regulation of expression of genes critical to transformation pathways. Regarding DNA methylation, the low level of CpG methylation in tumours compared with that in their normal-tissue counterparts was one of the first epigenetic alterations to be found in human cancer this let us to think that the cancer cells have a specific epigenome [46]. Hypomethylation in cancer cells is associated with a number of adverse products, including chromosome instability, activation of transposable elements, and loss of genomic imprinting [47].

Breast cancer has traditionally been staged by histopathological standards that are based on size, level of invasiveness and lymph node infiltration, and by immunochemical characterization of cell surface receptors, including oestrogen receptor (ER), the progesterone receptor (PR) and the human epidermal growth factor receptor 2 (HER2). However, in many instances staging breast cancer fails to predict prognosis or therapeutic response because of the heterogeneity of the disease. Changes in gene expression that reset a cell program from a normal to a diseased state involve multiple genetic circuitries, creating a characteristic signature of gene expression that defines the cell's unique identity and to classify subtypes of breast cancers [48]. Detailed knowledge of the DNA methylation status of all cytosines (the methylome) is paramount for understanding the mechanisms and functions underlying DNA methylation and led to extend our ability to classify breast cancer and the outcome prediction. DNA methylation is a forceful biomarker, greatly more stable than proteins or RNA, and is therefore a promising target for the development of new approaches for diagnosis and prognosis of breast cancer and other diseases. Because DNA methylation is critical in gene expression programming, a change in methylation from a normal to diseased state should be similarly reflected in a signature of DNA methylation that involves multiple gene pathways. Whole-genome approaches have been used with different levels of success to distinguish breastcancer-specific DNA methylation signatures, and to test whether they can classify breast cancer and whether they could be associated with specific clinical outcomes [48].

Application of DNA methylation profiling becomes important for breast cancer diagnosis and prognosis only if it provides additional classification value to other currently used methods like immunohistochemistry and mRNA expression analysis. A recent whole-genome DNA methylation analysis by using the Illumina 27 K arrays suggests that DNA methylation profiling might expand current classifications of breast cancer subtypes [49,50]. The analysis of 248 breast cancer tumour samples, comprising a 'main set' of 123 samples (4 normal and 119 infiltrating ductal carcinomas (IDCs)), and a 'validation set' of 125 samples (8 normal and 117 IDCs), revealed an immune 'signature' in a mixed tumour stromal population, as also reported [51]. Methylome analysis performed on frozen primary tumour samples, led to the identification of six different methylation clusters [52]. It was shown for the first time that DNA methylation profiles can reflect the cell-type composition of the tumour microenvironment, with a T lymphocyte infiltration of these tumours in particular in HER2-enriched and basal-like tumours. High expression of certain immune-related genes were found to be associated with improved relapse-free survival providing further insight into the importance of the immune system and tumour microenvironment in certain breast cancer subtypes [53].

Furthermore, aberrations in DNA methylation patterns of the CpG islands in the promoter regions of tumour-suppressor genes are accepted as being a common feature of human cancer [54]. CpG island promoter hypermethylation affects genes from a wide range of cellular pathways, such as cell cycle, DNA repair, toxic catabolism, cell adherence, apoptosis, and angiogenesis, among others [54], and may occur at various stages in the development of cancer [55]. The CpG-island-containing gene promoters are usually unmethylated in normal cells to maintain euchromatic structure, which is the transcriptionally active conformation allowing gene expression. Yet, during cancer development, many of these genes are hypermethylated at their CpG-island-containing promoters to inactivate their expression by changing open euchromatic structure to compact heterochromatic structure [56,57]. These genes are selectively hypermethylated in tumourigenesis for inactivation owing to their functional involvement in various cellular pathways that prevent cancer formation. Some of the methylated genes identified in human cancers are classic tumour suppressor genes in which one mutationally inactivated allele is inherited. According to Knudson's (2000) two-hit model, complete inactivation of a tumour suppressor gene requires loss-of-function of both gene copies [58]. Epigenetic silencing of the remaining wild-type allele of the tumour suppressor gene, thus, can be considered as the second hit in this model. For example, some well-known tumour suppressor genes, such as the cyclin-dependent kinase inhibitorp16INK4a, APC and BRCA1, are mutationally inactivated in the germline occasionally lose function of the remaining functional allele in breast epithelial cells through DNA hypermethylation [59].These advances in the knowledge of the breast methylome strongly indicate that DNA hypermethylation mechanism plays a crucial role in initiation, promotion and maintenance of breast carcinogenesis, which cooperatively and synergistically interact with other genetic alterations to promote the development of breast cancer. In addition to cell-cycle regulatory genes, DNA methylation-mediated silencing of DNA repair genes, such as BRCA1 and MGMT, could result in further inactivation of tumour suppressor genes or activation of oncogenes, which further drive breast tumourigenesis [60]. The genes that function as inhibitors of WNT oncogenic pathway such as SFRP1 and WIF1 have been found to be frequently hypermethylated in primary breast tumours [61]. Accordingly, epigenetic gene silencing is another mechanism that fosters malignant transformation of the mammary gland by aberrantly activating oncogenic signalling pathways in addition to the genetic mutation-mediated mechanism [62].

In vitro experiments showed that decreased BRCA1expression in cells led to increased levels of tumour growth, while increased expression of BRCA1 led to growth arrest and apoptosis. The magnitude of the decrease of functional BRCA1 protein correlates with disease prognosis [63]. Phenotypically, BRCA1-methylated tumours are similar to tumours from carriers of germline BRCA1 mutations. BRCA1 promoter hypermethylation was observed in one of two tumours from BRCA1 carriers lacking LOH [64]. In other study of population-based ovarian tumours, two of eight tumours with germline BRCA1mutations showed neither LOH nor promoter methylation [65]. Another study of 47 breast tumours from hereditary breast cancer families identified three BRCA1 carriers of which two showed BRCA1 promoter methylation in their tumours [66]. All these investigated studies suggest that methylation of BRCA1 may be serve as a second hit in tumours from a subset of BRCA1 mutation carriers [67].Tumours with BRCA1 mutations are usually more likely to be higher-grade, poorly differentiated, highly proliferative, ER negative, and PR negative, and p53 mutations. BRCA1 mutated breast cancers are also associated with poor survival in some studies [68]. BRCA1 promoter methylation was more frequent in invasive than in situ carcinoma and there were no correlation between BRCA1 promoter methylation and ER/PR status in a subset population [69]. However, they also found a higher prevalence of BRCA1 promoter methylation in cases with at least one node involved and with tumour size greater than 2cm. Based on their findings higher methylation levels may correlate with more advanced tumour stage at diagnosis. They also observed a 45% increase in mortality of individuals with BRCA1 methylation positive tumours compared those who had unmethylated BRCA1 promoters [69]. Another study conducted a familial breast cancer based study and found contradicting results. They found no overall correlation of ER, PR, or grade with hypermethylation of BRCA1 in the tumours from BRCA1 mutation negative families. However, seven individuals had both promoter hypermethylation and LOH; the majority of these tumours had a basal-like phenotype and were triple negative [70].

In addition, discriminate between tumour and normal or histologically non-malignant breast tissue has been applied widely by genome wide DNA methylation. One of the first genome wide DNA methylation studies in breast cancer developed methylation-specific digital karyotyping (MSDK) to assess epithelial, myoepithelial, and stromal fibroblasts from normal abreast and cancer tissues [71]. Furthermore, genome wide DNA methylation studies in breast cancer identified gene families that were commonly identified as differentially methylated between non-malignant and tumour included transcription factors (FOX, KLF, PRDM, ZBTB, and ZNF) and gene families involved in cell transport of proteins or vesicles(RAB and SLC) or involvement in cell adhesion (CDH and PCDH) [71-74]. The pathways and gene families do not appear to have a strong link to hormone metabolism or signalling, it is likely that these genes are not drivers of cancer but rather are secondary events that occur as part of the tumourigenic process [75,76].

Genome wide DNA methylation studies have supported correlation between DNA methylation and gene expression, particularly the association between CpG islands DNA hypermethylation and gene repression [49,74,77,78]. Using familial breast cancers and BRCA1/2-mutated tumours combined DNA methylation profiles that alone predicted BRCA status, with gene expression and copy number variation (CNV) and found that genes with reduced expression were more likely to be in genomic regions with loss of heterozygosity and/or high levels of DNA methylation. It has also been shown that the combination of gene dosage in breast cancer cell lines, allelic status, and DNA methylation explains more gene expression changes than either genomic element alone [79]. Combining DNA methylation profiling with CNV and gene expression can be promising tool to facilitate the identification of critical genes involved in tumourigenesis. In genome wide methylation analysis, several platforms have been recently developed to allow genome wide methylation analysis. The Golden Gate methylation array was the first platform which allowed methylation of 1536 CpG loci to be investigated. The Infinium Human Methylation 27 increased CpG investigation with the use of 27,578 probes. Most recently was the Infinium Human Methylation 450K array, designed by Illumina. This array utilises florescence microarray hybridisation technique, often associated with expression studies, to provide a methylation profile of 485,764 CpG loci including CpG associated in CpG islands, shores, shelves and the isolated loci in the open sea regions of the genome and promoter regionshave used Illumina Infinium Human Methylation 27 Bead Chip to analyse normal breast tissues from ten healthy individuals and compared this to 62 breast tumour samples (19 were inflammatory breast cancer) [73].

Further studies have also compared tumour to non-malignant tissue and the number of genes identified that discriminates the two depends on the filtering or analyses utilized. For instance, Kim et al. (2012) used several filtering processes to identify six genes [80], whereas, Faryna et al, (2012) identified 214 CpG islands but only one CpG island (TAC1) was methylated in all ten cancer samples [81]. The DNA methylation profiles divided the samples into three groups based on high, intermediate, and low DNA methylation levels, with the normal samples having low DNA methylation levels. When comparing DNA methylation between normal and tumour samples, 1352 CpG loci (1134 genes) were differentially methylated [73]. There was significantly greater methylation in tumours compared with normal and 77% of these are CpG loci. Another study using the same technology found 6309 CpGs differentially methylated between 119 tumours and four normal breast tissue samples identified several hundred differentially methylated loci between 11 adjacent non-malignant breast tissues and 108 tumours [49;74]. Kim et al, (2011) pooled DNA from ten cancers and ten non-malignant matched adjacent tissues and identified 1181 differentially methylated CpGs (corresponding to 1043 genes) with the vast majority (972) hypermethylated [82]. Another study found 291 probes (264 genes) hypermethylated in breast cancer (n=39) compared with non-malignant breast tissue (n=4) after removal of imprinted genes and X chromosome genes [83].

In addition, numbers of studies have investigated whether genome wide DNA methylation profiling can cluster breast cancers into hormone receptor status (ER/PR positive or negative) or subtype (luminal A or B, basal or HER2). These investigations differentiate hormone receptor-positive breast cancers from hormone receptor-negative cases using DNA methylation profiles [49,77,83-85]. The majority of genome wide DNA methylation studies have found that ER+PR+tumours have higher levels of DNA methylation compared with ER−PR− tumours [77,82,85,86]. Li et al, (2010) found 148 altered CpG sites (93 hypermethylated and 55 hypomethylated) in ER+PR+breast cancers relative to ER−PR− tumours [85]. Other study have identified 40 CpG probes that had an overall specificity of 89% and sensitivity of 90% for classifying ER+from ER− tumours [86].

Moreover, Hill et al, (2011) have used cluster analysis to show that ER+PR+tumours had high methylation, whereas triple-negative breast cancers had low methylation status [83]. Breast cancer cell lines have also shown clustering according to hormone receptor status based on DNA methylation levels [78]. Thus, all these genome wide DNA methylation studies demonstrate that an adequately results of appropriate clinical samples should identify methylation differences based on hormone receptor status. These studies may serve with additional future studies as a basis for the development of an improved clinical test to identify the hormone status of breast cancers.

In addition, in DNA methylation cluster analysis found that one cluster was predominantly luminal A (22/30 samples), the second cluster was highly correlated with basal-like (7/8 samples), and the third cluster contained a mixture of subtypes [74]. Recently, the Cancer Genome Atlas (TCGA) [87] and genome-wide profiling of DNA methylation has been also performed in primary breast tumours and revealed genes whose hypermethylation was significantly correlated with relapse-free survival, including RECK, SFRP2 and ACADL. Tumour specificity of methylation was confirmed for these genes by sequencing of an independent set of normal/breast tumour samples. Other investigation observed that the reduction of RECK methylation has been associated with worst prognosis in other tumours [88]. Genome-wide analysis has also been employed to characterize the DNA methylation profile of primary breast cancer with different metastatic potential. A global breast CpG island methylation phenotype (B-CIMP) was identified as an epigenetic profile associated with low risk of metastasis. Parallel gene expression analyses identified genes with both significant hypermethylation and down-regulation in B-CIMP tumours, including those involved in epithelial-mesenchymal transition (EMT), such as LYN, MMP7, KLK10 and WNT6 and the genes in the B-CIMP repression signature showed genes whose differential expression correlated with prognosis across several BC cohorts [89].

6. HDAC inhibitors and breast cancer

As we mentioned previously, abnormal HDAC activity has been documented in a variety of tumour types and led to the development of HDAC inhibitors as anticancer therapeutics. Currently available HDAC inhibitors target a variety of HDAC isoenzymes with class 1 (HDAC 1, 2, 3 and 8), class 2 (HDAC 4–7 and 9–10), and class 4 (HDAC 11) activity. Modest clinical benefits were previously reported with relatively weak HDAC inhibitors such as valproic acid and phenylbutyrate in advanced solid tumours or hematologic malignancies [89]. Laboratory research conducted to date supports the investigation of HDAC inhibitors for the treatment of breast cancer. Recently, vorinostat as HDAC inhibitor induces differentiation or arrests growth of a wide variety of human carcinoma cells including breast cancer cells [90].Vorinostat also reduced tumour incidence in NMU-induced rat mammary tumourigenesis by 40 % [91]. In vitro studies demonstrated that vorinostat inhibits clonogenic growth of both ER-positive and ER-negative breast cancer cell lines by inducing G1 and G2/M cell cycle arrest and subsequent apoptosis [92].

The ability of the HDAC inhibitors to relieve transcriptional repression in preclinical breast cancer models has also been investigated. The accumulation of acetylated H3 and H4 histone tails in conjunction with re-expression of a functional ER in ER-negative breast cancer cell lines has been observed with a novel HDAC inhibitor known as scriptaid [93].Treatment of ER-negative breast cancer cell lines with vorinostat is associated with reactivation of silenced ER, as well as down regulation of DNMT1 and EGFR protein expression [94]. The significance of an epigenetically reactivated ER was demonstrated when tamoxifen sensitivity was restored in the ER-negative MDA-MB-231 breast cancer cells following treatment with both HDAC (trichostatin A) and DNMT inhibitors (DAC) [95]. Entinostat has been shown to induce not only re-expression of ERα, but also the androgen receptor and the aromatase enzyme (CYP19) both in vitro and in triple-negative breast cancer xenografts [96]. In addition, the combination ofletrozole and entinostat resulted in a significant and durable reduction in the xenograft tumour volume when compared to treatment with either agent alone. These experiments have provided the strong rationale for combining epigenetic modifiers with hormonal therapy in breast cancer clinical trials [96]. Interestingly, many of these studies also indicate that a strategy which combines HDAC and DNMT inhibitors is more efficacious than either agent alone with respect to both re-expression of silenced genes and restoration of response to tamoxifen and aromatase inhibitors [93,97].

Moreover, pretreatment of various tumour cell lines with HDAC inhibitors increases the cytotoxicity of chemotherapy. Administering the HDAC inhibitor after chemotherapy did not achieve the same results, suggesting that pretreatment with these agents may open the chromatin structure and thus facilitate an enhanced anti-cancer effect of chemotherapy drugs that target DNA [98]. In breast cancer cell lines with amplification and overexpression of HER2, HDAC inhibitor use depleted HER2 by attenuation of its mRNA levels and promotion of proteosomal degradation. HDAC inhibition also had been reported to enhance apoptosis induction by trastuzumab, docetaxel, epothilone B, and gemcitabine [99]. HDAC inhibitors also significantly enhance trastuzumab-induced growth inhibition in trastuzumab-sensitive, HER2-overexpressing breast cancer cells, providing a strong rationale for clinical studies with this combination in patients with HER2-positive disease [100].

Additionally, HDAC inhibitors such as entinostat or valproic acid, have been tested in breast cancer cells and efficiently restored both ERα expression and letrozole sensibility in ER$^-$BC in vitro and in vivo [101,102].The association of HDAC inhibitors or 5-azadeoxycytidine with a treatment inducing overexpression of TFAP2C might improve ESR1 expression in ER$^-$patients. A combined HDAC inhibitors and 5-azadeoxycytidine treatment induces the most significant increase in ERα content. Surprisingly however, addition of tamoxifen does not produce a tumourigenic response in ER-BC cells demonstrated that a better response to tamoxifen in BC cells, correlated with a lower level of the RNA-stabilizing HuR protein [103]. Tamoxifen treatment increased HuR content, and contributed to its own resistance while HDAC inhibitors /5-azadeoxycytidine decreased HuR. Preliminary treatment with HDAC inhibitors /5-azadeoxycytidine was given before delivering tamoxifen to attempt to obtain the best tamoxifen sensitivity. The precise roles of tamoxifen are complex: although it competes with 17β-estradiol to bind to ERα, ERα bound to tamoxifen is still able to target the TFF1 (also called pS2) promoter without constitutive activation of gene transcription. The loss of transcriptional activity of the tamoxifen-ERα complex is mediated by changes in the balance of co-activators/co-repressors and ERα-interacting partners [104].

7. DNMTs inhibitors and breast cancer

The human DNMTs 1, 3A, and 3B coordinate mRNA expression in normal tissues and overexpression in tumours and the expression levels of these DNMTs are reportedly elevated in breast cancer [105,106]. The mean levels of DNMT1, DNMT3a, and DNMT3b overexpression have turned out to be quite similar among different tumour types. The DNMT3b gene has shown the highest range of expression (81.8 for DNMT3a compared with 16.6 and 14 for DNMT1 and DNMT3a, respectively). About 30% of patients revealed overexpression of DNMT3b in the tumour tissue as compared to normal breast tissue. Taking only these overexpressing tumours into account, the DNMT3b expression change was 82-fold, thus being significantly higher [106]. Interestingly, DNMT1 and DNMT3a were overexpressed in only 5 and 3% of breast carcinomas [107]. As a result of these studies, DNMT3b plays the predominant role over DNMT3a and DNMT1 in breast tumourigenesis. This is consistent with a recent study in breast cancer cell lines, which demonstrated a strong correlation between total DNMT activity and overexpression of DNMT3b, but not with the expression of DNMT3a or DNMT1 [107,108].

Cancer was the first group of diseases to be associated with DNA methylation and to be considered for DNA-methylation-targeted therapeutics, and it serves as a prototype for determining the role of DNA methylation and DNA-methylation-targeted therapeutics in other diseases [109]. As we mentioned previously, several types of aberration in DNA methylation and in the proteins involved in DNA methylation occur in cancer: hypermethylation of tumour suppressor genes, aberrant expression of DNMT1 and other DNMTs, and hypomethylation of unique genes and repetitive sequences [110,111]. Silencing of tumour suppressor genes by DNA methylation provides a powerful molecular mechanism by which DNA methylation can trigger cancer, and also provides a rationale for therapeutics aimed at inhibition of DNA methylation and re-expression of silenced tumour suppressor genes. Multiple genes are hypermethylatedin breast cancer compared to non-cancerous tissue [112]. These include genes involved in evasion of apoptosis (RASSF1A, HOXA5, TWIST1), limitless replication potential (CCND2, p16, BRCA1, RARβ), growth (ERα, PGR), and tissue invasion and metastasis (CDH1) [113]. These genes are not only hypermethylated in tumour cells, but show increased epigenetic silencing in normal epithelium surrounding the tumour site.

Unlike genetic alterations which are almost impossible to revert, DNA methylation is a reversible event. Reactivation of hypermethylated tumour-suppressor genes can be considered as a possible therapeutic target which will lead to develop pharmacological inhibitors of DNA methylation. Moreover, the use of DNMT inhibitors is good tools for cancer treatment because the restoration of expression of tumour-suppressor genes could restore the protective effect of these genes on tumour divisions [114]. The nucleoside analogues, 5-azacytidine (vidaza or AZA,) and 5-aza-2′-deoxycytidine (decitabine or DAC) are two DNMT inhibitors that are effective hypomethylating agent that inhibit cell proliferation [115]. These two drugs represent the two most prominent DNMT inhibitors being under preclinical and clinical investigation for over 30 years [116]. Moreover, these agents are pro-drugs that need to be incorporated into DNA to act as inhibitors of DNMTs [116]. The nucleoside analogues are first phosphorylated to the triphosphate nucleotide and incorporated into DNA during DNA synthesis. DNMT1 forms a covalent bond with the carbon at position 6 of the cytosine as well as 5-aza-cytosine ring. Under normal conditions, as mentioned previously, the enzyme transfers the methyl group from SAMe to the fifth carbon position of the cytosine ring. This enables the release of the enzyme from its covalent bond with cytosine. When a 5′-aza-cytosine ring replaces cytosine in the DNA, the methyl transfer does not take place and the DNMT is trapped on the DNA (Figure 3). The replication fork progresses in the absence of DNMT1 resulting in passive loss of DNA methylation in the nascent strand but not the template [116].

Because they are cytidine analogues, both agents are incorporated into DNA after activation to a triphosphate moiety. After formation of an irreversible complex with DNMT1, degradation of the enzyme occurs [117]. This prevents methylation of daughter DNA in CpG islands during DNA replication. In addition, AZA (but not DAC) is converted into a ribonucleoside moiety and is incorporated into RNA, interfering with protein translation. At low concentrations (e.g. 30nM DAC, 300nM AZA), these inhibitors exhibit potent DNA hypomethylation properties, whereas high concentrations (≈3–10 μM) are cytotoxic [119]. The doses of AZA and DAC that were employed in many of the early clinical trials in solid tumours were cytotoxic, reflecting maximum tolerated doses, which likely accounts for the excessive toxicity, and possibly also to lack of overall efficacy, observed in these studies [120]. Previous study indicated that the DNMT inhibitors were associated with response rates as high as 18% in breast cancer [120]. The doses of AZA that were employed in these studies, however, were far higher than doses used in clinical trials today and likely exerted cytotoxic activity as opposed to relief of transcriptional repression as an anti-cancer strategy [120].

Current clinical studies with administration of DNMT inhibitors at the presumed optimal epigenetic dose aim to elucidate the biological effects of these agents, and to assess clinical efficacy, alone or in combination with other anti-cancer agents. The ability of single agent AZA to induce expression of the ER and PR genes in patients with triple-negative breast cancer who are awaiting definitive breast cancer surgery is under investigation using a 75 mg/m^2/day dosing schedule [121]. Based on the preclinical evidence previously described which suggests that a combination of epigenetic modifiers may be more successful in re-expression of silenced genes and restoration of hormonal therapy responsiveness, patients with advanced triple-negative and hormone-resistant breast cancer are being enrolled in an ongoing multi-center phase 2 clinical trial and receive the combination of low dose AZA (40 mg/m^2) on days 1–5 and 8–10, and entinostat 7 mg on days 3 and 10 of a 28 day cycle. Tumour biopsies prior to and after therapy are collected to assess modulation of candidate gene methylation and expression, such as the ER gene. Patients may transition to an optional continuation phase at the time of disease progression in which the same epigenetic therapy is administered with the addition of hormonal therapy [122].

The DNMT inhibitors combination with standard chemotherapy has not been extensively evaluated in the breast cancer setting and preclinical evidence have shown the AZA could overcome platinum resistance through DNA hypomethylation, patients with both platinum resistant and refractory ovarian cancer received the combination of AZA and carboplatin after being enrolled [122,123]. Since DNMT inhibitors like AZA and DAC are known to be effective in the clinic for diseases like myelodys plastic syndromes that may result in part from transcriptional dysregulation due to epigenetic changes, there is interest in developing novel DNMT inhibitors that would be more effective and less toxic. One such putative agent is zebularine, a cytidine which has been reported to prevent early tumour development and also to inhibit growth of mammary gland tumours and breast cancer cells lines [124,125]. Zebularine is a novel DNMT inhibitor, which was developed as a more stable and less toxic drug [126]. Zebularine, similar to AZA-CR and 5-AZA-CdR, incorporates into DNA and forms a covalent irreversible complex with DNMT preventing the enzyme from methylating position 5 of cytosines clustered in regulatory CpG islands [127]. Recent studies showed the ability of zebularine to sustain the demethylation state of the 5′ region of the tumour suppressor gene CDKN2A/p16 and other methylated genes in T24, HCT15, CFPAC-1, SW48, and HT-29 cells [127]. It was also reported that zebularine inhibits growth of cancer cell lines but not normal cells [128].

Zebularine acts as a cytidine analogue containing a 2-(1H)-pyrimidinone ring that was originally developed as a cytidine deaminase inhibitor to prevent deamination of nucleoside analogues [129,130]. Zebularine is also a versatile starting material for the synthesis of complex nucleosides and is a mechanism based DNA cytosine methyltransferase inhibitor [131]. It acts primarily as a trap for DNMT protein by forming tight covalent complexes between DNMT protein and zebularine-substituted DNA [132]. In contrast, to other DNMT inhibitors, it has low toxicity in most tested cell lines and is quite stable with a half-life of 510 h at pH 7.4 [131, 133,134]. Because of its low toxicity, continuous administration of effective doses of zebularine alone or in combination with other DNMT inhibitors is feasible and this can result in the enhanced re-expression of epigenetically silenced genes in cancer cells [128].

Zebularine treatment led to increased p21 protein expression coupled with decreased cyclin B and D protein expression in MCF-7 cells and an increased percentage of cells in S-phase that indicates a zebularine induced S-phase arrest [135].This finding suggests errors in chromatin assembly that contribute to genomc instability [136]. S-phase arrest can also be triggered by repression of histone synthesis in human cells [137]. The genomic instability induced by DNMT1 down regulation and repression of histone synthesis triggers the activation of S-phase

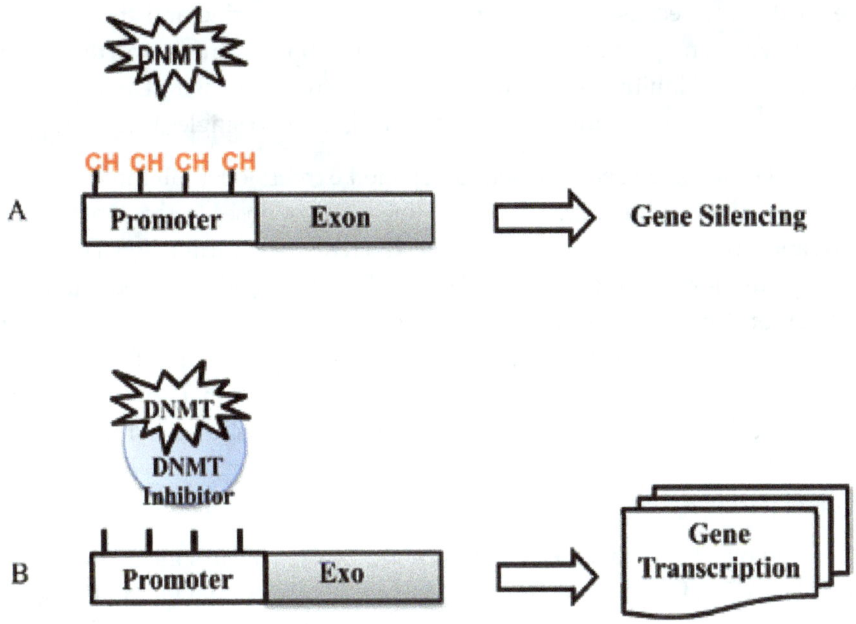

Figure 3. Activation of gene expression by nucleoside analogues, 5-azacytidine (vidaza or AZA,) and 5-aza-2′-deoxycytidine (decitabine or DAC), both are DNMTs inhibitors. (A) In active transcription is characterized by the presence of methylated cytosines within CpG dinucleotides (CH_3) which is sustained by DNMTs. (B) When a 5′-aza-cytosine ring replaces cytosine in the DNA, the methyl transfer does not take place and the DNMT is trapped on the DNA and the gene expression could restored again.

check point proteins like p21 (in MCF-7 cells) and/or down regulates cyclin-D to permit DNA repair before entering G2 phase.

The zebularine-mediated decrease in expression of global acetylated histones observed in our studies further supports our hypothesis. Several preclinical studies have evaluated zebularine as a possible therapeutic in cancer cell lines. Zebularine preferentially incorporates into DNA, leading to cell growth inhibition and increased expression of cell cycle regulatory genes in cancer cell lines compared with normal fibroblasts [135]. Additionally, to determine the ability of zebularine to prevent or treat breast cancer, Min et al, 2012 tested if daily oral treatment with zebularine affects mammary tumour growth in these MMTV-PyMT mice [124]. They observed a significant delay in tumour growth and a reduction of total tumour burden in the zebularine-treated mice. They have reported that the depletion of DNMTs in tumours excised from zebularine-treated mice and identified upregulation of 12 genes previously characterized as silenced by DNA hypermethylation. Zebularine treatment was shown to be associated with a dose-dependent depletion of DNMT1, DNMT3a, and DNMT3b proteins in the breast cancer cell lines MCF-7 and MDA-MB-231 [124]. Zebularine also depletes DNMT1 in T24 bladder carcinoma cells after 24 hours of treatment and partially depletes DNMT3b after 3 days of drug exposure [128]. Recently, Chen et al, (2012) have proofed in in vivo study that DNMT1 was depleted, and DNMT3b was significantly lowered (50% depletion) in the mammary tumours derived from zebularine-treated mice as compared with untreated mice [138]. Regardless of the mechanism of tumour growth inhibition, tumour cells eventually develop resistance to zebularine treatment. Because it has been shown that zebularine and the HDAC inhibitor depsipeptide have a synergistic effect on the inhibition of breast cancer growth a combinatorial treatment with DNMT inhibitors and a combinatorial treatment with DNMT inhibitors and HDAC inhibitors may be warranted to overcome resistance to single-drug therapy.

Moreover, zebularine have been reported to depleted expression of all three DNMT proteins post-transcriptionally in both breast cancer cell lines at most doses tested. It has been reported that human cancer cells lacking DNMT1 or DNMT3b retain significant global methylation and gene silencing, but those lacking both DNMT1 and DNMT3b had >95% reduction in genomic DNA methylation and virtually absent DNMT activity [135]. The zebularine treatment specifically targets DNMT1, and reduced DNMT 3a and 3b protein expression, implying that treated cells may still retain substantial methylation [139]. Another study observed similar results in T24 bladder cancer cells continuously treated with zebularine for 40 days. In these cells zebularine had no effect on the expression of DNMT1, 3a or 3b mRNA but complete loss of DNMT1 and partial depletion of DNMT 3a and 3b protein were observed [128].

Previous findings observed that ER can be epigenetically silenced in some human breast cancer cell lines and HDAC or DNMT inhibitors could reexpress functional ER in ER negative breast cancer cells [140,141]. Further investigation demonstrated that treatment of ER negative MDA-MB-231 breast cancer cells with zebularine results in functional ER reactivation as manifested by expression of ER mRNA and its target gene, PR. This has been reported with a dose as low as 50μM, far lower than doses that induced apoptosis. Chromatin immunoprecipitation analysis of the ER promoter in zebularine-treated cells showed characteristics of an active chromatin as manifested by accumulation of acetylated H3 and H4 and release of DNMT1, 3a and 3b from the ER promoter region. Although reexpression of ER with zebularine was not as robust as with 5-azaDc, the low toxicity could enable continuous administration for sustained re-expression of ER cells [141].

However, several studies have shown that zebularine has some potential limitations such as less potent than the two FDA-approved DNMT inhibitors, azaC and 5-azaDc [133]. It is hypothesized that the reduced inhibitor potency is due to sequestration of the drug by cytidine deaminase, competitive inhibition of zebularine incorporation into DNA by increased cytidine and deoxycytidine that accumulate as a consequence of its cytidine deaminase properties, and preferential incorporation of zebularine into RNA over DNA [142]. For these reasons, the drug is effective only at very high doses, making administration more problematic. Its efficacy combined with a low toxicity profile makes it an attractive agent for combination or sequential therapy with other DNMT or HDAC inhibitors [143].

8. Combination of DNMT inhibitors

Based on the preclinical evidence previously described which suggests that a combination of epigenetic modifiers may be more successful in re-expression of silenced genes and restoration of hormonal therapy responsiveness, we have mentioned previously that the patients with advanced triple-negative and hormone-resistant breast cancer are being enrolled in an ongoing multi-center phase 2 clinical trial and receive the combination of low dose of AZA [122]. Tumour biopsies prior to and after therapy are collected to assess modulation of candidate gene methylation and expression, such as the ER. Patients may transition to an optional continuation phase at the time of disease progression in which the same epigenetic therapy is administered with the addition of hormonal therapy [123]. Indeed, in a recently published trial exploring the combination of AZA and entinostat in advanced non-small cell lung cancer patients, investigators observed that the regimen was well tolerated and associated with a number of objective responses [144]. These included a complete response as well as a partial response in a patient without progression of disease for 2 years after completing the clinical trial. Interestingly, a number of patients were found to have unexpected major objective responses to subsequent anti-cancer strategies, raising the question as to whether these agents may prime tumour cells to respond to subsequent therapies. A phase 1/2 Canadian trial investigating the combination of decitabine and vorinostat in patients with advanced solid tumours or hematologic malignancies has also indicated clinical activity. Stabilization of disease for 4 or more cycles was observed in 29 % evaluable patients; two of these patients had metastatic breast cancer [145].

Moreover, cytidine deaminase destabilizes DNMT inhibitors like 5-azaDc, resulting in complete loss of their antineoplastic ability [146]. Hence administration of cytidine deaminase inhibitors like zebularine should theoretically potentiate therapeutic effects of 5-azaDc by slowing its degradation and stabilizing activity. Indeed, the combination of 5-aza-Dc and zebularine produced greater inhibition in cell proliferation and clonogenicity than either drug alone in leukemic L1210 and HL-60 cell lines [147]. Similarly, treatment of the AML-193 acute myeloid leukemic cell line, which has a densely methylated p15INK4B CpG island, with zebularine followed by the HDAC inhibitor, trichostatin-A, synergistically enhanced p15INK4B expression [134]. Consistent with these results, the combination of 50μMzebularine and 1μM 5-azaDc in breast cancer cells significantly inhibited cell proliferation compared with either drug alone. Similarly, zebularine significantly inhibited cell proliferation and colony formation in combination with low doses of vorinostat. Cheishvili et al, (2014) have investigated the combination of methylated DNA binding protein 2 (MBD2) depletion and DNMT inhibitor 5-azaCdR in breast cancer cells results in a combined effect in vitro and in vivo, enhancing tumour growth arrest on one hand while inhibiting invasiveness triggered by 5-azaCdR on the other hand. The combined treatment of MBD2 depletion and 5-azaCdR suppresses and augments distinct gene networks that are induced by DNMT inhibition alone. These data point to a potential new approach in targeting the DNA methylation machinery by combination of MBD2 and DNMT inhibitors [148].

The combination of DNMT inhibitors with standard chemotherapy has not been extensively evaluated in the breast cancer setting. Based on strong preclinical evidence that the addition of AZA could overcome platinum resistance through DNA hypomethylation, patients with both platinum resistant and refractory ovarian cancer received the combination of AZA and carboplatin after being enrolled into a phase 1b/2 study. The overall response rate of 22 % was observed in the platinum-resistant patients (disease progression within 6 months of platinum, n=18) suggesting that further evaluation of the combination was warranted [149]. Whether combining DNMT inhibitors with standard therapies or novel agents will result in clinical benefit for patients with breast cancer remains to be seen. In the meantime, robust preclinical data should support the development of new concepts in order to maximize the chance of success with these agents in the solid tumour arena.

9. Conclusion

Future studies need to include a more detailed investigation of the methylation differences between breast cancer subtypes to determine whether there is a methylation signature that can identify breast cancer subtypes. It is also possible that DNA methylation subtypes are different to the subtypes identified by gene expression and may provide additional information that assists in the clinical setting. Further research is required to delineate these options and determine how subtypes identified by DNA methylation profiling differ to subtypes identified by gene expression. Laboratory studies have shown that AZA and DAC optimally inhibit DNA methylation when used at lower than cytotoxic doses with prolonged exposures. The exact impact of using epigenetic modifiers at an optimally epigenetic dose instead of a cytotoxic dose is yet unknown in solid tumours, despite the supposition that anti-cancer activity will be enhanced. Ongoing clinical trials in breast cancer patients aim to elucidate this question. Optimizing the use of the clinically available epigenetic modifiers is clearly important. An oral form of AZA is currently in development which may be far more convenient for patients than the intravenous and subcutaneous routes employed at this time. A number of new agents are also in development which may circumvent some of the limitations of the currently available drugs such as their in vivo deamination by cytidine deaminase and tendency to be subject to drug resistance.

Author details

Majed S. Alokail[1*] and Amal M. Alenad[2]

*Address all correspondence to: malokail@ksu.edu.sa

1 Biomarker Research Group, Biochemistry Department, College of Science, King Saud University, Riyadh, Saudi Arabia

2 School of Biological Sciences, Life Science Building, University of Southampton, Southampton, UK

References

[1] Waddington CH. Selection of the genetic basis for an acquired character. Nature 1952;169:625-626.

[2] Waddington CH. Evolutionary adaptation. Perspectives in Biology and Medicine1959;2:379-401.

[3] Wolffe AP, Matzke MA. Epigenetics: regulation through repression. Science 1999;286:481-486.

[4] Wolffe AP, Matzke MA. Epigenetics: regulation through repression. Science 1999;286:481-486.

[5] Bird A. Perceptions of epigenetics. Nature2007;447:396-398.

[6] Vaissiere T, Sawan C, Herceg Z. Epigenetic interplay between histone modifications and DNA methylation in gene silencing. Mutation Research 2008;659:40-48.

[7] Klose RJ, Bird AP. Genomic DNA methylation: the mark and its mediators. Trends in Biochemical Scinces 2006;31:89-97.

[8] RazinA, Szyf M. DNA methylation patterns. Formation and function. Biochimical et Biophysical Acta 1984;782(4):331-342.

[9] Fuks F. DNA methylation and histone modifications: teaming up to silence genes. Current Opinion in Genetics & Development 2005;15:490-495.

[10] Robertson KD, Jones PA. DNA methylation: past, present and future directions. Carcinogenesis 2000;21:461-467.

[11] Singal R, Ginder GD. DNA methylation. Blood 1999;93:4059-4070.

[12] Straussman R, Nejman D, Roberts D, Steinfeld I, Blum B, et al,. Developmental programming of CpG island methylation profiles in the human genome. Nature Structural & Molecular Biology2009;16:564-571.

[13] Bird AP. CpG-rich islands and the function of DNA methylation. Nature 1986;321:209-213.

[14] Jin B, Li Y, Robertson KD. DNA methylation: superior or subordinate in the epigenetic hierarchy? Genes & Cancer 2011;2:607–17.

[15] Bestor TH. Activation of mammalian DNA methyltransferase by cleavage of a Zn binding regulatory domain. The European Molecular Biology Organization Journal 1992;11:2611-2617.

[16] Buryanov YI, Shevchuk TV. DNA methyltransferases and structural-functional specificity of eukaryotic DNA modification. Biochemistry (Mosc) 2005;70: 730-742.

[17] Lauster R, Trautner TA, and Noyer-Weidner M. Cytosine-specific type II DNA methyltransferases. A conserved enzyme core with variable target-recognizing domains. Journal Molecular Biology 1989;206: 305-312.

[18] Subramaniam D, Thombre R, Dhar A, Anant S. DNA methyltransferases: a novel target for prevention and therapy.Frontiers in Oncology2014;1(4):80.

[19] Lei H, Oh SP, Okano M, Juttermann R, Goss KA, Jaenisch R, Li E. De novo DNA cytosine methyltransferase activities in mouse embryonic stem cells. Development 1996;122:3195-3205.

[20] Buryanov YI, Shevchuk TV. DNA methyltransferases and structural-functional specificity of eukaryotic DNA modification. Biochemistry (Mosc) 2005;70: 730-742.

[21] Ghoshal K, BaiS. DNA methyltransferases as targets for cancer therapy. Drugs of today (Barcelona)2007;43: 395–422.

[22] Li H, Rauch T, Chen ZX, Szabo PE, Riggs AD, Pfeifer GP. The histone methyltransferase SETDB1 and the DNA methyltransferase DNMT3A interact directly and localize to promoters silenced in cancer cells. Journal of Biological Chemistry 2006;281:19489–19500.

[23] Jones PA,Takai D. The role of DNA methylation in mammalian epigenetics 2001;93(5532):1068-1070.

[24] Macleod D, Charlton J, Mullins J, Bird AP. Sp1 sites in the mouse aprt gene promoter are required to prevent methylation of the CpG island. Genes & Development1994;8: 2282-2292.

[25] Miller CA, Sweatt JD. Covalent modification of DNA regulates memory formation. Neuron 2007;53: 857-869.

[26] Kornberg RD, Lorch Y. Chromatin-modifying and-remodeling complexes.Current Opinion in Genetics and Development1999;9(2):148-151.

[27] Zhang Y, Reinberg D. Transcription regulation by histone methylation: interplay between different covalent modifications of the core histone tails.Genes & Development 2001;15(18):2343-2360.

[28] Nakayama T, Watanabe M, Yamanaka M, Hirokawa Y, Suzuki H, et al. The role of epigenetic modifications in retinoic acid receptor beta2 gene expression in human prostate cancers. Laboratory Investigation2001;81:1049-1057.

[29] Strahl BD, Briggs SD, Brame CJ, Caldwell JA, Koh SS, et al. Methylation of histone H4 at arginine 3 occurs in vivo and is mediated by the nuclear receptor coactivator PRMT1.Current Biology 2001;11(12):996-1000.

[30] Turner BM. Histone acetylation and an epigenetic code. Bioessays 2000;22: 836-845.

[31] Connolly R, Stearns V. Epigenetics as a Therapeutic Target in Breast Cancer.Journal of Mammary Gland Biology and Neoplasia 2012;17(3-4):191–204.

[32] Jones PA, Baylin SB. The fundamental role of epigenetic events in cancer.Nature Review Genet 2002;3:415–428.

[33] Arts J, de Schepper S, Van Emelen K. Histone deacetylase inhibitors: from chromatin remodeling to experimental cancer therapeutics. Current Medicinal Chemistry2003;10:2343–2350.

[34] Prince HM, Bishton MJ, Harrison SJ. Clinical studies of histone deacetylase inhibitors. Clinical Cancer Research 2009;15:3958–3969.

[35] Grant PA. A tale of histone modifications. Genome Biology 2001;2(4): reviews0003-reviews0003.6

[36] Allfrey VG, Faulknerr R, Mirsky AE. Acetylation and methylation the histones and their possible role in the regulation of RNA synthesis. Proceedings of the National Academy of Sciences of the United States of America1964;51: 786-794.

[37] Roth SY, Denu JM, Allis CD. Histone acetyltransferases. Annual Review in Biochemistry 2001; 70: 81-120.

[38] Hong L, Schroth GP, Matthews HR, Yau P, Bradbury EM. Studies of the DNA binding properties of histone H4 amino terminus. Thermal denaturation studies reveal that acetylation markedly reduces the binding constant of the H4 "tail" to DNA. Journal of Biological Chemistry1993;268: 305-314.

[39] Kim Y, Tanner KG, Denu JM. A continuous, nonradioactive assay for histone acetyltransferases.Analytical Biochemistry 2000;280(2):308-314.

[40] Glaser KB. HDAC inhibitors: clinical update and mechanism-based potential. Biochemical Pharmacology 2007;74:659-671.

[41] Vigushin DM, Ali S, Pace PE, Mirsaidi N, Ito K.Trichostatin A is a histone deacetylase inhibitor with potent antitumor activity against breast cancer in vivo. Clinical Cancer Research 2001;7: 971-976.

[42] Kyrylenko S, Kyrylenko O, Suuronen T, Salminen A. Differential regulation of the Sir2 histone deacetylase gene family by inhibitors of class I and II histone deacetylases. Cellular and molecular life sciences2003;60: 1990-1997.

[43] Crabb SJ, Howell M, Rogers H, Ishfaq M, Yurek-George A, et al. C,aracterisation of the in vitro activity of the depsipeptide histone deacetylase inhibitor spiruchostatin A. Biochemical Pharmacology 2008;76: 463-475.

[44] Szyf M. The dynamic epigenome and its implications in toxicology. Toxicology Science 2007;100: 7-23.

[45] Sharma S, Kelly TK, Jones PA. Epigenetics in cancer. Carcinogenesis 2010;31:27-36.

[46] Feinberg AP, Vogelstein B. Hypomethylation distinguishes genes of some human cancers from their normal counterparts. Nature 1983;301:89–92.

[47] BerdascoM,Esteller M. Aberrant epigenetic landscape in cancer: how cellular identity goes awry. Developmental cell 2010;19:698-711.

[48] Szyf M. DNA methylation signatures for breast cancer classification and prognosis. Genome Medicine 2012;4(3): 26.

[49] Dedeurwaerder S, Desmedt C, Calonne E, Singhal SK, Haibe-Kains B, et al. DNA methylation profiling reveals a predominant immune component in breast cancers.EMBO Molecular Medicine2011;3(12):726-741

[50] Dedeurwaerder S, Fumagalli D, Fuks F. Unravelling the epigenomic dimension of breast cancers.Current Opinion in Oncology2011;23(6):559-565.

[51] Kristensen VN, Vaske CJ, Ursini-Siegel J, Van Loo P, Nordgard SH. Et al. Integrated molecular profiles of invasive breast tumors and ductal carcinoma in situ (DCIS) reveal differential vascular and interleukin signaling. Proceedings of the National Academy of Sciences of the USA 2012;109(8):2802-2807.

[52] Cornacchia E, Golbus J, Maybaum J, Strahler J, Hanash S. et al.Hydralazine and procainamide inhibit T cell DNA methylation and induce autoreactivity. Journal of Immunology 1988;140(7):2197-200.

[53] Mi XB, Zeng FQ. Hypomethylation of interleukin-4 and-6 promoters in T cells from systemic lupus erythematosus patients. ActaPharmacologicaSinica 2008;29(1): 105-112.

[54] Esteller M. Epigenetics in cancer. New England Journal of Medicine 2008;358(11): 1148-1159.

[55] Berdasco M, Esteller M. Aberrant epigenetic landscape in cancer: how cellular identity goes awry. Developmental cell 2010;19:698-711.

[56] EstellerM.Epigenetic gene silencing in cancer: the DNA hypermethylome. Human molecular genetics 2007;16: R50–R59.

[57] Jones PA, Baylin SB. The epigenomics of cancer. Cell 2007;128:683–692.

[58] Knudson AG. Chasing the cancer demon. Annual Review of Genetic 2000; 34:1–19.

[59] Birgisdottir V, Stefansson OA, Bodvarsdottir SK, Hilmarsdottir H, JonassonJG.Epigenetic silencing and deletion of the BRCA1 gene in sporadic breast cancer. Breast Cancer Research 2006;8:R38.

[60] Esteller M. Epigenetic lesions causing genetic lesions in human cancer: promoter hypermethylation of DNA repair genes. European Journal of Cancer 2000;36:2294–2300.

[61] Lo PK, Mehrotra J, D'CostaA.Fackler MJ, Garrett-Mayer E. Epigenetic suppression of secreted frizzled related protein 1 (SFRP1) expression in human breast cancer. Cancer Biology and Therapeutics 2006;5:281–286.

[62] Lo PK, Sukumar S. Epigenomics and breast cancer. Pharmacogenomics 2008;12:1879–1902.

[63] Mirza S, Sharma G, Prasad CP, Parshad R, Srivastava, A et al. Promoter hypermethylation of TMS1, BRCA1, ERalpha and PRB in serum and tumor DNA of invasive ductal breast carcinoma patients. Life Science 2007; 81:280–287.

[64] Esteller M, Corn PG, Baylin SB, Herman JG. A gene hypermethylation profile of human cancer. Cancer Research 2001; 61:3225–3229.

[65] Press JZ, De Luca A, Boyd N, Young S, Troussard A. et al. Ovarian carcinomas with genetic and epigenetic BRCA1 loss have distinct molecular abnormalities. BMC Cancer 2008;8:17.

[66] Birgisdottir V, Stefansson OA, Bodvarsdottir SK, Hilmarsdottir H, Jonasson JG. et al. Epigenetic silencing and deletion of the BRCA1 gene in sporadic breast cancer. Breast Cancer Research 2006;8: R38.

[67] Dworkin AM, Huang TH-M, Tolandbcd AE. Epigenetic alterations in the breast: Implications for breast cancer detection, prognosis and treatment. Seminar in Cancer Biology 2009;3:165-171.

[68] ChappuisPO, Kapusta L, Begin LR, Wong N, Brunet JS, et al. Germline BRCA1/2 mutations and p27(Kip1) protein levels independently predict outcome after breast cancer. Journal of Clinical Oncology 2000;18:4045–4052.

[69] Xu X, Gammon MD, Zhang Y, Bestor TH, Zeisel SH. Et al. BRCA1 promoter methylation is associated with increased mortality among women with breast cancer. Breast cancer research and treatment 2009;115:397-404.

[70] Honrado, E., Osorio, A., Milne, RL., Paz MF, Melchor L, et al. Immunohistochemical classification of non-BRCA1/2 tumors identifies different groups that demonstrate the heterogeneity of BRCAX families. Modern Pathology 2007;20:1298–1306.

[71] Hu M, Yao J, Cai L, Bachman KE, van den Brule F, et al. Distinct epigenetic changes in the stromal cells of breast cancers. Nature Genetics 2005;37:899–905.

[72] Tommasi S, Karm DL, Wu X, Yen Y, Pfeifer GP. Methylation of homeobox genes is a frequent and early epigenetic event in breast cancer. Breast Cancer Research 2009;11: R14.

[73] Van der Auwera I, Yu W, Suo L, Van Neste L, van Dam P, et al., Array-based DNA methylation profiling for breast cancer subtype discrimination. PLOS ONE 2010;5: e12616.

[74] Kamalakaran S, Varadan V, GierckskyRussnes HE, Levy D, Kendall J. DNA methylation patterns in luminal breast cancers differ from non-luminal subtypes and can identify relapse risk independent of other clinical variables. Molecular Oncology 2011;5: 77–92.

[75] DayTK, Bianco-MiottoT. Common gene pathways and families altered by DNA methylation in breast and prostate cancers. Endocrine Related Cancer 2013; 20(5):R215-32.

[76] Alokail MS; Epigenetic and breast cancer. In: Gunduz M and Gunduz E. (ed.) Breast Cancer (Focusing tumor microenvironment, stem cells and metastasis). Rijeka: InTech; 2011. p291-320.

[77] Fang F, Turcan S, Rimner A, Kaufman A, Giri D, et al. Breast cancer methylomes establish an epigenomic foundation for metastasis. Science Translational Medicine 2011;3: 75ra25.

[78] Sun Z, Asmann YW, Kalari KR, Bot B, Eckel-Passow JE, et al. Integrated analysis of gene expression, CpG island methylation, and gene copy number in breast cancer cells by deep sequencing. PLOS ONE 2011;6: e17490.

[79] Chari R, Coe BP, Vucic EA, Lockwood WW and Lam WL An integrative multi-dimensional genetic and epigenetic strategy to identify aberrant genes and pathways in cancer. BMC Systems Biology 2010;4: 67.

[80] Kim MS, Lee J, Oh T, Moon Y, Chang E, et al.Genome-wide identification of OTP gene as a novel methylation marker of breast cancer. Oncology Reports 2012;27:1681–1688.

[81] Faryna M, Konermann C, Aulmann S, Bermejo JL, Brugger M, et al. Genome-wide methylation screen in low-grade breast cancer identifies novel epigenetically altered genes as potential biomarkers for tumor diagnosis. FASEB Journal 2012;26:4937–4950.

[82] Kim JH, Dhanasekaran SM, Prensner JR, Cao X, Robinson D, et al. Deep sequencing reveals distinct patterns of DNA methylation in prostate cancer. Genome Research 2011;21:1028–1041.

[83] Hill VK, Ricketts C, Bieche I, Vacher S, Gentle D, etal.Genome-wide DNA methylation profiling of CpG islands in breast cancer identifies novel genes associated with tumorigenicity. Cancer Research 2011;71: 2988–2999.

[84] Slater AA, Alokail M, Gentle D, Yao M, Kovacs G. et al. DNA methylation profiling distinguishes histological subtypes of renal cell carcinoma. Epigenetics 2013;8(3): 252-267.

[85] Li L, Lee KM, Han W, Choi JY, Lee JY, et al.Estrogen and progesterone receptor status affect genome-wide DNA methylation profile in breast cancer. Human Molecular Genetics 2010;19:4273–4277.

[86] Fackler MJ, Umbricht CB, Williams D, Argani P, Cruz LA, et al.Genome-wide methylation analysis identifies genes specific to breast cancer hormone receptor status and risk of recurrence. Cancer Research 2011;71:6195–6207.

[87] Trape AP, Gonzalez-AnguloAM. Breast Cancer and Metastasis: On the Way Toward Individualized Therapy. Cancer Genomics Proteomics 2012;9(5):297-310.

[88] Van't Veer LJ, Dai H, van de Vijver MJ, He YD, et al Gene expression profiling predicts clinical outcome of breast cancer. Nature 2002;415: 530–536.

[89] Smid M, Wang Y, Klijn JG, Sieuwerts AM, Zhang Y, et al. Genes associated with breast cancer metastatic to bone. Journal Clinical Oncology 2006;24:2261–2267.

[90] Jenuwein T, Allis CD. Translating the histone code.Science. 2001;293:1074–1080.

[91] Olsen EA, Kim YH, Kuzel TM, Pacheco TR, Foss FM, et al. Phase IIbmulticenter trial of vorinostat in patients with persistent, progressive, or treatment refractory cutaneous T-cell lymphoma. Journal of Clinical Oncology 2007;25:3109–3115.

[92] Munster PN, Troso-Sandoval T, Rosen N, Rifkind R, Marks PA, et al. The histone deacetylase inhibitor suberoylanilidehydroxamic acid induces differentiation of human breast cancer cells. Cancer Research 2001;61:8492–8497.

[93] Cohen LA, Amin S, Marks PA, Rifkind RA, Desai D, et al. Chemoprevention of carcinogen-induced mammary tumorigenesis by the hybrid polar cytodifferentiation agent, suberanilohydroxamic acid (SAHA) Anticancer Research 1999;19:4999–5005.

[94] Huang L, Pardee AB. Suberoylanilidehydroxamic acid as a potential therapeutic agent for human breast cancer treatment. Molecular Medicine 2000;6:849–866.

[95] Keen JC, Yan L, Mack KM, Pettit C, Smith D, et al. A novel histone deacetylase inhibitor, scriptaid, enhances expression of functional estrogen receptor alpha (ER) in ER negative human breast cancer cells in combination with 5-aza 2′-deoxycytidine. Breast Cancer Research and Treatment 2003;81:177–186.

[96] Zhou Q, Shaw PG, Davidson NE. Inhibition of histone deacetylase suppresses EGF signaling pathways by destabilizing EGFR mRNA in ER-negative human breast cancer cells. Breast Cancer Research and Treatment 2009;117(2):443–451.

[97] Sharma D, Saxena NK, Davidson NE, Vertino PM. Restoration of tamoxifen sensitivity in estrogen receptor-negative breast cancer cells: tamoxifen-bound reactivated ER recruits distinctive corepressor complexes. Cancer Research 2006;66:6370–6378.

[98] Kim MS, Blake M, Baek JH, Kohlhagen G, Pommier Y, et al. Inhibition of histone deacetylase increases cytotoxicity to anticancer drugs targeting DNA. Cancer Research 2003;63:7291–7300.

[99] Fuino L, Bali P, Wittmann S, Donapaty S, Guo F, et al. Histone deacetylase inhibitor LAQ824 down-regulates Her-2 and sensitizes human breast cancer cells to trastuzumab, taxotere, gemcitabine, and epothilone B. Molecular Cancer Therapeutics 2003;2:971–984.

[100] Bali P, Pranpat M, Swaby R, Fiskus W, Yamaguchi H, et al. Activity of suberoylanilidehydroxamic Acid against human breast cancer cells with amplification of her-2. Clinical Cancer Research 2005;11:6382–6389.

[101] Yang X, Phillips DL, Ferguson AT, Nelson WG, Herman JG, et al. Synergistic activation of functional estrogen receptor (ER)-alpha by DNA methyltransferase and histone deacetylase inhibition in human ER-alpha-negative breast cancer cells. Cancer Research 2001;61:7025–7029.

[102] Sabnis GJ, Goloubeva O, Chumsri S, Nguyen N, Sukumar S, et al. Functional activation of the estrogen receptor-alpha and aromatase by the HDAC inhibitor entinostat sensitizes ER-negative tumors to letrozole. Cancer Research 2011;71:1893–1903.

[103] Hostetter CL, Licata LA, Keen JC. Timing is everything: order of administration of 5-aza 2′ deoxycytidine, trichostatin A and tamoxifen changes estrogen receptor mRNA expression and cell sensitivity. Cancer Letters 2009;275:178–84.

[104] Hervouet E, Cartron PF, Jouvenot M, a Delage-Mourroux R. Epigenetic regulation of estrogen signaling in breast cancer. Epigenetics. 2013;8(3):237–245.

[105] Robertson KD, Uzvolgyi E, Liang G, Talmadge C, Sumegi J, et al. The human DNA methyltransferases (DNMTs) 1, 3a and 3b: coordinate mRNA expression in normal tissues and overexpression in tumors. Nucleic Acids Research 1999;27(11):2291.

[106] Girault I, Tozlu S, Lidereau R, Bieche I. Expression analysis of DNA methyltransferases 1, 3A, and 3B in sporadic breast carcinomas. Clinical Cancer Research 2003;9(12): 4415–4422.

[107] Subramaniam D, Thombre R, Dhar A, Anant S. DNA Methyltransferases: A Novel Target for Prevention and Therapy Frontiers in Oncology 2014; 4: 80.

[108] Roll JD, Rivenbark AG, Jones WD, Coleman WB. DNMT3b overexpression contributes to a hypermethylator phenotype in human breast cancer cell lines. Molecular Cancer 2008;7:15

[109] Gokul G, Gautami B, Malathi S, Sowjanya AP, Poli UR, et al. DNA methylation profile at the DNMT3L promoter: a potential biomarker for cervical cancer. Epigenetics 2007;2(2):80.

[110] Minami K, Chano T, Kawakami T, Ushida H, Kushima R, et al. DNMT3L is a novel marker and is essential for the growth of human embryonal carcinoma. Clinical Cancer Research 2010;16(10):2751.

[111] Naishadham D, Lansdorp-Vogelaar I, Siegel R, Cokkinides V, Jemal A. State disparities in colorectal cancer mortality patterns in the United States. Cancer Epidemiology Biomarkers & Prevention 2011;20(7):1296

[112] Agrawal A, Murphy RF, Agrawal DK. DNA methylation in breast and colorectal cancers. Modern Pathology2007;(7):711-721.

[113] Widschwendter M, Jones PA. DNA methylation and breast carcinogenesis.Oncogene. 2002;21(35):5462-5482.

[114] Esteller M. Epigenetics in Biology and Medicine. Boca Raton: In CRC: 2009.

[115] Jones PA, Taylor SM. Cellular differentiation, cytidine analogs and DNA methylation.Cell. 1980;20(1):85-93.

[116] Wu JC, SantiDV.On the mechanism and inhibition of DNA cytosine methyltransferases. Progress Clinical and Biological Research 1985;198:119–129.

[117] el-Deiry WS, Nelkin BD, Celano P, Yen RW, Falco JP, et al. High expression of the DNA methyltransferase gene characterizes human neoplastic cells and progression stages of colon cancer. Proceedings of the National Academy of Sciences USA 1991;88(8):3470–3410.

[118] Patra SK, Patra A, Zhao H, Dahiya R. DNA methyltransferase and demethylase in human prostate cancer. Molecular Carcinogenesis 2002;33(3):163.

[119] Girault I, Tozlu S, Lidereau R, Bieche I. Expression analysis of DNA methyltransferases 1, 3A, and 3B in sporadic breast carcinomas. Clinical Cancer Research 2003;9(12): 4415–4422.

[120] Broske AM, Vockentanz L, Kharazi S, Huska MR, Mancini E, et al. DNA methylation protects hematopoietic stem cell multipotency from myeloerythroid restriction. Nature Genetics 2009; 41(11):1207–1510.

[121] Sen GL, Reuter JA, Webster DE, Zhu L, Khavari PA. DNMT1 maintains progenitor function in self-renewing somatic tissue. Nature 2010;463(7280):563–710.

[122] Fu S, Hu W, Iyer R, Kavanagh JJ, Coleman RL,et al. Phase 1b-2a study to reverse platinum resistance through use of a hypomethylating agent, azacitidine, in patients with platinum-resistant or platinum-refractory epithelial ovarian cancer. Cancer 2011;117:1661–1669.

[123] Connolly R, Stearns V. Epigenetics as a therapeutic target in breast cancer. Journal of Mammary Gland Biology and Neoplasia 2012; 17(3-4):191–204.

[124] Chen M, Shabashvili D, Nawab A, Yang SX, Dyer LM, et al. DNA methyltransferase inhibitor, zebularine, delays tumor growth and induces apoptosis in a genetically engineered mouse model of breast cancer. Molecular Cancer Therapeutics2012;11(2): 370-382.

[125] Billam M, Sobolewski MD, Davidson NE. Effects of a novel DNA methyltransferase inhibitor zebularine on human breast cancer cells. Breast Cancer Research Treatment 2010;120:581–592.

[126] Yoo CB, Cheng JC, Jones PA.Zebularine: a new drug for epigenetic therapy. Biochemical Society Transactions 2004;32:910–912.

[127] Cheng JC, Yoo CB, Weisenberger DJ, Chuang J, Wozniak C, et al. Preferential response of cancer cells to zebularine. Cancer Cell 2004;6:151–158. Cheng JC, Weisenberger DJ, Gonzales FA, Liang G, Xu GL. et al. Continuous zebularine treatment effectively sustains demethylation in human bladder cancer cells. Molecular and Cellular Biology 2004;24:1270–1278.

[128] Kim CH, Marquez VE, Mao DT, Haines DR, McCormack JJ.Synthesis of pyrimidin-2-one nucleosides as acid-stable inhibitors of cytidinedeaminase. Journal of Medicinal Chemistry 1986;29:1374–1380.

[129] Laliberte J, Marquez VE, Momparler RL.Potent inhibitors for the deamination of cytosine arabinoside and 5-aza-2′-deoxycytidine by human cytidinedeaminase.Cancer Chemotherapy and Pharmacology 1992;30:7–11.

[130] Marquez VE, Barchi JJ, Jr, Kelley JA, Rao KV, Agbaria R, et al. Zebularine: a unique molecule for an epigenetically based strategy in cancer chemotherapy. The magic of its chemistry and biology.Nucleosides Nucleotides Nucleic Acids 2005;24:305–318.

[131] Hurd PJ, Whitmarsh AJ, Baldwin GS, Kelly SM, Waltho JP, et al. Mechanism-based inhibition of C5-cytosine DNA methyltransferases by 2-H pyrimidinone.Journal of Molecular Biology 1999;286:389–401.

[132] Cheng JC, Matsen CB, Gonzales FA, Ye W, Greer S, et al. Inhibition of DNA methylation and reactivation of silenced genes by zebularine. Journal of the National Cancer Institute 2003;95:399–409.

[133] Scott SA, Lakshimikuttysamma A, Sheridan DP, Sanche SE, Geyer CR, et al. Zebularine inhibits human acute myeloid leukemia cell growth in vitro in association with p15INK4B demethylation and reexpression. Experimental Hematology 2007;35:263–273.

[134] Billam M, Sobolewski MD, and Davidson NE. Effects of a novel DNA methyltransferase inhibitor zebularine on human breast cancer cells Breast Cancer Research Treatment 2010;120(3): 581–592.

[135] Ye X, Franco AA, Santos H, Nelson DM, Kaufman PD, et al. Defective S phase chromatin assembly causes DNA damage, activation of the S phase checkpoint, and S phase arrest. Molecular Cell 2003;11(2):341-351.

[136] Nelson DM, Ye X, Hall C, Santos H, Ma T, et al. Coupling of DNA synthesis and histone synthesis in S phase independent of cyclin/cdk2 activity. Molecular and Cellular Biology 2002;22(21):7459-7472.

[137] Chen Molecular Cancer Therapeuticsmct.aacrjournals.org

[138] Published OnlineFirst December 27, 2011; doi: 10.1158/1535-7163.MCT-11-0458 M, Shabashvili D,Nawab A, Yang SX, Dyer LM, Brown KD, et al., DNA Methyltransferase Inhibitor, Zebularine, Delays Tumor Growth and Induces Apoptosis in a Genetically Engineered Mouse Model of Breast Cancer. Published OnlineFirst December 27, 2011; doi: 10.1158/1535-7163.MCT-11-0458 Molecular Cancer Therapeutics 2012;11; 370.

[139] Rhee I, Bachman KE, Park BH, Jair KW, Yen RW, et al. DNMT1 and DNMT3b cooperate to silence genes in human cancer cells. Nature 2002;416:552–556.

[140] Sharma D, Blum J, Yang X, Beaulieu N, Macleod AR, et al. Release of methyl CpG binding proteins and histone deacetylase 1 from the Estrogen receptor alpha (ER) promoter upon reactivation in ER-negative human breast cancer cells. Molecular Endocrinology 2005;19(7):1740-1751.

[141] Yang X, Ferguson AT, Nass SJ, Phillips DL, Butash KA, et al. Transcriptional activation of estrogen receptor alpha in human breast cancer cells by histone deacetylase inhibition. Cancer Research 2000;60(24):6890-6894.

[142] Ben-Kasus T, Ben-Zvi Z, Marquez VE, Kelley JA, AgbariaR.Metabolic activation of zebularine, a novel DNA methylation inhibitor, in human bladder carcinoma cells. Biochemical Pharmacology 2005;70(1):121-133.

[143] Yoo CB, Chuang JC, Byun HM, Egger G, Yang AS, et al. Long-term epigenetic therapy with oral zebularine has minimal side effects and prevents intestinal tumors in mice.Cancer Prevention Research 2008;1(4):233-240.

[144] Juergens RA, Wrangle J, Vendetti FP, Murphy SC, Zhao M, et al. Combination epigenetic therapy has efficacy in patients with refractory advanced non–small cell lung cancer. Cancer Discovery 2011;1(7):598–607.

[145] Stathis A, Hotte SJ, Chen EX, Hirte HW, Oza AM, et al Phase I study of decitabine in combination with vorinostat in patients with advanced solid tumors and non-Hodgkin's lymphomas. Clinical Cancer Research 2011;17:1582–1590.

[146] Eliopoulos N, Cournoyer D, Momparler RL. Drug resistance to 5-aza-2′-deoxycytidine, 2′, 2′-difluorodeoxycytidine, and cytosine arabinoside conferred by retroviral-mediated transfer of human cytidinedeaminasecDNA into murine cells.Cancer Chemotherapy and Pharmacology 1998;42:373–378.

[147] Lemaire M, Momparler LF, Bernstein ML, Marquez VE, MomparlerRL.Enhancement of antineoplastic action of 5-aza-2′-deoxycytidine by zebularine on L1210 leukemia. Anticancer Drugs 2005;16:301–308.

[148] Cheishvili D, Chik F, Li CC, Bhattacharyya B, Suderman M et al. Synergistic effects of combined DNA methyltransferase inhibition and MBD2 depletion on breast cancer cells; MBD2 depletion blocks 5-aza-2'-deoxycytidine triggered invasiveness. Carcinogenesis 2014 Sep 1.

[149] Fu S, Hu W, Iyer R, Kavanagh JJ, Coleman RL, et al. Phase 1b-2a study to reverse platinum resistance through use of a hypomethylating agent, azacitidine, in patients with platinum-resistant or platinum-refractory epithelial ovarian cancer. Cancer 2011;117:1661–1669.

6

Bioinformatics in Breast Cancer Research

Beyzanur Yigitoglu, Eyyup Uctepe,
Ramazan Yigitoglu, Esra Gunduz and
Mehmet Gunduz

1. Introduction

Developments both in computer hardware and software allowed for storing, distributing, and analyzing data obtained from biological experimentation, the very definition of bioinformatics. From this standpoint, bioinformatics can be narrowly defined as a field at the crossroads of biology and computer engineering, responsible for the storage, distribution, and analysis of biological information.[1] The term of bioinformatics relatively refers to the formation and advancement of algorithms, computational and statistical techniques, and theory to solve formal and practical problems posed by or inspired from the management and analysis of biological data.[2,3]

Since its emergence as an independent discipline in the 1980s, bioinformatics has been rapidly developing, keeping up with the expansion of genome sequence data. Whereas it is safe to say that 20 years ago, publishing computationally-derived results was a challenge and experimental observations were considered the only way of making progress[1]; after the famous Clinton-Blair handshake for the completion of the human genome in April 2003 [4], headlines such as "the laboratory rat is giving way to the computer mouse" arose.[5] The importance of bioinformatics methods has further increased following the technological improvement of large-scale gene expression analysis using DNA microarrays and proteomics experiments. Wet experiments and the use of bioinformatics analyses go hand in hand in today's biological and clinical research.[6] Undeniably, it is almost inconceivable that a high-impact research publication in biology does not contain some elements of computing.[1]

To date, the genome, transcriptome and proteome are investigated with large-scale and high-throughput techniques to suggest treatment and predict outcomes. With the availability of high-throughput sequencing in hypothesis driven science, various sequence-based techniques are originated, namely expressed sequence tags (ESTs)[7], serial analysis of gene expression (SAGE)[8], massively parallel signature sequencing (MPSS)[9], the 'HapMap' project proceeding by means of individual SNPs (single nucleotide polymorphisms) to link specific genotypes to diseases.[10,11] Aside from sequencing techniques, microarray technology is one of the high-throughput techniques, possibly the most promising one. As for protein analysis techniques, tissue arrays[12] and proteomics can be named.

On the one hand, microarrays are microscope slides or chips with immobilized probes, usually cDNA (complementary DNA), BAC (bacterial artificial chromosome), or oligo probes.[13] There are very large numbers of spots on an array, each containing a huge number of identical DNA molecules. Two important applications of microarray technology are gene expression monitoring and Single Nucleotide Polymorphisms (SNP) detection.[14] This technique is widely applicable because less RNA is used to analyze thousands of genes. Despite its increasing use around the world, microarray analysis has some limitations if used as a single method for exploring tumor biology. An obvious weakness is that a microarray represents a single snapshot of the patient.[15] But there are a large number of elements leading to disturbed gene function[16], such as large and small deletions or single base substitutions, mutations that affect promoter regions or splice-sites, as well as epigenetic silencing. Those factors may influence the result but may go undetected as well, depending on the exact type of lesion as well as its location with respect to the area hybridizing with the probe.[17] Furthermore, differentially expressed genes do not necessarily translate into varying protein levels with functional implications; so, it does not always show a correlation between the expression of a gene and the amount of translated protein.[18] Also, compared to RT-PCR (reverse transcription polymerase chain reaction), microarray signals are less sensitive, accurate and not able to resolve smaller differences in gene expression.[19] In addition to its comparative simplicity, microarray technology requires better understanding of the limitations and careful attention to experimental design and data analysis for meaningful results.

Bioinformatics applications are used in analysis of entire gene expression profiles to approach the disease at genome level and pose new hypotheses regarding certain mechanisms including but not limited to signaling pathways governing the process of formation, maintenance and expansion of tumor.[20] Bioinformatics analyses can also be applied to miRNA, DNA copy-number, SNPs, sequence, and methylation data[21] along with the field of medical sciences to know the pathways for diagnosing which genomic changes could give rise to each known inherited disease, i.e., identification of the gene causing disease, and also genetic therapies that can reverse disease phenotype.[14] Different Browser and Databases has been developed to analyze and process this huge quantity of data (Table 1.0 and Table 2.0).

Kept in mind that the discovery of complete protein classes is still in progress, e.g., the kinases of the human genome[22], the classification of proteins with related structure and function[23] will preserve its significance in the molecular dissection of human health and disease. In the future, bioinformatics is expected to continue its fascinating interplay with the field of genomics in cancer research, that is cancer bioinformatics and oncogenomics.[24]

2. Bioinformatics in various cancers

Cancer is one of the prevalent diseases that bring about death worldwide. Given that Scientists have sequenced the human genome[25], now it is time to use these genomic data, and the high-throughput technology developed to generate them, to tackle major health problems such as cancer.[24] Cancer molecular mechanisms are more successfully examined considering the genes and proteins interaction and network. Bioinformatics tools are vital for acquiring a more holistic view of cancer and analyzing the intricate data, speeding up the research process including biomarker discovery. Moreover, cancer clinical bioinformatics is critical to reach systems clinical medicine by combining clinical measurements and signs with human cancer tissue-generated bioinformatics, understanding clinical symptoms and signs, disease development and progress, and therapeutic strategy.[26,27,28]

The leading cause of cancer death is lung cancer but still awaits reliable molecular markers. Kim et al.[29] used multiple clinical samples and combined the bioinformatics analysis of the public gene expression data with clinical validation to identify biomarker genes for non–small-cell lung cancer, which shows poor prognosis and recurrence. They meta-analyzed the SAGE and EST data and chose 20 genes for experimental validation through semiquantitative RT-PCR. Then, applied quantitative RT-PCR to 7 genes (CBLC, CYP24A1, ALDH3A1, AKR1B10, S100P, PLUNC, and LOC147166) identified as potential diagnostic markers, leading to 2 highly probable novel biomarkers (CBLC and CYP24A1).

Liver cancer is the most common type, subsequent to lung cancer, responsible for cancer-related deaths. Sawey et al.[30] performed a forward genetic screen, using a mouse hepatoblast model and RNAi, guided by human hepatocellular carcinoma amplification data. They found that the amplification led to the selective sensitivity to FGF19 inhibition. Hence, FGF19 is an equally important driver gene of 11q13.3 amplicon as CCND1 in liver cancer, which means 11q13.3 amplification could be an effective biomarker for patients predicted to respond to anti-FGF19 therapy.

In a recent study[31], an individualized bioinformatics analysis strategy was applied to previously-established transcriptome data for clear cell renal cell carcinoma (ccRCC) to identify and reposition 8 FDA-approved drugs with negative correlation and P-value <0.05 for anticancer therapy. Authors demonstrated that pentamidine is effective against RCC cells in culture, and slows tumor growth in a RCC xenograft mouse model so it might be a new therapeutic agent to be combined with current standard-of-care regimens for patients with metastatic RCC.

With regard to leukemia, diagnosis and subclassification is mostly based on the application of various techniques like cytomorphology, cytogenetics, fluorescence in situ hybridization, multiparameter flow cytometry, and PCR-based methods which are time-consuming and cost-intensive, also require expertise in central reference laboratories. Therefore, microarray analysis represents a novel promising method to be used as a diagnostic tool.[14] A key determinant in the prognosis of chronic lymphocytic leukemia (CLL) is the mutational status of the immunoglobulin heavy chain variable region (IGHV) genes.[32] For the correct delineation of the mutational status, the patient's leukemic cells and closest germline counterpart should be compared. Unfortunately, public web-based databases are commonly used instead of the patient's germline DNA sequence from non-leukemic cells. Several of these reference databases involve VBASE, GenBank/IgBLAST and the international ImMunoGeneTics information systems that employ different software types, amount of natural IGHV polymorphism and criteria used to map the complementarity determining regions and framework regions. As a result, the correct interpretation of the IGHV mutational status in CLL may be affected.[33]

Because of the heterogeneity of many tumors, it is a very challenging work to identify good molecular targets. For instance, resistant subclones of overexpressed and mutated genes may prevent them from being good molecular targets. Therefore, best target is a 'red dot' gene whose mutation occurs early in oncogenesis and dysregulates a key pathway that drives tumor growth in all of the subclones. Examples include mutations in the genes ABL, HER-2, KIT, EGFR and probably BRAF, in chronic myelogenous leukemia, breast cancer, gastrointestinal stromal tumors, non-small-cell lung cancer and melanoma, respectively. For efficacious therapeutics; identification of red-dot targets, development of drugs that inhibit the red-dot targets, and diagnostic classification of the related pathways are a must.[34]

3. Bioinformatics and breast cancer

Breast cancer occurs in both men and women, yet male breast cancer is less common. Although a cure for each stage of breast cancer has not yet been found, identifying the genetic mutations that cause the disease can play an important role and this is said by scientists to be like looking for needles in a haystack, and after finding the needles or coding regions, they must find disease-related sequences within them.[3,6] Bioinformatics sets the stage for searching 3 billion base pairs to detect genetic defects.

Allinen et al. described the comprehensive gene expression profiles of each cell type composing normal breast tissue and in situ and invasive breast carcinomas performing SAGE (serial analysis of gene expression) and utilizing cell-type specific cell surface markers and magnetic beads for the rapid sequential isolation. Their results suggest that considerable transcriptional alterations happen in all cell populations while genetic changes were detected only in epithelial cells among myoepithelial, endothelial and stromal cells, myofibroblasts and lymphocytes.[35] To continue with another study, based upon a systematic Sanger sequencing analysis of 13,023 genes in 11 human breast cancers, individual tumors accumulate an average of approximately 90 point mutations in gene coding regions, but only a tiny number of these were recurrent and were in significant genes of breast cancer, including p53 and PIK3CA. A much larger number of the genes do not necessarily contribute to the carcinogenesis.[36] Considering the genomic landscape of breast cancer, these more common mutations resemble "mountains" while the vast majority of genes reflect "hills" that are infrequently mutated. We need to elucidate mechanisms involved in the disease to understand the heterogeneity of human cancers and utilize personal genomics for tumor diagnosis and new therapeutic strategies.[37]

As widely accepted, early detection of breast cancer has an enormous impact on patient's survival. Seeing that genome-wide expression patterns of tumors mirror the biology of the tumors, relating gene expression patterns to clinical outcomes sheds light on the biological diversity of the tumors.[38] In the discovery of genes and pathways that are specifically activated or inactivated during tumor progression, high throughput genome-wide array based techniques like array comparative genomic hybridization (aCGH) and transcriptional profiling can be used.[13] A molecular classification of breast cancer, with more than five reproducible subtypes (basal-like, ERBB2, normal-like, luminal A, luminal B) was defined through gene expression profiling and microarray analysis.[38,39,17] In addition, performing the gene set enrichment analysis (GSEA), a gene set linked to the growth factor (GF) signaling was observed to be significantly enriched in the luminal B tumors.[40] Another study states that multiple pathways were identified by mapping gene sets defined in Gene Ontology Biological Process (GOBP) for estrogen receptor positive (ER+) or estrogen receptor negative (ER-); and among them, in a separate set, pathways related to apoptosis and cell division or G-protein coupled receptor signal transduction are associated with the metastatic capability of ER+or ER-tumors, respectively.[41] Additionally, in a study, it is supported that breast cancer is initiated with mutated stem cells/progenitors, also called "breast cancer stem cells" because they are sufficient to sustain oncogenesis and tumor growth.[42] To identify genetic changes in the progression of breast carcinoma, Yao et al. [43] used aCGH and SAGE combined for ductal carcinoma in situ (DCIS), invasive breast carcinomas, and lymph node metastases. They identified 49 minimal commonly amplified regions and reported that the overall frequency of copy number alterations was more in invasive tumors than in DCIS, with several of them present only in invasive cancer. In breast cancer, gene amplification happens recurrently on some chromosomal locations (e.g. 1q, 8p12, 8q24, 11q13, 12p13, 12q13, 17q21-q23, 20q13) [43,44], which points to the activation of some oncogenes at high frequency during the growth of tumor. Amplification is a mechanism causing the gene expression constitutively enhanced above the level of physiologically normal variation, so the significance of oncogene amplification in tumorigenesis had originated from expression profiling of tumor cells by oncogene arrays.[45]

Bioinformatics is also crucial in the realm of pharmacogenomics. There became a need to develop accurate tools for the effective treatment relying on biological characterization of each patient's tumor. Gene-expression profiling of tumors with DNA microarrays is a powerful tool for pharmacogenomics targeting of treatments. Oncotype DX™ assay (Genomic Health) is a good example, which was described for identifying the subset of node-negative estrogen-receptor-positive breast cancer patients who do not require adjuvant chemotherapy.[46,34] A recent research demonstrated that microarray analysis with qRT-PCR validation reveals distinct pathways of resistance to bevacizumab (BEV) in xenograft models of human ER+breast cancer, showing Follistatin (FST) and NOTCH as the top signaling pathways associated with resistance in VEGF-driven tumors ($P < 0.05$). According to the gene expression analysis, the level of VEGF expression affects the response to BEV therapy and gene pathways.[47] Using appropriate bioinformatics tools, such findings may elucidate the matter of resistance to drugs for individual patients and provide a deeper understanding of treatments and risk factors, opening the door from novel targets and disease-related biomarkers to right drugs.

Last but not least, the effect of epigenetic changes on breast cancer etiology is beyond doubt. In spite of quite a number of DNA methylation research manifesting diverse patterns including tumor suppressor genes and oncogenes, only a small fraction of them connect the epigenome data with the transcriptome. In a recent study by Minning and coworkers[48], DNA methylation and gene expression profiling of primary breast tumor tissues and adjacent non-cancerous breast tissues was carried out. They preferred MS-MLPA or MS-qPCR for validation of results. The overlapping genes between DNA methylation and gene expression datasets were further mapped to the KEGG database to identify the molecular pathways linking the used genes together and supervised hierarchical clustering was used for data analysis. The authors found that most of the overlapping genes belong to the focal adhesion and extracellular matrix-receptor interaction that play important roles in breast carcinogenesis. The more gene signature data is acquired by different studies, the better understanding of epigenetic regulation of gene expression and remedial intervention will be possible.

Advances in bioinformatics and its application are much possible by multidisciplinary teams pursuing focused research. The sensitivity, specificity and combination of tools, methodologies, and databases should be evaluated in a complete matter. On top of that, findings must be confirmed with several molecular techniques before translation into clinical practice.

Database Group	Database	Originator	Web Adress
Nucleotide Sequence	GenBank	US National Center for Biotechnology Information (NCBI)	www.ncbi.nlm.nih.gov/genbank
	EMBL	Europian Bioinformatics Institute	www.ebi.ac.uk/
	DDBJ	National Institute of Genetic, Japan	www.ddbj.nig.ac.jp/
	dbEST		www.ncbi.nlm.nih.gov/dbEST
Protein Sequence	SWISS-PROT	Swiss Institute of Bioinformatics, Geneva	web.expasy.org/docs/swiss-prot_guideline.html
		European Bioinformatics Institute	www.ebi.ac.uk/swissprot/
	TREMBLE	EBI (translation of coding sequences from the EMBL database that have not yet been deposited in SWISS-PROT)	www.ebi.ac.uk/tremble
	UniProt	Bioinformatics Institute (EMBL-EBI), Swiss Institute of Bioinformatics (SIB) and the Protein Information Resource (PIR).	www.uniprot.org
	PIR	US National Biomedical Research Foundation (NBRF)	pir.georgetown.edu
		Japan International Protein Information Database (JIPID)	www.ddbj.nig.ac.jp
		Munich Information Center for Protein Sequences (MIPS)	mips.gsf.de

Table 1. Major electronic nucleotide and protein databases

Genome Browser	Originator	Web Adress
Ensemble	Wellcome Trust Sanger Institute/ Europian Bioinformatics Institute(EBI)	www.ensembl.org/
NCBI Map Viewer	US National Center for Biotechnology Information(NCBI)	www.ncbi.nlm.nih.gov/mapview/
UCSC genome browser	Genome Bioinformatics Group of UC Santa Cruz	http://genome.ucsc.edu/
Genomes Compilations		
EBI Genomes	Europian Bioinformatics Institute(EBI)	www.ebi.ac.uk/genomes
GOLD	Genomes Online Database	www.genomesonline.org/

Table 2. Commonly used genom browser and databases

Author details

Beyzanur Yigitoglu[1], Eyyup Uctepe[1], Ramazan Yigitoglu[2], Esra Gunduz[1*] and Mehmet Gunduz[1]

*Address all correspondence to: mehmet.gunduz@gmail.com

1 Department of Medical Genetics, Faculty of Medicine, Turgut Ozal University, Ankara, Turkey

2 Medical Biochemistry, Faculty of Medicine, Turgut Ozal University, Ankara, Turkey

References

[1] Ouzounis, C. The Emergence of Bioinformatics: Historical Perspective, Quick Overview and Future Trends. in *Bioinformatics in Cancer and Cancer Therapy* (ed. Gordon, G.J.) 1-11 (Humana Press, 2009).

[2] Sims, A.H. Bioinformatics and breast cancer: what can high-throughput genomic approaches actually tell us? *J Clin Pathol* 62, 879-85 (2009).

[3] Maryam Gholizadeh, S.A.P., Reza Pasandideh. Proteomics and Bioinformatics Approaches for Breast Cancer Researches. *International Journal of Agriculture and Crop Sciences* 5, 1863-1868 (2013).

[4] Ouzounis, C.A. Rise and demise of bioinformatics? Promise and progress. *PLoS Comput Biol* 8, e1002487 (2012).

[5] Economist, T. The race to computerise biology. *The Economist* (2002).

[6] Daisuke Kihara, Y.D.Y., Troy Hawkins. Bioinformatics resources for cancer research with an emphasis on gene function and structure prediction tools. *Cancer Informatics* 2, 25-35 (2006).

[7] Adams M.D., K.J.M., Gocayne J.D., Dubnick M., Polymeropoulos M.H., Xiao H., Merril C.R., Wu A., Olde B., Moreno R.F., et al. Complementary DNA sequencing: expressed sequence tags and human genome project. *Science* 252, 1651-1656 (1991).

[8] Velculescu V.E., Z.L., Vogelstein B., Kinzler K.W. Serial analysis of gene expression. *Science* 270, 484-487 (1995).

[9] Sydney Brenner, M.J., John Bridgham, George Golda, David H. Lloyd, Davida Johnson, Shujun Luo, Sarah McCurdy, Michael Foy, Mark Ewan, Rithy Roth, Dave George, Sam Eletr, Glenn Albrecht, Eric Vermaas, Steven R. Williams, Keith Moon, Timothy Burcham, Michael Pallas, Robert B. DuBridge, James Kirchner, Karen Fearon, Jen-i Mao, Kevin Corcoran. Gene expression analysis by massively parallel signature sequencing (MPSS) on microbead arrays. *Nature Biotechnology* 18, 630-634 (2000).

[10] Lon R. Cardon, G.R.A. Using haplotype blocks to map human complex trait loci. *Trends in Genetics* 19, 135-140 (2003).

[11] Andrew G. Clark, R.N., James Signorovitch, Tara C. Matise, Stephen Glanowski, Jeremy Heil, Emily S. Winn-Deen, Arthur L. Holden, Eric Lai. Linkage Disequilibrium and Inference of Ancestral Recombination in 538 Single-Nucleotide Polymorphism Clusters across the Human Genome. *American Journal of Human Genetics* 73, 285-300 (2003).

[12] Hector, B. The multitumor (sausage) tissue block: novel method for immunohistochemical antibody testing. *Laboratory Investigation* 55, 244-248 (1986).

[13] Rennstam, K. & Hedenfalk, I. High-throughput genomic technology in research and clinical management of breast cancer. Molecular signatures of progression from benign epithelium to metastatic breast cancer. *Breast Cancer Res* 8, 213 (2006).

[14] Vidya Vaidya, S.D. A Review of Bioinformatics Application in Breast Cancer Research. *Journal of Advanced Bioinformatics Applications and Research.* 1, 59-68 (2010).

[15] Yang, X., Ai, X. & Cunningham, J.M. Computational prognostic indicators for breast cancer. *Cancer Manag Res* 6, 301-12 (2014).

[16] Lonning, P.E., Knappskog, S., Staalesen, V., Chrisanthar, R. & Lillehaug, J.R. Breast cancer prognostication and prediction in the postgenomic era. *Ann Oncol* 18, 1293-306 (2007).

[17] Per Eystein Lønning, R.C., Vidar Staalesen, Stian Knappskog, Johan Lillehaug3. Adjuvant treatment: the contribution of expression microarrays. *Breast Cancer Research* 9, S14 (2007).

[18] Jaluria, P., Konstantopoulos, K., Betenbaugh, M. & Shiloach, J. A perspective on microarrays: current applications, pitfalls, and potential uses. *Microb Cell Fact* 6, 4 (2007).

[19] Dominick Sinicropi, M.C., Mei-Lan Liu. Gene Expression Profiling Utilizing Microarray Technology and RT-PCR. in *BioMEMS and Biomedical Nanotechnology* (eds. Ferrari, M., Ozkan, M. & Heller, M.) 23-46 (Springer US, 2007).

[20] Eroles, P., Bosch, A., Perez-Fidalgo, J.A. & Lluch, A. Molecular biology in breast cancer: intrinsic subtypes and signaling pathways. *Cancer Treat Rev* 38, 698-707 (2012).

[21] Schiavon, G. *et al.* Heterogeneity of Breast Cancer: Gene Signatures and Beyond. 13-25 (2012).

[22] Manning G, W.D., Martinez R, Hunter T, Sudarsanam S. The Protein Kinase Complement of the Human Genome. *Science* 298, 1912-1934 (2002).

[23] Christos A. Ouzounis, R.M.R.C., Anton J. Enright, Victor Kunin & José B. Pereira-Leal. Classification schemes for protein structure and function. *Nature Reviews Genetics* 4, 508-519 (2003).

[24] Strausberg RL, S.A., Old LJ, Riggins GJ. Oncogenomics and the development of new cancer therapies. *Nature* 429, 469-74 (2004).

[25] Human Genome Research Institute, The Human Genome Project Completion. http://www.genome.gov/11006943National.

[26] Duojiao Wu, C.M.R., Xiangdong Wang. Cancer bioinformatics: A new approach to systems clinical medicine. *BMC Bioinformatics* 13(2012).

[27] Wang, X. & Liotta, L. Clinical bioinformatics: a new emerging science. *J Clin Bioinforma* 1, 1 (2011).

[28] Wang, X. Role of clinical bioinformatics in the development of network-based Biomarkers. *J Clin Bioinforma* 1, 28 (2011).

[29] Kim, B. *et al.* Clinical validity of the lung cancer biomarkers identified by bioinformatics analysis of public expression data. *Cancer Res* 67, 7431-8 (2007).

[30] Sawey, E.T. *et al.* Identification of a therapeutic strategy targeting amplified FGF19 in liver cancer by Oncogenomic screening. *Cancer Cell* 19, 347-58 (2011).

[31] Zerbini LF, B.M., de Vasconcellos JF, Paccez JD, Gu X, Kung AL, Libermann TA. Computational repositioning and preclinical validation of pentamidine for renal cell cancer. *Molecular cancer therapeutics* 13, 1929-1941.

[32] Ghia, P. *et al.* ERIC recommendations on IGHV gene mutational status analysis in chronic lymphocytic leukemia. *Leukemia* 21, 1-3 (2007).

[33] Davi, F., Rosenquist, R., Ghia, P., Belessi, C. & Stamatopoulos, K. Determination of IGHV gene mutational status in chronic lymphocytic leukemia: bioinformatics advances meet clinical needs. *Leukemia* 22, 212-4 (2008).

[34] Simon., R. Bioinformatics in cancer therapeutics--hype or hope? *Nature Clinical Practice Oncology* 2, 223 (2005).

[35] Allinen, M. *et al.* Molecular characterization of the tumor microenvironment in breast cancer. *Cancer Cell* 6, 17-32 (2004).

[36] Sjöblom T, J.S., Wood LD, Parsons DW, Lin J, Barber TD, Mandelker D, Leary RJ, Ptak J, Silliman N, Szabo S, Buckhaults P, Farrell C, Meeh P, Markowitz SD, Willis J, Dawson D, Willson JK, Gazdar AF, Hartigan J, Wu L, Liu C, Parmigiani G, Park BH, Bachman KE, Papadopoulos N, Vogelstein B, Kinzler KW, Velculescu VE. The consensus coding sequences of human breast and colorectal cancers. *Science* 314, 268-274 (2006).

[37] Wood L.D., P.D.W., Jones S., Lin J., Sjöblom T., Leary R.J., Shen D., Boca S.M., Barber T., Ptak J., Silliman N., Szabo S., Dezso Z., Ustyanksky V., Nikolskaya T., Nikolsky Y., Karchin R., Wilson P.A., Kaminker J.S., Zhang Z., Croshaw R., Willis J., Dawson D., Shipitsin M., Willson J.K., Sukumar S., Polyak K., Park B.H., Pethiyagoda C.L., Pant P.V., Ballinger D.G., Sparks A.B., Hartigan J., Smith D.R., Suh E., Papadopoulos N., Buckhaults P., Markowitz S.D., Parmigiani G., Kinzler K.W., Velculescu V.E., Vogelstein B. The genomic landscapes of human breast and colorectal cancers. *Science* 318, 1108-1113 (2007).

[38] Sorlie, T. *et al.* Gene expression patterns of breast carcinomas distinguish tumor subclasses with clinical implications. *Proc Natl Acad Sci U S A* 98, 10869-74 (2001).

[39] Christos Sotiriou, S.-Y.N., Lisa M. McShane, Edward L. Korn, Philip M. Long, Amir Jazaeri, Philippe Martiat, Steve B. Fox, Adrian L. Harris, Edison T. Liu. Breast cancer classification and prognosis based on gene expression profiles from a population-based study. *Proc Natl Acad Sci U S A* 100, 10393-8 (2003).

[40] Loi, S. *et al.* Gene expression profiling identifies activated growth factor signaling in poor prognosis (Luminal-B) estrogen receptor positive breast cancer. *BMC Med Genomics* 2, 37 (2009).

[41] Jack X Yu, A.M.S., Yi Zhang, John WM Martens, Marcel Smid, Jan GM Klijn, Yixin Wang, John A Foekens. Pathway analysis of gene signatures predicting metastasis of node-negative primary breast cancer. *BMC Cancer* 7, 182 (2007).

[42] Behbod, F. & Rosen, J.M. Will cancer stem cells provide new therapeutic targets? *Carcinogenesis* 26, 703-11 (2005).

[43] Yao, J. *et al.* Combined cDNA array comparative genomic hybridization and serial analysis of gene expression analysis of breast tumor progression. *Cancer Res* 66, 4065-78 (2006).

[44] Frank Courjal, M.C., Joelle Simony-Lafontaine, Genevieve Louason, Paul Speiser, Robert Zeillinger, Carmen Rodriguez, and Charles Theilet. Mapping of DNA Amplifications at 15 Chromosomal Localizations in 1875 Breast Tumors: Definition of Phenotypic Groups. *cancer research* 57, 4360-4367 (1997).

[45] Larissa Savelyeva, M.S. Amplification of oncogenes revisited: from expression profiling to clinical application. *Cancer Letters* 167, 115-123 (2001).

[46] Soonmyung Paik, M.D., Steven Shak, M.D., Gong Tang, Ph.D., Chungyeul Kim, M.D., Joffre Baker, Ph.D., Maureen Cronin, Ph.D., Frederick L. Baehner, M.D., Michael G. Walker, Ph.D., Drew Watson, Ph.D., Taesung Park, Ph.D., William Hiller, H.T., Edwin R. Fisher, M.D., D. Lawrence Wickerham, M.D., John Bryant, Ph.D., Norman Wolmark, M.D. A Multigene Assay to Predict Recurrence of Tamoxifen-Treated, Node-Negative Breast Cancer. *The new england journal of medicine* 351, 2817-2826 (2004).

[47] Gokmen-Polar, Y. *et al.* Gene Expression Analysis Reveals Distinct Pathways of Resistance to Bevacizumab in Xenograft Models of Human ER-Positive Breast Cancer. *J Cancer* 5, 633-45 (2014).

[48] Chin Minning, N.M.M., Norlia Abdullah, Rohaizak Muhammad, Nor Aina Emran, Siti Aishah Md Ali, Roslan Harun, Rahman Jamal. Exploring breast carcinogenesis through integrative genomics and epigenomics analyses. international Journal of Oncology, 1959-1968 (2014).

7

Plasminogen Activator System — Diagnostic, Prognostic and Therapeutic Implications in Breast Cancer

Catherine Leurer and Shafaat Ahmed Rabbani

1. Introduction

As tumor metastasis to distant organs (lungs, liver, brain, bone) continues to be the leading cause of cancer associated morbidity and mortality, including breast cancer patients, therapies targeting genes involved in the metastatic cascade are a potentially effective strategy for blocking breast cancer progression and improving survival [1]. Previous 'one size fits all' cancer therapies, which have been used to treat a wide variety of cancers, are inefficient and often cause much unnecessary treatment-related toxicity. Thus, there is a huge unmet need in the research and medical community towards the characterization of cancers into more specific subcategories, which can then be used for prognosis and identifying potential therapies. However, this process requires the use of specific biomarkers to act as signatures for the different subcategories [2,3]. In breast cancer, the most commonly used biomarkers are the estrogen receptor (ER), the progesterone receptor (PR), and the epidermal growth factor 2 (HER2) oncogene [4]. More recently, the plasminogen activator (PA) system and its associated genes are being used as biomarkers to identify potential aggressive cancers, including in breast cancer. The urokinase-type plasminogen activator (uPA) and its inhibitor, the plasminogen activator inhibitor 1 (PAI-1), are proteins of the PA system which are distinguished among cancer biomarkers as being the first to attain level-of-evidence 1 (LOE-1). Thus, assessment of uPA and PAI-1 levels by ELISA assay has been a recommendation of the American Society of Clinical Oncology (ASCO) for assessment of the risk of reoccurrence in breast cancer patients since 2007 [5]. Elevated expression of uPA and its receptor (uPAR) are correlated with poor prognosis and are associated with advanced cancers, including occurrence of metastasis [6]. uPAR is unique as it is rarely expressed in normal quiescent tissue whereas its expression is uniformly high in several tumor tissues, identifying it as a good indicator of malignancy [7].

These characteristics and many more make the PA system an excellent biomarker for breast cancer diagnosis, and a promising target for future breast cancer therapies.

In this chapter, we will discuss the current state of knowledge and ongoing efforts to establish uPA-uPAR system as a diagnostic, prognostic and therapeutic target in breast cancer.

2. Molecular characterization of breast cancer

The wide variety of breast cancer-targeting therapies which exists is due in large part to the diversity in the manifestations of breast cancer. When characterizing these cancers into subtypes, in order to identify patterns, morphology remains the cornerstone for diagnosis [4]. However, molecular classification of breast cancers is being used more and more as an additional tool for prognosis and prediction of disease progression. Prognostic factors identify the severity of the disease, forecasting the outcome of the cancer in an untreated individual. Predictive factors are used to identify treatment options, given the characteristics of the cancer, and predict how beneficial a given treatment might be [8]. The most commonly used bio-markers for molecular classification of breast cancer are ER, PR, and HER 2, levels of expression of which are routinely determined by immunohistochemistry [4]. In addition to these, the nuclear protein Ki-67 is a good indicator of cell proliferation; higher levels of Ki-67 expression are associated with poor prognosis and identifies a point at which a patient is at an increased risk of developing distant metastases [9]. In order to establish a stronger prognostic test which takes into account breast cancer cell proliferation, the percentage of Ki-67-positive tumor cells has been combined with the HER2, ER, and PR scores to form the "IHC4". This prognostic test is powerful when used for ER-positive breast cancers [10]. In addition to immunohistochemical studies identifying key biomarker proteins, newer assays have been developed which use expression levels of mRNA to characterize breast cancers into different subsets [4,11-15].

3. Skeletal metastasis in breast cancer

Metastasis accounts for 90% of deaths in cancer patients [16]. In breast cancer specifically, 70% of patients dying of the disease show presence of bone metastases in their post mortem examination [17]. Cancer metastasis is the spread of cancerous cells to distant tissues, where the cells then go on to form colonies independent of the original source. The original source could be the primary tumor, or the circulating tumor cells could have originated from another metastatic tumor [18]. The process of metastasis is not a spontaneous event, but rather a concerted evolution, in which one cell or population of cells undergoes a series of alteration or mutations which render the cells their invasive and metastatic phenotype [19]. Breast cancer metastasis to the skeleton is a non-random metastatic process; the location of distant metastasis is not based on vasculature or blood circulation. Rather, it is known that certain tumors have an increased 'preference' towards metastasis in certain organs as first describe in the "seed and soil hypothesis" by Paget in 1889 [20]. In addition to breast cancer, cancers of the prostate, lungs, kidney, liver, and thyroid, all show predilections towards skeletal metastasis [1,21]. Thus, there is a continuous search to identify genes and proteins which are involved in initiation and progression of skeletal metastasis in breast cancer and which can be targeted to develop innovative therapies. Bisphosphonates are analogs of pyrophosphate, with a carbon atom replacing the central oxygen atom of the pyrophosphate molecule [22]. Bisphosphonates are rapidly deposited on the bone surface, where they are subsequently ingested by osteoclasts as the cells degrade the bone matrix. Once inside the osteoclast, they interfere with the resorption process by inducing a toxic apoptotic effect. Bisphosphonates can also inhibit osteoclast differentiation and maturation [22]. Due to these effects on bone remodeling they are routinely used in patient with osteoporosis. Bisphosphonates have also been shown to be effective in reducing the incidence and number of skeletal metastases in women with breast cancer who were seen as at-risk of developing distant metastases [23]. Phase II clinical trials have shown that the use of bisphosphonate therapy in conjunction with standard anti-cancer therapy is more effective in reducing the number and persistence of disseminated tumor cells than standard therapy alone [24]. There is also evidence which points to antiangiogenic activity of zoledronic acid, a commonly used bisphosphonate, supporting the rationale for its use in breast cancer therapy [25].

Another drug which targets osteoclast activity is Denosumab, an inhibitor of the receptor activator for nuclear factor kappa-b ligand (RANKL). RANKL is a key regulator of bone resorption which is secreted by osteoblasts and binds to the receptor activator for nuclear factor kappa-b (RANK) on osteoclast progenitor cells, thereby stimulating osteoclast activation and maturation [26]. Osteoblasts also secrete osteoprotogerin (OPG), which can bind to RANKL, acting as a soluble decoy receptor and preventing RANKL-induced osteoclast activation. Thus, osteoblasts have the ability to regulate the rate of bone resorption through the control of osteoclast activity [27]. RANKL levels have been found to be elevated in breast cancer cells, which results in excessive bone resorption [1]. It has also been shown that RANKL promotes the migration of RANK-expressing tumor cells to bone [28]. Denosumab is a fully humanized anti-RANKL monoclonal antibody, acting like OPG to block RANKL binding to RANK and thus preventing osteoclast activation and maturation [29]. Denosumab was originally developed as a treatment against osteoporosis in postmenopausal women, although it is now approved to treat skeletal related events in cancer patients as well [30]. Integrin $\alpha v\beta 3$ is a cell surface receptor found on osteoclasts which stimulates intracellular signaling of the c-Src cascade [31]. Preclinical studies have demonstrated that $\alpha v\beta 3$ integrin-inhibiting drugs can successfully blocked tumor growth and osteolysis [32,33]. Members of the integrin family including $\alpha v\beta 3$, are significant due to their interaction with the uPA-uPAR system.

4. Proteases and breast cancer

Cancer mortality is usually a result of the metastatic spread of the cancer to distant vital organs, as opposed to growth of the original tumor [34]. As such, it is crucial to understand the progression from the localized to an invasive cancer, and eventually a metastatic cancer. Along with growth factors and cytokines, proteases play a major role in this progression, causing the degradation of the basement membrane and surrounding extracellular matrix. Proteases play a crucial role in this first step, as they digest the basal lamina components, and allow for cell movement through the extracellular matrix (ECM) [34]. Matrix metalloproteinases (MMPs) are a family of zinc-dependent endopeptidases whose primary role is the degradation of ECM proteins, dissolving connective tissue [35]. There are a total of 28 identified MMPs, of which 14 have been implicated in breast cancer development and progression [36]. MMPs are synthesized by the tumor itself as well as the surrounding peritumoral stromal cells [37]. In the area surrounding a tumor, the major source of MMP activity is the stromal cells, with the tumor cells likely stimulating production of MMPs via the local fibroblasts [38]. In order for the cancer to move beyond its original location and invade into a nearby duct, MMP activity must break down the basement membrane and stromal matrix, facilitating ECM remodeling [34].

The PA system in general and uPAR in particular play a significant due to its ability to localize the proteolytic effects of uPA which can activate latent growth factors and proteases to effect angiogenesis, matrix degradation, adhesion, activation intracellular signalling pathways, tumor cell invasion and metastasis depicted in Figure 1.

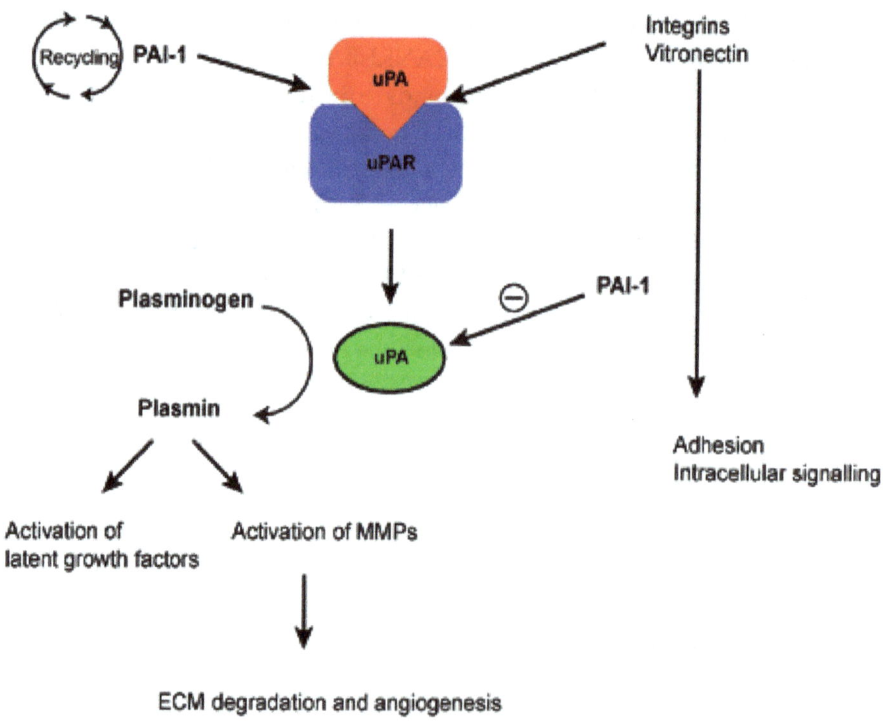

Figure 1. Central role of uPA and uPAR in tumor progression. uPA is localized to the tumor cells via its binding to domain 1 of uPAR. uPA can activate inactive zymogen plasminogen to plasmin, which can activate matrix metalloproteases (MMPs) and activate or release growth factors. Via its domains 2 and 3, uPAR can interact with integrins ($\alpha v\beta 3$, $\alpha v\beta 5$) and vitronectin. PAI-1 binding to the uPA-uPAR complex inhibits the activation of plasminogen by uPA, and promoted internalization of the uPA-uPAR-PAI-1 complex and recycling of uPAR back to the cell surface. Collectively, the uPA/uPAR system plays a central role in matrix degradation, angiogenesis, adhesion, intracellular signalling, tumor invasion and metastasis.

5. Plasminogen Activator (PA) system

The plasminogen activator (PA) system is a key regulator of the tumor microenvironment, and is heavily implicated in the metastatic process in breast and other common cancers. It is involved in tumor recruitment of inflammatory cells, tumor cell growth and survival, angiogenesis, and tumor invasion and migration [39,40]. The PA system of enzymes comprises two plasminogen activators, tissue type plasminogen activator (tPA) which converts plasminogen to plasmin during clot lysis, and uPA which is used therapeutically as a fibrinolytic agent. tPA is present in normal and some malignant tissues, whereas uPA is more commonly associated with malignancies and plays a major role in pericellular proteolysis during cell migration and tissue remodelling (Figure 1) [41]. Within the PA system three key peptide members: uPA, uPAR and PAI-1 and 2 have now emerged as a viable and effective diagnostic, prognostic and therapeutic target in breast cancer patients [6]. uPA and uPAR expression have been shown to enhance tumor growth and metastasis [42,43]. Expression of uPA and uPAR is also correlated with poor prognosis, being associated with late stage disease, including metastasis [6]. This section will examine the members of the PA system, discussing their structures and functions, and will describe the important role this system plays in the progression of breast cancer.

5.1. Urokinase-type Plasminogen Activator (uPA) and plasmin

uPA is a serine protease expressed as a single chain zymogen, pro-uPA, which undergoes cleavage to form two-chain high molecular weight uPA (HMW uPA) [44]. After an additional proteolytic step, HMW-uPA is converted into an amino terminal fragment (ATF) containing the receptor-binding growth factor domain (GFD), and a proteolytically-active low molecular weight uPA (LMW-uPA) which retains its plasminogen activator (PA) function [45]. In previous studies, we identified the ATF of uPA as a selective mitogen for cells of the osteoblast phenotype [46-49]. uPA is composed of three domains: a kringle domain, a growth factor-like domain, and a serine protease domain [50]. The serine protease domain of uPA shows high specificity for its substrate, the inactive zymogen plasminogen, which it cleaves to form the activated protease plasmin; plasmin is responsible for the breakdown of various component of the ECM, exerting uPA's pro-invasive and pro-metastatic effects [51,52]. Plasmin is also a serine protease, and catalyzes the process of fibrinolysis, in which fibrin and other components of the ECM are degraded to allow for cell invasion, migration, and dissemination [52]. Plasmin promotes further tumor cell invasion through the conversion of pro-MMPs to enzymatically active MMPs. Plasmin can also promote tumor cell proliferation by activating latent growth factors. Thus, plasmin can also activate ECM degradation both directly and indirectly [53]. Interestingly, plasmin promotes a positive feedback loop in the ECM degradation process, as plasmin also cleaves pro-uPA to create HMW-uPA [52]. uPA synthesis and/or release can be induced by a variety of cytokines and growth factors, including EGF, VEGF, and TNF-α [54,55].

There is speculation regarding which enzyme is responsible for the cleaved activation of pro-uPA into uPA. It is hypothesized that plasmin may be the activator, however, this theory results in ambiguity concerning whether uPA or plasmin is first activated and how [56]. Other enzymes, such as kallikreins, cathepsins, and matriprase, have been shown to be capable of cleaving single chain uPA (scuPA) *in vitro* and are speculated as potential 'first activators' [57]. Interestingly, *in vitro* experiments have shown that binding of pro-uPA to uPAR allows for activation of plasminogen into plasmin, despite pro-uPA not having been converted into it active form. It is thus believed that binding of pro-uPA to uPAR causes a conformational change that confers protease abilities to the single-chain molecule [58]. This is not entirely surprising, as a known role of uPAR is increasing the catalytic efficiency of uPA; in vivo, binding of uPA to uPAR greatly increases the efficiency of plasminogen conversion by as much as 50-fold [59].

Elevated expression levels of uPA in tumor tissue as compared with normal tissue have long been noted [60-62]. In both primary and metastatic tumors, uPA is localized to the invading front, which supports the theory that uPA plays an important role in tumor cell invasion and migration [63]. In breast cancer, increased levels of uPA are correlated with poor relapse-free and overall survival [64]. Increased expression of uPA is seen in patients several common cancers (breast, prostate, lung, colon, thyroid, glioma) where it promotes metastasis and indicates poor prognosis [65-70].

5.2. Plasminogen Activator Inhibitors (PAI)

The effects of uPA are neutralized by plasminogen activator inhibitors 1 and 2 (PAI-1 and 2), produced by stromal cells surrounding the tumor cells. PAI-1 and PAI-2 are involved in the tight control of proteolysis, causing the uPA-uPAR complex to be internalized [71]. Increased PAI-1 expression is associated with higher metastasis whereas PAI-2 has a protective role [72]. PAI-1 binding maintains the active conformation of the uPA-uPAR-vitronectin (VN) complex, interferes with cell matrix interactions, and acts as a detachment factor to promote tumor metastasis [73]. The uPA-PAI-1-uPAR complex is internalized via clathrin-mediated endocytosis, with help from the very low-density lipoprotein receptor (VLDLR) related protein LRP. Inside the cell, the uPA-PAI-1 complex dissociated from uPAR, and is trafficked to the lysosome for degradation. The unbound uPAR is then recycled to the cell surface [71,74]. Interest in PAI-1 as a target in malignancy was revealed in studies where an anti-PAI-1 antibody showed anti-invasive effects on melanoma and fibrosarcoma cells [75]. High-throughput screening led to the identification of small molecule inhibitors of PAI-1 with anti-angiogenic and polyp-formation inhibition activities, thereby identifying PAI-1 as a viable novel target for cancer [76,77].

5.3. uPA Receptor (uPAR)

The role of uPAR within the PA system goes beyond localizing the proteolytic activity of uPA. Rather, uPAR itself plays an important role in tumor progression, interacting with many key signaling molecules, a surprising discovery as uPAR is devoid of a transmembrane domain. Rather, uPAR is a three-domain protein covalently linked to the outer layer of the cell membrane by a glysocylphosphatidylinositol (GPI) anchor [6]. uPAR is important in localizing uPA to the cell surface, which is necessary for uPA's activation of plasminogen to plasmin [59]. All three domains (D1, D2, D3) are involved in the binding of uPA to uPAR, however only domains D2 and D3 are thought to play a role in uPAR's interactions with other cell surface proteins [6]. uPAR alters cell adhesion and signaling through the interaction with various cell surface proteins, such as integrins (including $\alpha v\beta 3$, $\alpha v\beta$, $\alpha 5\beta 1$, and $\alpha 3\beta 1$), G-protein coupled receptors (GPCR), VLDLR, and receptor tyrosine kinases (including epithelial growth factor receptor (EGFR) and platelet-derived growth factor receptor (PDGFR)) [7,78-80]. It is hypothesized that uPAR is part of a larger complex of signaling molecules, called a 'signalosome', which uses signaling effectors such as Src, Akt, and focal adhesion kinase (FAK) [81]. Many of these signaling effectors have been implicated in breast cancer progression, including Src, integrins/FAK, Ras/ERK, and Akt as depicted in Figure 2 [82]. As discussed in a later section, these effectors have become important drug targets for the inhibition of uPA/uPAR-induced breast cancer progression. uPAR is rarely expressed in physiologically normal tissue, although its expression can be up regulated during some pathological processes, such as wound healing or inflammatory response to infection [83,84]. It is involved in normal hemostasis, as plasmin plays an important role in fibrin clot lysis. Under those circumstances, plasmin proteolyzes ECM components either directly or through the activation of MMPs [85,86]. Importantly, uPAR is highly expressed in cancers, and can be expressed by the tumor cells themselves, as well as by tumor-associated cells such as stromal cells, endothelial cells, and infiltrating inflammatory cells [56]. uPAR-expressing tumors generally fall into two categories: those in which both tumor cells and tumor-associated cells express uPA and uPAR, and those in which only the tumor-associated cells express uPAR [56].

uPA and uPAR are not expressed homogeneously throughout the tumor, but instead are generally associated with the interface of tumor tissue-benign tissue or tumor and vascular tissue [87]. uPAR is generally expressed on the migrating or invading edge of cancer cells, restricting the region of proteolytic activity and providing directionality. Thus, a path is created through the ECM, in the direction of movement. A chemical gradient is also created for the invading cancer cells to follow, as chemotactic ECM fragments and latent growth factors are released in the path of ECM destruction [88]. The PA system is responsible for not only the migration of tumor cells, but is also implicated in the migration of tumor-associated macrophages. Binding of uPA to uPAR has different effects depending on the state of maturation of the monocytic cells. uPA-uPAR binding stimulates migration in less mature, more monocyte-like cells; this is would induce the cells to follow the uPA gradient towards the tumor site. On more mature, more macrophage-like cells, uPA-uPAR binding instead induces adhering; thus, a macrophage which arrives at the tumor site will remain [89,90]. uPA has also been implicated in angiogenesis, initially observed in models of corneal vascularization [91]. uPA proteolytic activity is required for endothelial cell migration, one of the earliest steps in angiogenesis, and is also required for the earliest stages in tube formation [92,93]. Thus, the PA system plays an important role in the progression of breast cancer, promoting proliferation through angiogenesis, and enabling metastasis through the induction of tumor cell invasion and migration.

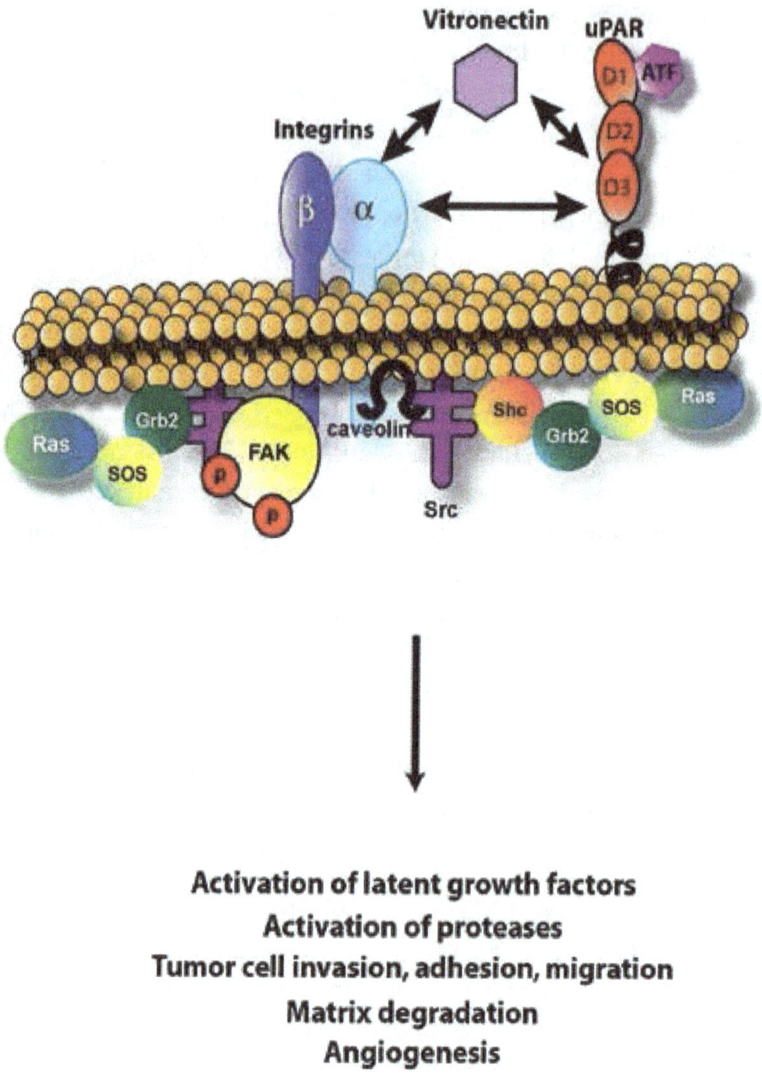

Figure 2. Schematic diagram of pathway involved in the uPA/uPAR signalling. Through its amino terminal fragment (ATF), uPA can bind to domain (D) 1 of its receptor uPAR. Via D2, D3, uPAR can interact vitronectin and members of the integrin family. Through its glycophosphatidyl inositol (GPI) anchor on D3, uPAR is associated to cell membrane. Collectively uPA/uPAR interaction can activate a number of key intracellular signalling pathways to 1) activate latent growth factors, 2) activate proteases, 3) promote tumor cell invasion, adhesion and migration, 4) facilitate matrix degradation and 5) promote angiogenesis.

6. Transcriptional regulation of uPA

Cancer development and progression to the metastatic stage involve the coordinated activation and deactivation of many specific genes. For a long time, cancer was regarded as primarily a genetic disease, with mutation in the DNA sequence being ascribed as the cause for the change in gene expression throughout cancer progression. However, it has now been established that epigenetic changes may also play a key role in the differential gene expression in cancer [94]. The epigenome is dynamic, with some parts of the epigenome being inherited or established during embryonic development, while other aspects are in a state of flux throughout life [95,96].

Epigenetic modifications can be made through various methods, including DNA methylation, nucleosome positioning, post-translational modification of histone tails, and non-coding RNA [97]. The protein machinery which is responsible for implementing these modifications consists of methyl-DNA binding proteins (MBDs), DNA methyltransferases (DNMTs), chromatin remodeling complexes, histone modifiers, and proteins which interact with histone modifications [95]. One of the most closely studied aspects of epigenetics is DNA methylation.

We were the first to identify the epigenetic regulation of uPA by examining the correlation between hormone (estrogen) sensitivity and expression of uPA in normal human mammary epithelial cells (HMEC), early stage hormone-responsive breast cancer cells lines (MCF-7 and T-47D), and late stage hormone-insensitive breast cancer cells (MDA-MB-231). uPA expression was only observed in the highly invasive MDA-MB-231 cells. Expression of various members of the PA system is shown in different human breast cancer cell lines in Table 1. Upon examination of the DNA methylation status of the uPA gene via Southern blot analysis using methylation sensitive enzymes, it was observed that CpG islands within the uPA gene are methylated in normal breast cells and early stage breast cancer cells. Conversely, the CpG islands of the uPA gene are hypomethylated in the highly invasive breast cancer cell line. Treatment of early stage MCF-7 cells with 5′ azacytidine (5-aza-C), a cytosine DNA methyltransferase inhibitor, caused demethylation of the uPA CpG islands and a dose-dependent expression of uPA mRNA [98]. Thus, this study was the first to demonstrate that expression of uPA in invasive vs. non-invasive breast cancers is regulated by DNA methylation of CpG islands within the gene and that this regulation is reversible. In another study conducted by us, methylation-sensitive PCR was used to quantify the methylation status of the CpG islands in the uPA promoter, comparing non-invasive hormone-sensitive MCF-7 cells to highly-invasive hormone-insensitive MDA-MB-231 cells. 90% of the CpG islands in the uPA promoter were found to be methylated in the MCF-7 cells, whereas the MDA-MB-231 cells had fully demethylated CpGs. Luciferase reporter assays demonstrated that the Ets-1 transcription factor binding, which regulates uPA promoter activity, was inhibited by methylation [99]. In order to determine the cause of the differences in the methylation status of the uPA promoter between MCF-7 and MDA-MB-231 cells, our group examined the levels of DNA methylation machinery. Both maintenance DNMT (DNMT1) and DNA demethylase (DMase) activities were shown to correlate with the methylation status of the uPA gene. Thus, MCF-7 cells show high DNMT1 activity and low DMase activity, resulting in a methylated uPA promoter, whereas MDA-MB-231 cells show increased DMase activity and reduced DNMT1 activity, resulting in a demethylated uPA promoter. DNA methylation was confirmed as the dominant mechanism in the silencing of the uPA gene, as histone deacetylase inhibitor Trichostatin A induced uPA expression in MDA-MB-231 cells but not in MCF-7 cell [99]. Thus, this study collectively demonstrated that DNA methylation is critical in the regulation of uPA expression in breast cancer cells.

Cell lines	Early Stage				Late Stage		
	MCF-7	BT-474	ZR 75-1	T-47-D	MDA-MB-231	BT-549	HS-578T
Invasion	-	-	-	-	+	+	+
ER	+	+	+	+	-	-	-
PR	+/-	+/-	+/-	+/-	-	-	-
HER2	-	+	+	-	-	-	-
uPA	N/D	N/D	N/D	N/D	High	High	High
uPAR	Low	Low	Low	Low	High	High	High
PAI-1	N/D	N/D	N/D	N/D	High	High	High
PAI-2	Low	Low	Low	Low	High	High	High

Expression of members of the plasminogen activator (PA) system, urokinase-type plasminogen activator (uPA), its receptor (uPAR), PA inhibitor 1 (PAI-1] and 2 (PAI-2] in human breast cancer cell lines (MCF-7, BT-474, ZR-75-1, T-47-D, MDA-MB-231, BT-549, HS-578T). uPA and PAI-1 are only detectable in highly invasive, estrogen (ER), progesterone (PR) receptor and Her-2 negative human breast (MDA-MB-231, BT-549, HS-578T) cancer cell lines.

N/D: None detected

Table 1. Expression of members of the plasminogen activator (PA) system in human breast cancer cells.

In a later study, our group set out to test the hypothesis that hypomethylation of the uPA promoter plays a causal role in breast cancer metastasis. In order to test this hypothesis, highly invasive MDA-MB-231 breast cancer cells were treated with different doses of the methyl donor S-adenosyl-methionine (SAM) for six days. SAM has been shown to inhibit hypomethylation, either through the inhibition of active demethylation or through the enhancement of DNMT activity [100]. Treatment with SAM resulted in a marked inhibition of uPA mRNA expression, accompanied by the expected decrease in uPA enzymatic activity [101]. Reduction in uPA production was accompanied by a significant decrease in tumor cell invasive capacity as determined by Matrigel invasion assay. The methylating capacity of SAM in breast cancer cells was confirmed, as the SAM-treated cells showed hypermethylation of the uPA promoter. Subsequent treatment of the SAM-treated cells with demethylating agent 5-aza-C caused a reversal of the observed uPA silencing, demonstrating that the effect of SAM on uPA expression is mediated through promoter hypermethylation. In *in vivo* studies carried out in immune deficient mice, animals were injected with MDA-MB-231 cells treated with vehicle or SAM via mammary fat pad. Experimental animals inoculated with MDA-MB-231 cells treated with SAM showed the development tumors which were significantly smaller in volume as compared to control animals. These anti-tumors effects of SAM were accompanied by a significant decrease in the development of tumor cells metastatic ability, resulting in significantly fewer metastatic foci in lungs, liver, kidney, spleen and kidneys as compared to animals inoculated with control cells (Figure 3). Analyses of tumoral RNA demonstrated that the tumors derived from SAM-treated breast cancer cells expressed no detectable levels of uPA, while uPA mRNA was highly expressed in tumors derived from control breast cancer cells. Thus, this was the first report to describe a potential epigenetic based strategy to block the expression of pro-metastatic genes like uPA which resulted in decreased tumor growth and metastasis [101].

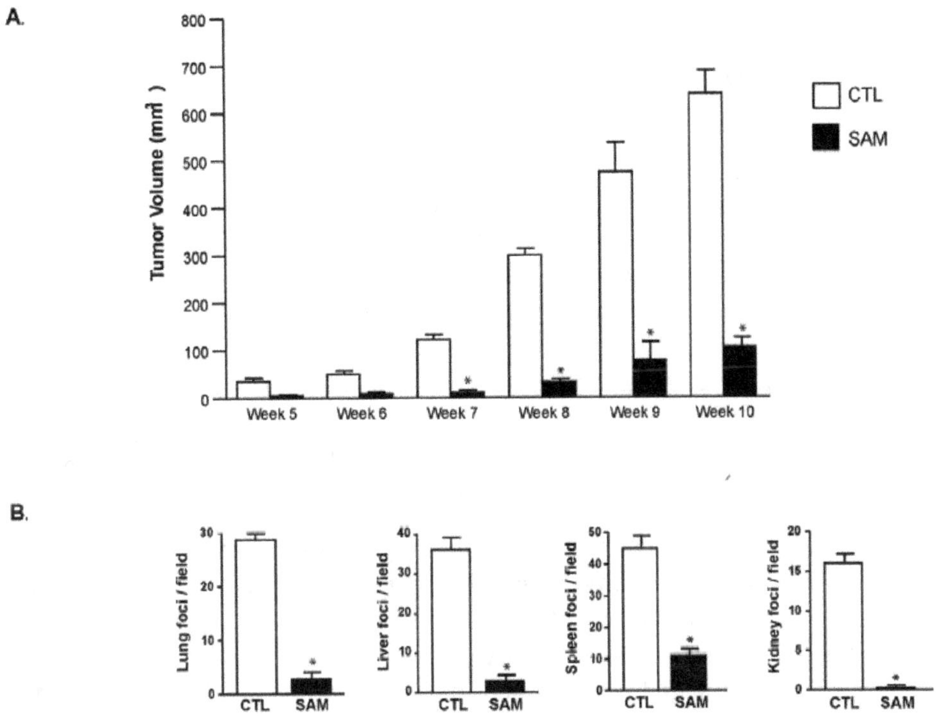

Figure 3. Effect of SAM on MDA-MB-231 tumor volume and metastasis. A: MDA-MB-231 cells treated with vehicle alone as control (CTL) or SAM were introduced into the mammary fat pad of female BALB/c nude mice. Tumor volumes were determined at weekly interval. **B**: At the end of these studies animals were sacrificed and fluorescent microscopic tumor foci in lungs, liver, spleen and kidneys were counted and compared with control group of animals. Significant difference from control is shown by an asterisk (P <0.05). (Adapted from Pakneshan P et al; Ref. 101)

Demethylation results in the activation of tumor suppressor genes, which has led to development of demethylating agent 5-aza-C (Vidaza) for myelodysplastic syndromes, and which is now being tested for its beneficial effects in solid tumors [102,103]. The anti-tumor effects of SAM led us to investigate whether combining 5-aza-C and SAM can have additive or synergetic effects by activating tumor suppressor genes and suppressing pro-metastatic genes. Using several human breast cancer cell lines we have recently shown that SAM inhibits global and gene specific demethylation, prevents potential activation of pro-metastatic genes like uPA and MMPs, and potentiates the activation of tumor suppressor genes by 5-aza-C. These results have led us to propose epigenetic based demethylation (5-aza-C) and methylation (SAM) based therapies at different stage of tumor progression [104].

While a large number of these studies were carried out in breast cancer, DNA methylation has also been shown to regulate uPA and PAI-1 expression in prostate cancer, laryngeal squamous cell carcinoma, meningioma, and gastric cancer, where these genes are also identified as epigenetic based prognostic and therapeutic targets [105,106]. However, large scale clinical studies still remain to be carried out to demonstrate the impact of uPA-PAI-1 methylation in cancer. These epigenetic based therapies can also influence the effects of radiotherapy and chemotherapeutic agents to alter metastatic behaviour [107,108].

7. Diagnostic approaches

The field of cancer research has moved away from the development of broad drug classes which aim to target all cancers, and is instead moving towards personalized medicine. The current goal is to subdivide patients into groups based on molecular characteristics, which then allows therapy options to be assessed and administered based on the molecular characteristics within that particular group [109]. The proteins uPA and PAI-1 are now clinically used biomarkers which are unique among cancer biomarkers because of the lack of contradictory evidence which exists. This is especially surprising, given the variety of demographics which are covered by uPA/PAI-1 diagnostic studies [110]. Notably, uPA and PAI-1 have achieved the highest LOE-1 score attainable according the Tumor Marker Utility Grading System. uPA/PAI-1 are the only breast cancer biomarkers to reach LOE-1 [111].

In 1985, the first comprehensive report examining uPA expression in breast cancer was published. O'Grady *et al.* measured uPA proteolytic activity in both benign tumors and primary breast cancer tissue. Although no measurement was made of actual uPA antigen levels, the study demonstrated significantly elevated levels of uPA enzymatic activity in malignant tumors as compared with benign tumors [112]. In 1988, Duffy *et al.* added further to this area of research, showing that elevated levels of uPA proteolytic activity in primary cancer tissue was correlated with shorter disease-free intervals [113]. Later on, Jänicke *et al.* were first to examine actual proteins levels of uPA in breast cancer tissue, and in 1989 published a study which used the immunoenzymometric test ELISA, showing significant correlation between elevated expression of the uPA antigen in primary tumor tissues and poor prognosis of breast cancer patients [114]. Later on, the same group found a similar correlation existing for the uPA inhibitor PAI-1 [115]. In 2007, uPA and PAI-1 were added to the Breast Cancer Treatment Guidelines of the ASCO as novel cancer biomarkers. They are now used to help determine appropriate adjuvant systemic therapies in primary breast cancers [116].

Today, ELISA remains the gold-standard for assessment of uPA/PAI-1 correlation with breast cancer outcomes. It is the only system examining uPA/PAI-1 in which clinically relevant, validated data have been obtained. When conducting ELISA analysis, either detergent-released tumor-tissue fractions or tumor-tissue cytosolic fractions can be used [117]. Analysis can be conducted on core needle biopsies, primary tumor biopsies, and cryostat sections [118]. Therefore, a major advantage of the use of ELISA tests is the requirement for only very small tissue extract samples [119]. Currently, there is a commercially available ELISA-based assay called FEMTELLE® which is used to assess the probability of breast cancer reoccurrence in newly diagnosed women with node-negative breast cancer. FEMTELLE classifies women into categories of high or low risk of reoccurrence, based on the quantitatively-determined levels of uPA and PAI-1 found in tumor-tissue extracts [52].

A major disadvantage of FEMTELLE, and other ELISA-based assays, is the requirement of fresh or fresh-frozen tissue samples [109]. Thus, other methods of uPA/PAI-1 quantification are under investigation for validation. Immunohistochemistry allows the use of fixed, archived, paraffin-embedded tissue samples for analysis. A roadblock in the development of this assay is that uPA and PAI-1 are present in both tumor and stromal cells, as well as being released into the tissue. Thus, it is extremely difficult to develop a reliable scoring system for uPA/PAI-1 in immunohistochemical analysis. Nevertheless, in 1990 Jänicke *et al.* published a comparison of uPA levels obtained using immunohistochemical scoring and ELISA. The study showed a statistically significant increase in staining intensity for uPA in immunohistochemistry which correlated with an increase in ELISA uPA values [120]. Reilly *et al.* later published the same correlation for PAI-1 [121]. Thus, much work is being done to develop immunohistochemistry as a validated, clinically relevant method of quantifying uPA/PAI-1 expression in breast cancer samples. It is important to note that significant correlation is yet to be established between plasma levels of uPA/PAI-1 with tissue expression of these proteins. Thus, expression of uPA/PAI-1 must be measured directly in the breast cancer tissue sample, and cannot be extrapolated from any plasma measurements [122].

Rather than measuring protein expression levels of uPA and PAI-1 in breast cancer tissue, much research is also invested in the assessment of uPA and PAI-1 biomarker expression at the transcriptional level. The highly sensitive quantitative reverse transcription-polymerase chain reaction (RT-PCR) does not require fresh or fresh-frozen tissue samples, as it can use formalin-fixed tissue specimens and only requires minute amount of mRNA for assessment [123]. Significant correlation between transcript and protein levels for uPA and PAI-1 have been found in breast cancer cell lines [123]. Unfortunately, no correlation was found when examining breast cancer tissue specimens. Spyratos *et al.* found no significant correlation when examining uPA expression, and found only a weak correlation in the case of PAI-1 [124]. Conversely, Lamy *et al.* was able to show high concordance between uPA/PAI-1 antigen expression, as assessed by ELISA, and mRNA expression as assessed by the novel technique nuclei acid sequence-based amplification (NASBA) [125]. However, the results of this study require future validation.

The final area of study which examines the correlation between uPA/PAI-1 expression and breast cancer prognosis is the examination of DNA methylation. As this is a DNA-based assessment, this form of analysis can be easily carried out in formalin-fixed, paraffin-embedded samples, using PCR-based or DNA array technology [109]. As described above, our lab demonstrated the correlation between uPA promoter methylation status in breast cancer [98]. In this study uPA promoter was methylated in normal mammary epithelial cells and in low invasive breast cancer cell lines. In contrast the uPA promoter was demethylated resulting in high levels of uPA expression. Using surgical biopsy specimens, uPA promoter demethylation was associated with advanced disease stage (Figure 4). This effect was independent of the hormone receptor status and results from this study demonstrated the determination of uPA promoter methylation can be developed as a reliable and early marker for uPA expression in breast cancer patents [126]. A similar correlation has also been demonstrated for the PAI-1 promoter [105]. Using surgical biopsy specimens from breast cancer patients, we demonstrated a correlation between uPA promoter methylation status and disease stage correlating with uPA mRNA expression which can serve as an early and reliable diagnostic and prognostic marker for breast cancer [126].

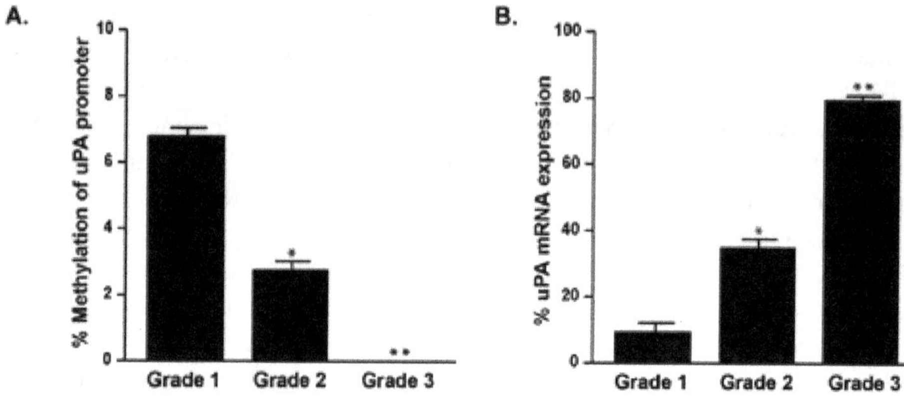

Figure 4. Reverse correlation between percentage of methylation of the urokinase promoter (uPA) and uPA mRNA expression in breast cancer. Percentage of methylation of the uPA promoter (A) and the uPA mRNA expression (B) in the biopsy samples of breast cancer patients were analyzed and graphed. Results are the mean ± SE of at least three independent analyses. Significant difference from grade 1 is shown by an asterisk, and significant difference from both grade 1 and 2 is shown by two asterisks ($P < 0.05$). (Adapted from Pakneshan P et al; Ref. 126)

8. uPAR as an imaging target in breast cancer

Continued development of novel targeted therapies and the effective use of current approaches for breast cancer are still not yielding optimum benefit due to poor strategies to monitor therapeutic efficacy. While diagnostic imaging is extensively used to stage cancers and assess therapy effectiveness, development of highly sensitive non-invasive imaging agents which can identify aggressive lesions while also identifying residual disease will prove to be highly beneficial. High levels of uPAR in cancer lesions as compared to adjacent tissue and normal hemostatic tissues provide a unique opportunity to target uPAR as an imaging target in several common malignancies [127-129]. These unique characteristics allowed the development of non-invasive approaches to detect invasive cancers and detect the presence of occult tumor metastases [130-132]. Our group was first to identify uPAR as an imaging target in cancer and towards these goals we used our well established syngeneic model of breast cancer, which led to the validation of uPAR as a viable target to detect the presence and progression of cancer [133]. In a series of studies, a species specific (rat) antibody directed against the rat (r)-uPAR was developed and characterized by immunofluorescence and Western blot analysis. Following ^{125}I-labelling of the antibody, the binding of r-uPAR-IgG was confirmed in rat prostate cancer cells (Dunning R3227 Mat Ly Lu) and breast cancer cells (Mat B-III) overexpressing (r)-uPAR (Mat B-III-uPAR). In *in vivo* studies, ^{125}I-rat (r)-PAR-IgG was injected on to rat breast and prostate cancer tumor-bearing animals. Uptake of this radiolabel was seen in primary tumors and in liver, spleen, lungs, and lymph nodes, which are common sites of tumor metastasis in these models. Minimal levels of radioactivity were seen in these organs in normal animals and tumor-bearing animals injected with ^{125}I-labeled pre-immune IgG. This study not only further confirmed uPAR as a therapeutic target but also validated it as an imaging target to monitor tumor progression and metastasis.

Following our report, a number of groups have actively pursued these goals; uPAR is now established as an excellent imaging target in cancer. Studies in this regard include the use of dual labelled nanoparticles conjugated to the ATF of uPA, which allowed the accumulation of dye in a xenograft model of pancreatic cancer [134]. Following its internalization, the use of nanoparticles was shown to increase dye retention in the primary tumor and metastatic sites.

The organic compound, 1,4,7,10-tetraazacyclododecane-1,4,7,10-tetraacetic acid (also known as DOTA) has medical application including its use as an imaging agent. DOTA was conjugated to the lead uPAR-targeted peptide (AE-105) and labelled with ^{64}Cu [135-137]. It was successfully shown to monitor the levels of uPAR-expressing tumor cells using positron emission tomography (PET) in a human glioma xenograft model. In this study, solid-based synthesis was carried out via Fmoc approach, followed by the elution and concentration of chelator used for labelling. The labelled reagent was characterized in a series of *in vitro* studies to determine its uptake followed by dynamic ET imaging in tumor-bearing mice. Use of gallium (Ga) based tracers and PET imaging with targeting peptide was shown to be highly effective due to its high radiochemical yield, purity, stability, cellular uptake and good tumor to background ratio using non-invasive PET-based imaging which will be highly useful in a clinical setting [135]. These investigators followed up by combining their findings with a therapeutic approach as well where AE105 was first labelled with ^{64}Cu and ^{177}Lu for its uses in PET-based imaging as well as radionuclide therapy in a xenograft model of colorectal cancer [136].

Various imaging modalities like plane film X-ray, bone scan, ultrasound, computed tomography (CT), magnetic resonance imaging (MRI), and PET are used alone or in combination. PET is a non-invasive imaging technique that offers substantial advantages over anatomic imaging modalities in oncology. Additionally, PET can often distinguish between benign and malignant lesions. Given that highly expressed receptors like uPAR or enzymes can be linked to prognosis in many cases, targeted imaging with highly specific probes may provide prognostic information concerning the level of differentiation of breast cancer, both at primary and metastatic sites.

Over the past few years, there has been a significant growth in the development of radiolabeled monoclonal antibodies (mAbs), which bind with high affinity to receptors frequently highly overexpressed on diverse human cancer cells, for diagnostic and therapeutic applications [138,139]. Characterization of the structure of ATN-658 and its demonstrated efficacy in several xenograft models has led to the initiation of clinical trials using ATN-658 as a therapeutic agent [140]. Availability of this selective anti-uPAR antibody provides us with the opportunity to evaluate it as an imaging agent using multiple radiolabels which can be effectively used to develop PET tracers.

Collectively, evidence continues to accumulate in multiple models, validating uPAR as a viable imaging target for future translational studies for the use of uPAR imaging agents in patients with various malignancies, where overexpression of uPA-uPAR system plays a major role in tumor progression.

9. Targeting the PA system in breast cancer

Since first identifying the PA system as an important player in breast cancer progression and metastasis, there have been many attempts made to target this system specifically. Early development focused on the inhibition of plasminogen activation, looking to inhibit uPA enzymatic activity. This could be accomplished either through the use of small molecules to block the active site of uPA, or by attempting to block the binding of uPA or scuPA to uPAR. Blocking the binding of uPA to uPAR proved to be a more challenging method, as uPAR's binding pocket is much larger than the enzymatic active site of uPA [56]. Many studies have been published which show early attempts at blocking proteolytic activation of plasminogen by uPA.

A common approach was to use small-molecule inhibitors of uPA to block its enzymatic activity, thereby reducing proliferation, invasion, and metastasis. Using this strategy we showed the use of one such uPA inhibitor (B-428) for its ability to block tumor metastases in a xenograft model of prostate cancer. Infusion of B-428 into syngeneic rats inoculated with rat (r) prostate cancer cells Mat LyLu which overexpressed r-uPA resulted in a significantly decreased tumor volume and smaller metastatic foci, as compared with control tumor bearing animals receiving vehicle alone [141]. Other serine protease inhibitors have also been used, and have even been advanced into clinical trials. Promising results have recently been reported with regard to a Phase Ib clinical trial using serine protease inhibitor WX-UK1 for treatment of breast cancer, as well as other solid tumors [142]. A similar agent, known as WX-671 (MESUPRON®), which is a pro-drug of WX-UK1 has also completed a Phase Ib trial for treatment of patients with head and neck cancer [143]. MESUPRON has now moved on to two Phase II clinical trials, currently underway, in which it is being given patients with advanced breast or pancreatic cancer. In both trials, patients are receiving MESUPRON alongside a traditional chemotherapy drug, Capecitabine and Gemcitabine for breast and pancreatic cancer, respectively [5].

Other methods which have been used to successfully block plasminogen activation through inhibition of the uPA system include peptide inhibitors of the uPA-uPAR interaction and anti uPA-uPAR antibodies [144,145]. A non-competitive antagonist of the uPA-uPAR interaction corresponding to the amino acid 136-143 was identified and this peptide (A6) was shown to inhibit endothelial cell migration and breast cancels invasion *in vitro* [146]. Treatment of breast cancer cells MDA-MB-231 tumor-bearing mice resulted in significant inhibition of tumor volume and metastasis (Figure 5). These experimental tumors also showed decreased factor

VIII-positive tumor micro vessel hot-spots, establishing the anti-angiogenic effects of A6. In studies carried out by Mishima *et al.* the antitumor and anti angiogenic effects of A6 were shown alone and in combination with chemotherapeutic agent Cisplatin in a glioblastoma model which led to the clinical evaluation of A6 [147,148]. Use of antibody based therapies has been established during the last decade, resulting in highly beneficial therapeutic approaches for various cancers [149]. The use of antibodies to block uPA-induced metastasis has met with some success, as described below. Using a polyclonal anti-rat uPAR antibody we targeted the ligand binding NH_2-terminal domain of rat uPAR we showed its ability to block breast cancer growth and metastasis *in vivo* [133]. More recently, we evaluated the potential of a highly selective monoclonal antibody against human uPAR (ATN-658). First we examined the efficacy of ATN-658 in blocking prostate cancer growth, invasion, migration, and skeletal metastasis. Examination of the effects of ATN-658 administration *in vitro* using human prostate cancer PC-3 cells showed its ability to cause a decrease in tumor cell invasion and migration by interference with downstream signaling molecules involved in mediating the effects of uPAR (Figure 6). In *in vivo* studies ATN-658 administration caused a significant decrease in tumor volume and number of skeletal metastatic foci [150]. Using ATN-658, Larengyl *et al.* showed its ability to block ovarian cancer metastasis by inducing apoptosis and u-PAR-α_5-integrin interaction [151]. Recently, we have examined the effect of ATN-658 alone and in combination with the bisphosphonate Zometa on skeletal metastasis associated with breast cancer. ATN-658 had a significant effect on reducing the number and area of skeletal lesions as determined by X-ray, however these effects were more pronounced when ATN-658 and Zometa were administered in combination (Rabbani *et al.*, unpublished observations).

A.

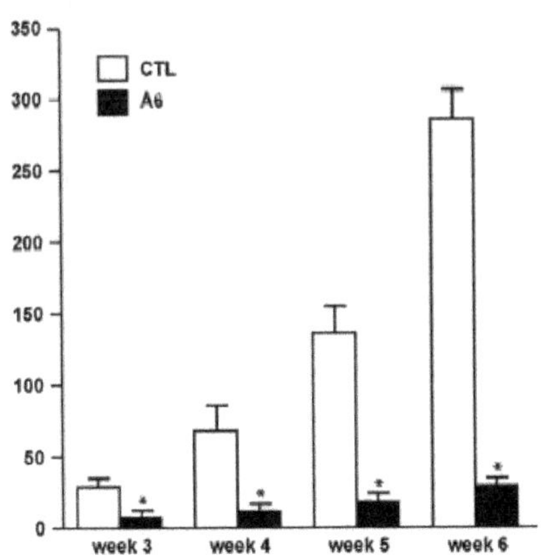

B.

	TISSUE	CONTROL	A6
Macroscopically (number of tumor foci)	LUNG	6 ± 2	3 ± 2
	AX. LYMPH NODES	5 ± 2	1 ± 1
Microscopically (tumor cells per field)	LUNG	4.23 ± 0.18	2.09 ± 0.30
	LIVER	18.83 ± 0.36	3.11 ± 0.14
	SPLEEN	35.67 ± 0.82	28.30 ± 2.80

Figure 5. Effect of Å6 on tumor growth and metastases. A: MDA-MB-231-GFP tumor-bearing BALB/c (nu/nu) mice were injected i.p. with Å6 or vehicle alone (CTL) and tumor volume was determined at weekly intervals. **B:** At the end of this study, control and experimental mice were sacrificed to count the number of macroscopic and microscopic fluorescent tumor foci in different organs. Significant difference from control tumor-bearing animals after treatment with Å6 is denoted by asterisks (P<0.05). (Adapted from Guo Y et al; Ref. 146)

Additional efforts towards therapeutic targeting of the PA system in breast cancer have focused on either decreasing uPA/uPAR/PAI-1 expression, or have focused on using uPA/

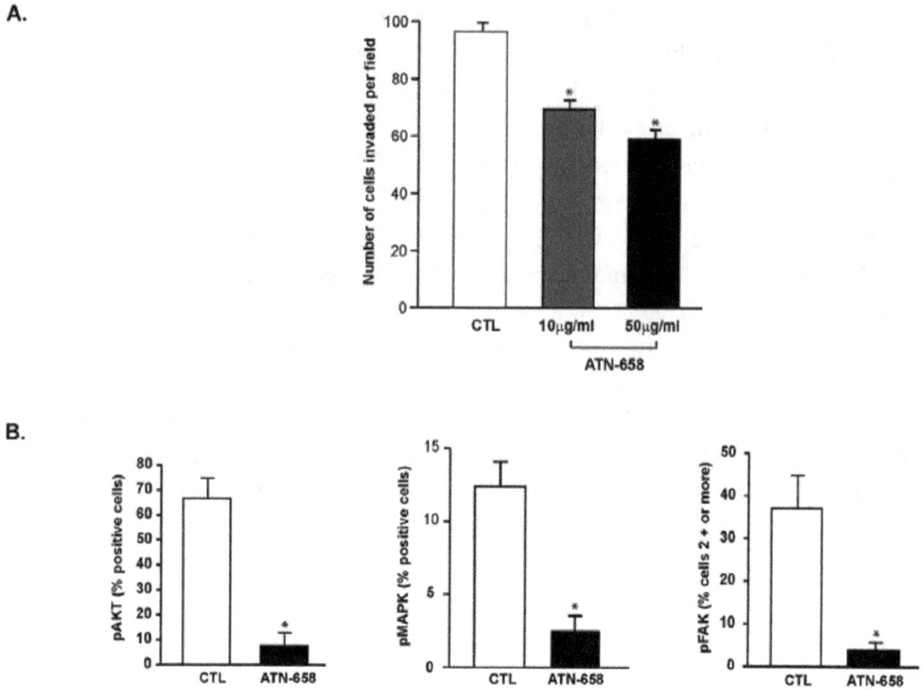

Figure 6. Effect of ATN-658 on tumor cells invasion in vitro and intracellular signaling pathways *in vivo*. A: Human prostate cancer cells PC-3 cell invasive capacity was evaluated after treating with control IgG or ATN-658 using a Boyden chamber Matrigel invasion assay. Number of cells invading is shown as bar diagram ± SEM. B: Male Fox chase SCID mice were inoculated with PC-3 cells through the intra tibial route of injection. Animals were treated with 10.0 mg/kg of control IgG (CTL) or ATN-658. At the end of these studies, animals were sacrificed, and tibias were removed, formalin-fixed, and subjected to immunohistochemical analysis to determine the effect on various intracellular signaling pathways. (Adapted from Rabbani SA et al; Ref. 150)

uPAR as homing mechanisms for cytotoxic drugs. Techniques which aim to reduce or block the expression of uPA/uPAR/PAI-1 include the use of antisense oligonucleotides, interference (RNAi), ribozymes, or DNAzymes [55,152-155]. Experiments using these techniques have shown significant effects on uPAR signaling and tumor behaviour. Anti-uPAR antisense oligonucleotides have been used to inhibit cancer cell proliferation and invasion *in vitro* using melanoma cells, while *in vivo* experiments also showed inhibition of tumor growth and metastasis [156]. Down regulation of uPA and uPAR expression using RNAi has also shown promise, and *in vitro* experiments using human glioma cells showed inhibition of pro-cancer signaling molecules, such as RAS-and MEK-mediated signaling, and resulted in activation of apoptosis [157]. As mentioned above, Pakneshan *et al.* have shown that treatment of highly invasive breast cancer MDA-MB-231 cells with SAM results in decreased expression of uPA, as well as decreased tumor proliferation, invasion, and metastasis [101]. While the exact mechanism through which SAM exerts its methylating actions is still being debated, SAM is a methyl donor and thus may increase the number of methyl groups available for the methyltransferase reaction [94]. SAM has also been shown to inhibit DNA demethylase activity, including MBD2 [100]. Thus, uPA/uPAR expression can be targeted at the transcriptional or at the translational level as well.

Not only is the PA system an excellent therapeutic target because of its pro-metastatic effects, but it is also an exciting group of proteins because of the specificity through which it is highly expressed in tumor cells and the surrounding stroma. This allows for therapeutic targeting of cytotoxic drugs to the tumor compartment through the use of uPA-derived or other uPAR-binding peptides. One example is the conjugation of the growth factor domain (GFD) of uPA to the chelator DOTA and 213-Bi, an α-emitter. With the GFD portion binding to uPAR, this combination has been shown to be cytotoxic to uPAR-expressing ovarian cancer cells *in vitro* [158]. It is also possible to use the amino terminal fragment (ATF) of uPA to deliver drugs to the tumor compartment. ATF binds uPAR with an affinity similar to that of the full sized uPA peptide, resulting in extremely effective delivery of the ATF-conjugated therapeutic payload. Many ATF-toxin fusions have been made, including a ATF-pseudomonas exotoxin (PE), which has been shown to be effective against a number of cancerous cell lines, and ATF-diphtheria toxin (DTAT), which has shown efficacy both *in vitro* and *in vivo* [159-161].

Another recent area of exploration is the use of nanobins, a novel liposomal nanoparticle drug encapsulation and formulation system. Nanobins take advantage of the 'enhanced permeability and retention effect' (EPR effect), in which molecules of certain sizes tend to accumulate in tumor tissue more so than in normal tissue [162]. Although nanobins were already designed to target the tumor environment, relying either entirely on the EPR effect or in conjunction with the use of a pH-responsive cross-linked polymer shell, it is also possible to conjugate nanobin technology with uPA/uPAR-targeting techniques. O'Halloran *et al.* describe their current efforts to combine the monoclonal anti-uPA antibody ATN-291 with nanobins, creating a product which can be internalized into tumor and tumor-associated cells for greater therapeutic strength. ATN-291 binds to the kringle domain of uPA and is able to bind uPA which is already bound to uPAR. Interestingly, the internalization of the ATN-291-uPA-uPAR complex is not dependent on the presence of PAI-1. The efficacy of this system is currently being evaluated in several xenograft models, with hopes of advancing this technology into clinical development sometime in the near future [6].

One caveat when studying any uPA/uPAR-targeted therapy is the high degree of species specificity of uPA and uPAR, such that human uPA has an extremely low binding capacity towards murine uPAR, and vice versa. This is especially relevant to the use of xenograft models, in which therapies which target human uPA/uPAR will only have an effect on tumor cells, and not on the surrounding stromal cells [56]. One result of this issue is that the efficacy of potential uPA/uPAR-targeted therapies may be underestimated in xenograft models. The second implication is that the toxicity profiles of these drugs may also be underestimated in xenograft models. However, toxicity concerns can be somewhat put to rest, as analysis of cadaveric human tissue has demonstrated very little tissue expression of uPAR [7].

Like uPA, several studies have been carried out targeting the PAI-1 as an anti-cancer therapy. Elevated levels of PAI-1 are a predictor of aggressive cancers, although that fact seems contradictory, given that PAI-1 is an inhibitor of uPA activity. However, it is now believed that PAI-1 may possess functions independent of uPA inhibition [163]. For example, expression of PAI-1 is necessary for cancer-induced angiogenesis in preclinical models [164]. In addition, PAI-1 is associated with insensitivity to chemotherapy treatment, while PAI-1 deficiency causes increased chemotherapy sensitivity [165]. A way of targeting these actions is to inactivate PAI-1, forcing the conversion of PAI-1 into its latent form. This can be done using the small peptide paionin-4-D1D2 or small-molecule inhibitor PAI-039 [166,167]. Another method under examination is the interference of the interaction between PAI-1 and vitronectin, an interaction which has been shown to cause detachment of tumor cells from the ECM, promoting the metastatic process [168]. RNA-aptamers SM-20 and WT-15 are effective in inhibiting this interaction without affecting the uPA-inhibiting activity of PAI-1 [155, 169].

Thus, the PA system represents a promising area of research for the development of targeted anti-cancer therapies. There are a wide variety of methods being examined, targeting any of the three key players within the PA system, and using several molecular, chemical, and immunological approaches which have already shown highly promising results, paving the way for their clinical evaluation.

10. Summary and future goals

Within the last 20 years, the PA system has been established as an important regulator of breast cancer progress, being directly involved in proliferation, invasion, and migration of tumor cells. As such, it has become a key target for clinical use in diagnostics, imaging, and therapeutics. Over the next few years, there will likely be many more important developments in this field of study. The exact nature of the signalosome relationship is still being elucidated, and several studies are underway to identify which proteins are directly bound to uPAR and are involved in its intracellular signaling. Although ELISA is currently being used as the gold-standard in measuring uPA/uPAR for diagnostic purposes, much work is being done to establish immunohistochemical protocols, so that fresh or fresh-frozen tissue samples are no longer required. Much research is being conducted to evaluate the potential regulation of uPA/uPAR/PAI-1 expression via epigenetics as well as antisense oligonucleotides and RNAi. In addition, technologies which use uPA and uPAR to target cytotoxic drug to the tumor compartment are only now in their earliest stages of development, thus, there are many avenues to explore in that area of research. Collectively, results from these studies will drive the clinical development of several PA targeted diagnostic and therapeutic agents which are either already in clinical trials are expected to enter in the near future. There is great optimism in these studies using targeted approaches which will lead to reduced morbidity and mortality in several common malignancies, including breast cancer.

Acknowledgements

This work was supported by a grant MOP 130410 from the Canadian Institutes for Health Research to SAR.

Author details

Catherine Leurer and Shafaat Ahmed Rabbani*

*Address all correspondence to: shafaat.rabbani@mcgill.ca

Department of Medicine, McGill University Health Center, Canada

References

[1] Rabbani SA, Mazar AP. Evaluating distant metastases in breast cancer: from biology to outcomes. Cancer metastasis reviews. 2007;26(3-4):663-74.

[2] Dowsett M, Dunbier AK. Emerging Biomarkers and New Understanding of Traditional Markers in Personalized Therapy for Breast Cancer. Clinical Cancer Research. 2008 December 15, 2008;14(24):8019-26.

[3] Duffy MJ, Crown J. A Personalized Approach to Cancer Treatment: How Biomarkers Can Help. Clinical Chemistry. 2008 November 1, 2008;54(11):1770-9.

[4] Cornejo KM, Kandil D, Khan A, Cosar EF. Theranostic and Molecular Classification of Breast Cancer. Archives of Pathology & Laboratory Medicine. 2014;138(1):4456.

[5] Schmitt M, Mengele K, Napieralski R, Magdolen V, Reuning U, Gkazepis A, et al. Clinical utility of level-of-evidence-1 disease forecast cancer biomarkers uPA and its inhibitor PAI-1. Expert review of molecular diagnostics. 2010;10(8):1051-67.

[6] O'Halloran T, Ahn R, Hankins P, Swindell E, Mazar A. The many spaces of uPAR: delivery of theranostic agents and nanobins to multiple tumor compartments through a single target. Theranostics. 2013;3(7):496-506.

[7] Mazar AP, Ahn RW, O'Halloran TV. Development of novel therapeutics targeting the urokinase plasminogen activator receptor (uPAR) and their translation toward the clinic. Current pharmaceutical design. 2011;17(19):1970-8.

[8] Italiano A. Prognostic or Predictive? It's Time to Get Back to Definitions! Journal of Clinical Oncology. 2011 December 10, 2011;29(35):4718.

[9] Goldhirsch A, Wood WC, Coates AS, Gelber RD, Thürlimann B, Senn H-J, et al. Strategies for subtypes—dealing with the diversity of breast cancer: highlights of the St Gallen International Expert Consensus on the Primary Therapy of Early Breast Cancer 2011. Annals of Oncology. 2011 August 1, 2011;22(8):1736-47.

[10] Cuzick J, Dowsett M, Pineda S, Wale C, Salter J, Quinn E, et al. Prognostic Value of a Combined Estrogen Receptor, Progesterone Receptor, Ki-67, and Human Epidermal Growth Factor Receptor 2 Immunohistochemical Score and Comparison With the

Genomic Health Recurrence Score in Early Breast Cancer. Journal of Clinical Oncology. 2011 November 10, 2011;29(32):4273-8.

[11] Cardoso F, Van't Veer L, Rutgers E, Loi S, Mook S, Piccart-Gebhart MJ. Clinical Application of the 70-Gene Profile: The MINDACT Trial. Journal of Clinical Oncology. 2008;26(5):729-35.

[12] Paik S. Development and Clinical Utility of a 21-Gene Recurrence Score Prognostic Assay in Patients with Early Breast Cancer Treated with Tamoxifen. The Oncologist. 2007;12(6):631-5.

[13] Toussaint J, Sieuwerts AM, Haibe-Kains B, Desmedt C, Rouas G, Harris AL, et al. Improvement of the clinical applicability of the Genomic Grade Index through a qRT-PCR test performed on frozen and formalin-fixed paraffin-embedded tissues. BMC genomics. 2009;10:424.

[14] Filipits M, Rudas M, Jakesz R, Dubsky P, Fitzal F, Singer CF, et al. A New Molecular Predictor of Distant Recurrence in ER-Positive, HER2-Negative Breast Cancer Adds Independent Information to Conventional Clinical Risk Factors. Clinical Cancer Research. 2011;17(18):6012-20.

[15] Ma X-J, Wang Z, Ryan PD, Isakoff SJ, Barmettler A, Fuller A, et al. A two-gene expression ratio predicts clinical outcome in breast cancer patients treated with tamoxifen. Cancer Cell. 2004;5(6):607-16.

[16] Bendre M, Gaddy D, Nicholas RW, Suva LJ. Breast cancer metastasis to bone: it is not all about PTHrP. Clinical orthopaedics and related research. 2003 (415 Suppl):S39-45.

[17] Coleman RE. Clinical Features of Metastatic Bone Disease and Risk of Skeletal Morbidity. Clinical Cancer Research. 2006;12(20):6243s-9s.

[18] Norton L, Massague J. Is cancer a disease of self-seeding? Nat Med. 2006;12(8):875-8.

[19] Yokota J. Tumor progression and metastasis. Carcinogenesis. 2000;21(3):497-503.

[20] Paget S. The distribution of secondary growths in cancer of the breast. The Lancet. 1889 3/23/;133(3421):571-3.

[21] Weilbaecher KN, Guise TA, McCauley LK. Cancer to bone: a fatal attraction. Nat Rev Cancer. 2011;11(6):411-25.

[22] Russell RGG. Bisphosphonates: The first 40 years. Bone. 2011;49(1):2-19.

[23] Diel IJ, Solomayer E-F, Costa SD, Gollan C, Goerner R, Wallwiener D, et al. Reduction in New Metastases in Breast Cancer with Adjuvant Clodronate Treatment. New England Journal of Medicine. 1998;339(6):357-63.

[24] Aft R, Naughton M, Trinkaus K, Watson M, Ylagan L, Chavez-MacGregor M, et al. Effect of zoledronic acid on disseminated tumour cells in women with locally ad-

vanced breast cancer: an open label, randomised, phase 2 trial. The Lancet Oncology. 2010;11(5):421-8.

[25] Vincenzi B, Santini D, Dicuonzo G, Battistoni F, Gavasci M, La Cesa A, et al. Zoledronic acid-related angiogenesis modifications and survival in advanced breast cancer patients. Journal of interferon & cytokine research : the official journal of the International Society for Interferon and Cytokine Research. 2005;25(3):144-51.

[26] Suda T, Takahashi N, Udagawa N, Jimi E, Gillespie MT, Martin TJ. Modulation of Osteoclast Differentiation and Function by the New Members of the Tumor Necrosis Factor Receptor and Ligand Families. Endocrine Reviews. 1999;20(3):345-57.

[27] Guise T. Examining the Metastatic Niche: Targeting the Microenvironment. Seminars in Oncology. 2010;37, Supplement 2(0):S2-S14.

[28] Jones DH, Nakashima T, Sanchez OH, Kozieradzki I, Komarova SV, Sarosi I, et al. Regulation of cancer cell migration and bone metastasis by RANKL. Nature. 2006;440(7084):692-6.

[29] Lacey DL, Boyle WJ, Simonet WS, Kostenuik PJ, Dougall WC, Sullivan JK, et al. Bench to bedside: elucidation of the OPG–RANK–RANKL pathway and the development of denosumab. Nat Rev Drug Discov. 2012;11(5):401-19.

[30] FDA. Denosumab (XGEVA®)-summary of product characteristics. http://www.accessdata.fda.gov/drugsatfda_docs/label/2010/125320s007lbl.pdf2011 [cited 2014 July 29 2014].

[31] Zou W, Kitaura H, Reeve J, Long F, Tybulewicz VLJ, Shattil SJ, et al. Syk, c-Src, the αvβ3 integrin, and ITAM immunoreceptors, in concert, regulate osteoclastic bone resorption. The Journal of Cell Biology. 2007;176(6):877-88.

[32] Clezardin P. Integrins in bone metastasis formation and potential therapeutic implications. Current cancer drug targets. 2009;9(7):801-6.

[33] Bäuerle T, Komljenovic D, Merz M, Berger MR, Goodman SL, Semmler W. Cilengitide inhibits progression of experimental breast cancer bone metastases as imaged noninvasively using VCT, MRI and DCE-MRI in a longitudinal in vivo study. International Journal of Cancer. 2011;128(10):2453-62.

[34] Davies KJ. The Complex Interaction of Matrix Metalloproteinases in the Migration of Cancer Cells through Breast Tissue Stroma. International Journal of Breast Cancer. 2014;2014:5.

[35] Duffy MJ, Maguire TM, Hill A, McDermott E, O'Higgins N. Metalloproteinases: role in breast carcinogenesis, invasion and metastasis. Breast cancer research : BCR. 2000;2(4):252-7.

[36] Kohrmann A, Kammerer U, Kapp M, Dietl J, Anacker J. Expression of matrix metalloproteinases (MMPs) in primary human breast cancer and breast cancer cell lines: New findings and review of the literature. BMC cancer. 2009;9:188.

[37] Lebeau A, Nerlich AG, Sauer U, Lichtinghagen R, Lohrs U. Tissue distribution of major matrix metalloproteinases and their transcripts in human breast carcinomas. Anticancer research. 1999;19(5B):4257-64.

[38] Reimers N, Zafrakas K, Assmann V, Egen C, Riethdorf L, Riethdorf S, et al. Expression of Extracellular Matrix Metalloproteases Inducer on Micrometastatic and Primary Mammary Carcinoma Cells. Clinical Cancer Research. 2004;10(10):3422-8.

[39] Hildenbrand R, Gandhari M, Stroebel P, Marx A, Allgayer H, Arens N. The urokinase-system--role of cell proliferation and apoptosis. Histology and histopathology. 2008;23(2):227-36.

[40] Mekkawy AH, Morris DL, Pourgholami MH. Urokinase plasminogen activator system as a potential target for cancer therapy. Future Oncology. 2009;5(9):1487-99.

[41] Collen D, Lijnen HR. Basic and clinical aspects of fibrinolysis and thrombolysis. Blood. 1991;78(12):3114-24.

[42] Frandsen TL, Holst-Hansen C, Nielsen BS, Christensen IJ, Nyengaard JR, Carmeliet P, et al. Direct Evidence of the Importance of Stromal Urokinase Plasminogen Activator (uPA) in the Growth of an Experimental Human Breast Cancer Using a Combined uPA Gene-Disrupted and Immunodeficient Xenograft Model. Cancer Research. 2001;61(2):532-7.

[43] Xing RH, Rabbani SA. Overexpression of urokinase receptor in breast cancer cells results in increased tumor invasion, growth and metastasis. Int J Cancer. 1996;67(3): 423-9.

[44] Gunzler WA, Steffens GJ, Otting F, Kim SM, Frankus E, Flohe L. The primary structure of high molecular mass urokinase from human urine. The complete amino acid sequence of the A chain. Hoppe-Seyler's Zeitschrift fur physiologische Chemie. 1982;363(10):1155-65.

[45] Appella E, Robinson EA, Ullrich SJ, Stoppelli MP, Corti A, Cassani G, et al. The receptor-binding sequence of urokinase. A biological function for the growth-factor module of proteases. J Biol Chem. 1987;262(10):4437-40.

[46] Koutsilieris M, Rabbani SA, Bennett HP, Goltzman D. Characteristics of prostate-derived growth factors for cells of the osteoblast phenotype. J Clin Invest. 1987;80(4): 941-6.

[47] Koutsilieris M, Rabbani SA, Goltzman D. Effects of human prostatic mitogens on rat bone cells and fibroblasts. The Journal of endocrinology. 1987;115(3):447-54.

[48] Rabbani SA, Desjardins J, Bell AW, Banville D, Mazar A, Henkin J, et al. An amino-terminal fragment of urokinase isolated from a prostate cancer cell line (PC-3) is mi-

togenic for osteoblast-like cells. Biochemical and Biophysical Research Communications. 1990;173(3):1058-64.

[49] Rabbani SA, Mazar AP, Bernier SM, Haq M, Bolivar I, Henkin J, et al. Structural requirements for the growth factor activity of the amino-terminal domain of urokinase. J Biol Chem. 1992;267(20):14151-6.

[50] Wang Y, Dang J, Johnson LK, Selhamer JJ, Doe WF. Structure of the human urokinase receptor gene and its similarity to CD59 and the Ly-6 family. European Journal of Biochemistry. 1995;227(1-2):116-22.

[51] Kwaan HC, Mazar AP, McMahon BJ. The Apparent uPA/PAI-1 Paradox in Cancer: More than Meets the Eye. Semin Thromb Hemost. 2013;39(04):382-91.

[52] Mengele K, Napieralski R, Magdolen V, Reuning U, Gkazepis A, Sweep F, et al. Characteristics of the level-of-evidence-1 disease forecast cancer biomarkers uPA and its inhibitor PAI-1. Expert review of molecular diagnostics. 2010;10(7):947-62.

[53] Kwaan HC, McMahon B. The role of plasminogen-plasmin system in cancer. Cancer treatment and research. 2009;148:43-66.

[54] Szabo H, Novak Z, Bauer H, Szatmari E, Farkas A, Wejksza K, et al. Regulation of proteolytic activity induced by inflammatory stimuli in lung epithelial cells. Cellular and molecular biology (Noisy-le-Grand, France). 2005;51 Suppl:OL729-35.

[55] Ulisse S, Baldini E, Sorrenti S, D'Armiento M. The urokinase plasminogen activator system: a target for anti-cancer therapy. Current cancer drug targets. 2009;9(1):32-71.

[56] Mazar AP. Urokinase plasminogen activator receptor choreographs multiple ligand interactions: implications for tumor progression and therapy. Clinical cancer research : an official journal of the American Association for Cancer Research. 2008;14(18):5649-55.

[57] Kilpatrick LM, Harris RL, Owen KA, Bass R, Ghorayeb C, Bar-Or A, et al. Initiation of plasminogen activation on the surface of monocytes expressing the type II transmembrane serine protease matriptase. Blood. 2006;108(8):2616-23.

[58] Higazi AA-R, Cohen RL, Henkin J, Kniss D, Schwartz BS, Cines DB. Enhancement of the Enzymatic Activity of Single-chain Urokinase Plasminogen Activator by Soluble Urokinase Receptor. Journal of Biological Chemistry. 1995;270(29):17375-80.

[59] Ellis V, Behrendt N, Danø K. Plasminogen activation by receptor-bound urokinase. A kinetic study with both cell-associated and isolated receptor. Journal of Biological Chemistry. 1991;266(19):12752-8.

[60] Svanberg L, Astedt B. Release of plasminogen activator from normal and neoplastic endometrium. Experientia. 1979;35(6):818-9.

[61] Markus G, Takita H, Camiolo SM, Corasanti JG, Evers JL, Hobika GH. Content and Characterization of Plasminogen Activators in Human Lung Tumors and Normal Lung Tissue. Cancer Research. 1980;40(3):841-8.

[62] Corasanti JG, Celik C, Camiolo SM, Mittelman A, Evers JL, Barbasch A, et al. Plasminogen activator content of human colon tumors and normal mucosae: separation of enzymes and partial purification. Journal of the National Cancer Institute. 1980;65(2):345-51.

[63] Kwaan HC, Keer HN, Radosevich JA, Cajot JF, Ernst R. Components of the plasminogen-plasmin system in human tumor cell lines. Semin Thromb Hemost. 1991;17(3):175-82.

[64] Look MP, van Putten WLJ, Duffy MJ, Harbeck N, Christensen IJ, Thomssen C, et al. Pooled Analysis of Prognostic Impact of Urokinase-Type Plasminogen Activator and Its Inhibitor PAI-1 in 8377 Breast Cancer Patients. Journal of the National Cancer Institute. 2002;94(2):116-28.

[65] Andres SA, Edwards AB, Wittliff JL. Expression of Urokinase-Type Plasminogen Activator (uPA), its Receptor (uPAR), and Inhibitor (PAI-1) in Human Breast Carcinomas and Their Clinical Relevance. Journal of Clinical Laboratory Analysis. 2012;26(2):93-103.

[66] Kumano M, Miyake H, Muramaki M, Furukawa J, Takenaka A, Fujisawa M. Expression of urokinase-type plasminogen activator system in prostate cancer: Correlation with clinicopathological outcomes in patients undergoing radical prostatectomy. Urologic Oncology: Seminars and Original Investigations. 2009;27(2):180-6.

[67] Skriver L, Larsson LI, Kielberg V, Nielsen LS, Andresen PB, Kristensen P, et al. Immunocytochemical localization of urokinase-type plasminogen activator in Lewis lung carcinoma. J Cell Biol. 1984;99(2):753-7.

[68] Halamkova J, Kiss I, Pavlovsky Z, Tomasek J, Jarkovsky J, Cech Z, et al. Clinical significance of the plasminogen activator system in relation to grade of tumor and treatment response in colorectal carcinoma patients. Neoplasma. 2011;58(5):377-85.

[69] Horvatic Herceg G, Herceg D, Kralik M, Kulic A, Bence-Zigman Z, Tomic-Brzac H, et al. Urokinase plasminogen activator and its inhibitor type-1 as prognostic factors in differentiated thyroid carcinoma patients. Otolaryngol Head Neck Surg. 2013;149(4):533-40.

[70] Hsu DW, Efird JT, Hedley-Whyte ET. Prognostic role of urokinase-type plasminogen activator in human gliomas. Am J Pathol. 1995;147(1):114-23.

[71] Nykjær A, Conese M, Christensen EI, Olson D, Cremona O, Gliemann J, et al. Recycling of the urokinase receptor upon internalization of the uPA:serpin complexes. The EMBO Journal. 1997;16(10):2610-20.

[72] Croucher DR, Saunders DN, Lobov S, Ranson M. Revisiting the biological roles of PAI2 (SERPINB2) in cancer. Nat Rev Cancer. 2008;8(7):535-45.

[73] Deng G, Curriden SA, Wang S, Rosenberg S, Loskutoff DJ. Is plasminogen activator inhibitor-1 the molecular switch that governs urokinase receptor-mediated cell adhesion and release? The Journal of Cell Biology. 1996;134(6):1563-71.

[74] Blasi F, Carmeliet P. uPAR: a versatile signalling orchestrator. Nat Rev Mol Cell Biol. 2002;3(12):932-43.

[75] Brooks TD, Slomp J, Quax PH, De Bart AC, Spencer MT, Verheijen JH, et al. Antibodies to PAI-1 alter the invasive and migratory properties of human tumour cells in vitro. Clinical & experimental metastasis. 2000;18(6):445-53.

[76] Leik CE, Su EJ, Nambi P, Crandall DL, Lawrence DA. Effect of pharmacologic plasminogen activator inhibitor-1 inhibition on cell motility and tumor angiogenesis. Journal of Thrombosis and Haemostasis. 2006;4(12):2710-5.

[77] Mutoh M, Niho N, Komiya M, Takahashi M, Ohtsubo R, Nakatogawa K, et al. Plasminogen activator inhibitor-1 (Pai-1) blockers suppress intestinal polyp formation in Min mice. Carcinogenesis. 2008;29(4):824-9.

[78] Kugler MC, Wei Y, Chapman HA. Urokinase receptor and integrin interactions. Current pharmaceutical design. 2003;9(19):1565-74.

[79] Hu J, Jo M, Cavenee WK, Furnari F, VandenBerg SR, Gonias SL. Crosstalk between the urokinase-type plasminogen activator receptor and EGF receptor variant III supports survival and growth of glioblastoma cells. Proceedings of the National Academy of Sciences. 2011;108(38):15984-9.

[80] Webb DJ, Nguyen DH, Gonias SL. Extracellular signal-regulated kinase functions in the urokinase receptor-dependent pathway by which neutralization of low density lipoprotein receptor-related protein promotes fibrosarcoma cell migration and matrigel invasion. Journal of Cell Science. 2000;113(1):123-34.

[81] Degryse B. The Urokinase Receptor and Integrins Constitute a Cell Migration Signalosome. In: Edwards D, Høyer-Hansen G, Blasi F, Sloane B, editors. The Cancer Degradome: Springer New York; 2008. p. 451-74.

[82] Friedl P, Wolf K. Tumour-cell invasion and migration: diversity and escape mechanisms. Nat Rev Cancer. 2003;3(5):362-74.

[83] Xia W, de Bock C, Murrell GAC, Wang Y. Expression of urokinase-type plasminogen activator and its receptor is up-regulated during tendon healing. Journal of Orthopaedic Research. 2003;21(5):819-25.

[84] Gyetko MR, Sud S, Kendall T, Fuller JA, Newstead MW, Standiford TJ. Urokinase Receptor-Deficient Mice Have Impaired Neutrophil Recruitment in Response to Pul-

monary Pseudomonas aeruginosa Infection. The Journal of Immunology. 2000;165(3): 1513-9.

[85] Roth D, Piekarek M, Paulsson M, Christ H, Bloch W, Krieg T, et al. Plasmin Modulates Vascular Endothelial Growth Factor-A-Mediated Angiogenesis during Wound Repair. The American Journal of Pathology. 2006;168(2):670-84.

[86] Kim MH. Flavonoids inhibit VEGF/bFGF-induced angiogenesis in vitro by inhibiting the matrix-degrading proteases. Journal of Cellular Biochemistry. 2003;89(3):529-38.

[87] Sullivan R, Graham C. Hypoxia-driven selection of the metastatic phenotype. Cancer Metastasis Rev. 2007;26(2):319-31.

[88] Waltz DA, Natkin LR, Fujita RM, Wei Y, Chapman HA. Plasmin and plasminogen activator inhibitor type 1 promote cellular motility by regulating the interaction between the urokinase receptor and vitronectin. The Journal of Clinical Investigation. 1997;100(1):58-67.

[89] Franco P, Iaccarino C, Chiaradonna F, Brandazza A, Iavarone C, Mastronicola MR, et al. Phosphorylation of Human Pro-Urokinase on Ser138/303 Impairs Its Receptor-dependent Ability to Promote Myelomonocytic Adherence and Motility. The Journal of Cell Biology. 1997;137(3):779-91.

[90] Jardí M, Inglés-Esteve J, Burgal M, Azqueta C, Velasco F, López-Pedrera C, et al. Distinct patterns of urokinase receptor (uPAR) expression by leukemic cells and peripheral blood cells. Thrombosis and haemostasis. 1996;76(6):1009-19.

[91] Berman M, Winthrop S, Ausprunk D, Rose J, Langer R, Gage J. Plasminogen activator (urokinase) causes vascularization of the cornea. Investigative Ophthalmology & Visual Science. 1982;22(2):191-9.

[92] Lu H, Mabilat C, Yeh P, Guitton J-D, Li H, Pouchelet M, et al. Blockage of urokinase receptor reduces in vitro the motility and the deformability of endothelial cells. FEBS Letters. 1996;380(1–2):21-4.

[93] Schnaper HW, Barnathan ES, Mazar A, Maheshwari S, Ellis S, Cortez SL, et al. Plasminogen activators augment endothelial cell organization in vitro by two distinct pathways. J Cell Physiol. 1995;165(1):107-18.

[94] Chik F, Szyf M, Rabbani SA. Role of epigenetics in cancer initiation and progression. Advances in experimental medicine and biology. 2010;720:91-104.

[95] Reik W, Dean W, Walter J. Epigenetic Reprogramming in Mammalian Development. Science. 2001;293(5532):1089-93.

[96] Kim GD, Ni J, Kelesoglu N, Roberts RJ, Pradhan S. Co-operation and communication between the human maintenance and de novo DNA (cytosine-5) methyltransferases. EMBO J. 2002;21(15):4183-95.

[97] Board E. Moving AHEAD with an international human epigenome project. Nature. 2008;454(7205):711-5.

[98] Xing RH, Rabbani SA. Transcriptional regulation of urokinase (uPA) gene expression in breast cancer cells: Role of DNA methylation. International Journal of Cancer. 1999;81(3):443-50.

[99] Guo Y, Pakneshan P, Gladu J, Slack A, Szyf M, Rabbani SA. Regulation of DNA Methylation in Human Breast Cancer: Effect on the urokinase-type plasminogen activator gene production and tumor invasion. Journal of Biological Chemistry. 2002;277(44):41571-9.

[100] Detich N, Hamm S, Just G, Knox JD, Szyf M. The Methyl Donor S-Adenosylmethionine Inhibits Active Demethylation of DNA: A candidate novel mechanism for the pharmacological effects of s-adenosylmthionine. Journal of Biological Chemistry. 2003;278(23):20812-20.

[101] Pakneshan P, Szyf M, Farias-Eisner R, Rabbani SA. Reversal of the hypomethylation status of urokinase (uPA) promoter blocks breast cancer growth and metastasis. The Journal of biological chemistry. 2004;279(30):31735-44.

[102] Falchook G, Fu S, Naing A, Hong D, Hu W, Moulder S, et al. Methylation and histone deacetylase inhibition in combination with platinum treatment in patients with advanced malignancies. Invest New Drugs. 2013 2013/10/01;31(5):1192-200. English.

[103] Bauman J, Verschraegen C, Belinsky S, Muller C, Rutledge T, Fekrazad M, et al. A phase I study of 5-azacytidine and erlotinib in advanced solid tumor malignancies. Cancer chemotherapy and pharmacology. 2012 2012/02/01;69(2):547-54. English.

[104] Chik F, Machnes Z, Szyf M. Synergistic anti-breast cancer effect of a combined treatment with the methyl donor S-adenosyl methionine and the DNA methylation inhibitor 5-aza-2′-deoxycytidine. Carcinogenesis. 2014;35(1):138-44.

[105] Gao S, Skeldal S, Krogdahl A, Sørensen JAS, Peter AA. CpG methylation of the PAI-1 gene 5'-flanking region is inversely correlated with PAI-1 mRNA levels in human cell lines. Thrombosis and haemostasis. 2005;94(9):651-60.

[106] Gao S, Nielsen BS, Krogdahl A, Sørensen JA, Tagesen J, Dabelsteen S, et al. Epigenetic alterations of the SERPINE1 gene in oral squamous cell carcinomas and normal oral mucosa. Genes, Chromosomes and Cancer. 2010;49(6):526-38.

[107] Ari F, Napieralski R, Ulukaya E, Dere E, Colling C, Honert K, et al. Modulation of protein expression levels and DNA methylation status of breast cancer metastasis genes by anthracycline-based chemotherapy and the demethylating agent decitabine. Cell Biochemistry and Function. 2011;29(8):651-9.

[108] Velpula KK, Gogineni VR, Nalla AK, Dinh DH, Rao JS. Radiation-induced hypomethylation triggers urokinase plasminogen activator transcription in meningioma cells. Neoplasia. 2013;15(2):192-203.

[109] Schmitt M, Mengele K, Gkazepis A, Napieralski R, Magdolen V, Reuning U, et al. Assessment of Urokinase-Type Plasminogen Activator and Its Inhibitor PAI-1 in Breast Cancer Tissue: Historical Aspects and Future Prospects. Breast Care. 2008;3(2):22.

[110] Harbeck N, Schmitt M, Paepke S, Allgayer H, Kates RE. Tumor-Associated Proteolytic Factors uPA and PAI-1: Critical Appraisal of Their Clinical Relevance in Breast Cancer and Their Integration into Decision-Support Algorithms. Critical Reviews in Clinical Laboratory Sciences. 2007;44(2):179-201.

[111] Hayes DF, Bast RC, Desch CE, Fritsche H, Kemeny NE, Jessup JM, et al. Tumor Marker Utility Grading System: a Framework to Evaluate Clinical Utility of Tumor Markers. Journal of the National Cancer Institute. 1996;88(20):1456-66.

[112] O'Grady P, Lijnen HR, Duffy MJ. Multiple Forms of Plasminogen Activator in Human Breast Tumors. Cancer Research. 1985;45(12 Part 1):6216-8.

[113] Duffy MJ, O'Grady P, Devaney D, O'Siorain L, Fennelly JJ, Lijnen HJ. Urokinase-plasminogen activator, a marker for aggressive breast carcinomas. Preliminary report. Cancer. 1988;62(3):531-3.

[114] Janicke F, Schmitt M, Ulm K, Gössner W, Graeff H. Urokinase-type plasminogen activator antigen and early relapse in breast cancer. The Lancet. 1989;334(8670):1049.

[115] Jänicke F, Schmitt M, Graeff H. Clinical Relevance of the Urokinase-Type and Tissue-Type Plasminogen Activators and of Their Type 1 Inhibitor in Breast Cancer. Semin Thromb Hemost. 1991;17(03):303-12.

[116] Harris L, Fritsche H, Mennel R, Norton L, Ravdin P, Taube S, et al. American Society of Clinical Oncology 2007 Update of Recommendations for the Use of Tumor Markers in Breast Cancer. Journal of Clinical Oncology. 2007;25(33):5287-312.

[117] Jänicke F, Pache L, Schmitt M, Ulm K, Thomssen C, Prechtl A, et al. Both the Cytosols and Detergent Extracts of Breast Cancer Tissues Are Suited to Evaluate the Prognostic Impact of the Urokinase-Type Plasminogen Activator and Its Inhibitor, Plasminogen Activator Inhibitor Type 1. Cancer Research. 1994;54(10):2527-30.

[118] Schmitt M, Sturmheit AS, Welk A, Schnelldorfer C, Harbeck N. Procedures for the quantitative protein determination of urokinase and its inhibitor, PAI-1, in human breast cancer tissue extracts by ELISA. Methods in molecular medicine. 2006;120:245-65.

[119] Thomssen C, Harbeck N, Dittmer J, Abraha-Spaeth SR, Papendick N, Paradiso A, et al. Feasibility of Measuring the Prognostic Factors uPA and PAI-1 in Core Needle Biopsy Breast Cancer Specimens. Journal of the National Cancer Institute. 2009;101(14): 1028-9.

[120] Jänicke F, Schmitt M, Hafter R, Hollrieder A, Babic R, Ulm K, et al. Urokinase-type plasminogen activator (u-PA) antigen is a predictor of early relapse in breast cancer. Fibrinolysis. 1990;4(2):69-78.

[121] Reilly D, Christensen L, Duch M, Nolan N, Duffy MJ, Andreasen PA. Type-1 plasminogen activator inhibitor in human breast carcinomas. Int J Cancer. 1992;50(2):208-14.

[122] Grebenchtchikov N, Maguire TM, Riisbro R, Geurts-Moespot A, O'Donovan N, Schmitt M, et al. Measurement of plasminogen activator system components in plasma and tumor tissue extracts obtained from patients with breast cancer: an EORTC Receptor and Biomarker Group collaboration. Oncology reports. 2005;14(1):235-9.

[123] Biermann JC, Holzscheiter L, Kotzsch M, Luther T, Kiechle-Bahat M, Sweep FC, et al. Quantitative RT-PCR assays for the determination of urokinase-type plasminogen activator and plasminogen activator inhibitor type 1 mRNA in primary tumor tissue of breast cancer patients: comparison to antigen quantification by ELISA. International journal of molecular medicine. 2008;21(2):251-9.

[124] Spyratos F, Bouchet C, Tozlu S, Labroquere M, Vignaud S, Becette V, et al. Prognostic value of uPA, PAI-1 and PAI-2 mRNA expression in primary breast cancer. Anticancer research. 2002;22(5):2997-3003.

[125] Lamy P-J, Verjat T, Servanton A-C, Paye M, Leissner P, Mougin B. Urokinase-type Plasminogen Activator and Plasminogen Activator Inhibitor Type-1 mRNA Assessment in Breast Cancer by Means of NASBA: Correlation With Protein Expression. American Journal of Clinical Pathology. 2007;128(3):404-13.

[126] Pakneshan P, Têtu B, Rabbani SA. Demethylation of urokinase promoter as a prognostic marker in patients with breast carcinoma. Clinical Cancer Research: 2004;10(9): 3035-41.

[127] Dublin E, Hanby A, Patel NK, Liebman R, Barnes D. Immunohistochemical Expression of uPA, uPAR, and PAI-1 in Breast Carcinoma: Fibroblastic Expression Has Strong Associations with Tumor Pathology. The American Journal of Pathology. 2000;157(4):1219-27.

[128] Illemann M, Bird N, Majeed A, Lærum OD, Lund LR, Danø K, et al. Two distinct expression patterns of urokinase, urokinase receptor and plasminogen activator inhibitor-1 in colon cancer liver metastases. International Journal of Cancer. 2009;124(8): 1860-70.

[129] Nielsen BS, Rank F, Illemann M, Lund LR, Danø K. Stromal cells associated with early invasive foci in human mammary ductal carcinoma in situ coexpress urokinase and urokinase receptor. International Journal of Cancer. 2007;120(10):2086-95.

[130] Jankun J, Merrick HW, Goldblatt PJ. Expression and localization of elements of the plasminogen activation system in benign breast disease and breast cancers. J Cell Biochem. 1993;53(2):135-44.

[131] Costantini V, Sidoni A, Deveglia R, Cazzato OA, Bellezza G, Ferri I, et al. Combined overexpression of urokinase, urokinase receptor, and plasminogen activator inhibi-

tor-1 is associated with breast cancer progression: an immunohistochemical comparison of normal, benign, and malignant breast tissues. Cancer. 1996;77(6):1079-88.

[132] Fisher JL, Field CL, Zhou H, Harris TL, Henderson MA, Choong PF. Urokinase plasminogen activator system gene expression is increased in human breast carcinoma and its bone metastases--a comparison of normal breast tissue, non-invasive and invasive carcinoma and osseous metastases. Breast cancer research and treatment. 2000;61(1):1-12.

[133] Rabbani SA, Gladu J. Urokinase receptor antibody can reduce tumor volume and detect the presence of occult tumor metastases in vivo. Cancer research. 2002;62(8): 2390-7.

[134] Yang L, Mao H, Cao Z, Wang YA, Peng X, Wang X, et al. Molecular Imaging of Pancreatic Cancer in an Animal Model Using Targeted Multifunctional Nanoparticles. Gastroenterology. 2009;136(5):1514-25.e2.

[135] Persson M, Madsen J, Østergaard S, Ploug M, Kjaer A. 68Ga-labeling and in vivo evaluation of a uPAR binding DOTA-and NODAGA-conjugated peptide for PET imaging of invasive cancers. Nuclear Medicine and Biology. 2012;39(4):560-9.

[136] Persson M, Rasmussen P, Madsen J, Ploug M, Kjaer A. New peptide receptor radionuclide therapy of invasive cancer cells: in vivo studies using 177Lu-DOTA-AE105 targeting uPAR in human colorectal cancer xenografts. Nuclear Medicine and Biology. 2012;39(7):962-9.

[137] Mortimer JE, Bading JR, Colcher DM, Conti PS, Frankel PH, Carroll MI, et al. Functional Imaging of Human Epidermal Growth Factor Receptor 2–Positive Metastatic Breast Cancer Using 64Cu-DOTA-Trastuzumab PET. Journal of Nuclear Medicine. 2014;55(1):23-9.

[138] DeNardo SJ, Kroger LA, DeNardo GL. A new era for radiolabeled antibodies in cancer? Current Opinion in Immunology. 1999;11(5):563-9.

[139] Massa S, Xavier C, De Vos J, Caveliers V, Lahoutte T, Muyldermans S, et al. Site-Specific Labeling of Cysteine-Tagged Camelid Single-Domain Antibody-Fragments for Use in Molecular Imaging. Bioconjugate Chemistry. 2014;25(5):979-88.

[140] Xu X, Cai Y, Wei Y, Donate F, Juarez J, Parry G, et al. Identification of a new epitope in uPAR as a target for the cancer therapeutic monoclonal antibody ATN-658, a structural homolog of the uPAR binding integrin CD11b (alphaM). PloS one. 2014;9(1):e85349.

[141] Rabbani SA, Harakidas P, Davidson DJ, Henkin J, Mazar AP. Prevention of prostate-cancer metastasisin vivo by a novel synthetic inhibitor of urokinase-type plasminogen activator (uPA). International Journal of Cancer. 1995;63(6):840-5.

[142] Goldstein LJ. Experience in Phase I Trials and an Upcoming Phase II Study with uPA Inhibitors in Metastatic Breast Cancer. Breast Care. 2008;3(Suppl. 2):25-8.

[143] Meyer JE, Brocks C, Graefe H, Mala C, Thäns N, Bürgle M, et al. The Oral Serine Protease Inhibitor WX-671 – First Experience in Patients with Advanced Head and Neck Carcinoma. Breast Care. 2008;3(Suppl. 2):20-4.

[144] Kobayashi H, Gotoh J, Fujie M, Shinohara H, Moniwa N, Terao T. Inhibition of metastasis of Lewis lung carcinoma by a synthetic peptide within growth factor-like domain of urokinase in the experimental and spontaneous metastasis model. Int J Cancer. 1994;57(5):727-33.

[145] Hu X-w, Duan H-f, Duan H-f, Pan S-y, Li Y-m, Xi Y, et al. Inhibition of tumor growth and metastasis by ATF-Fc, an engineered antibody targeting urokinase receptor. Cancer Biology & Therapy. 2008;7(5):651-9.

[146] Guo Y, Higazi AA-R, Arakelian A, Sachais BS, Cines D, Goldfarb RH, et al. A peptide derived from the nonreceptor binding region of urokinase plasminogen activator (uPA) inhibits tumor progression and angiogenesis and induces tumor cell death in vivo. The FASEB Journal. 2000;14(10):1400-10.

[147] Mishima K, Mazar AP, Gown A, Skelly M, Ji X-D, Wang X-D, et al. A peptide derived from the non-receptor-binding region of urokinase plasminogen activator inhibits glioblastoma growth and angiogenesis in vivo in combination with cisplatin. Proceedings of the National Academy of Sciences. 2000;97(15):8484-9.

[148] Gold MA, Brady WE, Lankes HA, Rose PG, Kelley JL, De Geest K, et al. A phase II study of a urokinase-derived peptide (A6) in the treatment of persistent or recurrent epithelial ovarian, fallopian tube, or primary peritoneal carcinoma: A Gynecologic Oncology Group study. Gynecologic Oncology. 2012;125(3):635-9.

[149] Scott AM, Wolchok JD, Old LJ. Antibody therapy of cancer. Nat Rev Cancer. 2012;12(4):278-87.

[150] Rabbani SA, Ateeq B, Arakelian A, Valentino ML, Shaw DE, Dauffenbach LM, et al. An anti-urokinase plasminogen activator receptor antibody (ATN-658) blocks prostate cancer invasion, migration, growth, and experimental skeletal metastasis in vitro and in vivo. Neoplasia. 2010;12(10):778-88.

[151] Kenny HA, Leonhardt P, Ladanyi A, Yamada SD, Montag A, Im HK, et al. Targeting the Urokinase Plasminogen Activator Receptor Inhibits Ovarian Cancer Metastasis. Clinical Cancer Research. 2011;17(3):459-71.

[152] Gondi CS, Rao JS. Therapeutic Potential of siRNA-mediated Targeting of Urokinase Plasminogen Activator, Its Receptor, and Matrix Metalloproteinases. In: Sioud M, editor. siRNA and miRNA Gene Silencing. Methods in Molecular Biology. 487: Humana Press; 2009. p. 1-15.

[153] Zhou H, Tang Y, Liang X, Yang X, Yang J, Zhu G, et al. RNAi targeting urokinase-type plasminogen activator receptor inhibits metastasis and progression of oral squamous cell carcinoma in vivo. International Journal of Cancer. 2009;125(2):453-62.

[154] Meryet-Figuières M, Resina S, Lavigne C, Barlovatz-Meimon G, Lebleu B, Thierry AR. Inhibition of PAI-1 expression in breast cancer carcinoma cells by siRNA at nanomolar range. Biochimie. 2007;89(10):1228-33.

[155] Blake CM, Sullenger BA, Lawrence DA, Fortenberry YM. Antimetastatic potential of PAI-1-specific RNA aptamers. Oligonucleotides. 2009;19(2):117-28.

[156] D'Alessio S, Margheri F, Pucci M, Del Rosso A, Monia BP, Bologna M, et al. Antisense oligodeoxynucleotides for urokinase-plasminogen activator receptor have anti-invasive and anti-proliferative effects in vitro and inhibit spontaneous metastases of human melanoma in mice. International Journal of Cancer. 2004;110(1):125-33.

[157] Gondi CS, Kandhukuri N, Dinh DH, Gujrati M, Rao JS. Down-regulation of uPAR and uPA activates caspase-mediated apoptosis and inhibits the PI3K/AKT pathway. International journal of oncology. 2007;31(1):19-27.

[158] Knör S, Sato S, Huber T, Morgenstern A, Bruchertseifer F, Schmitt M, et al. Development and evaluation of peptidic ligands targeting tumour-associated urokinase plasminogen activator receptor (uPAR) for use in α-emitter therapy for disseminated ovarian cancer. Eur J Nucl Med Mol Imaging. 2008;35(1):53-64. English.

[159] Rajagopal V, Kreitman RJ. Recombinant Toxins That Bind to the Urokinase Receptor Are Cytotoxic without Requiring Binding to the α2-Macroglobulin Receptor. Journal of Biological Chemistry. 2000;275(11):7566-73.

[160] Kounnas MZ, Morris RE, Thompson MR, FitzGerald DJ, Strickland DK, Saelinger CB. The alpha 2-macroglobulin receptor/low density lipoprotein receptor-related protein binds and internalizes Pseudomonas exotoxin A. Journal of Biological Chemistry. 1992;267(18):12420-3.

[161] Huang J, Li Y, Massague J, Sicheneder A, Vallera D, Hall W. Intracerebral infusion of the bispecific targeted toxin DTATEGF in a mouse xenograft model of a human metastatic non-small cell lung cancer. J Neurooncol. 2012;109(2):229-38.

[162] Maeda H, Wu J, Sawa T, Matsumura Y, Hori K. Tumor vascular permeability and the EPR effect in macromolecular therapeutics: a review. Journal of Controlled Release. 2000;65(1–2):271-84.

[163] Binder BR, Mihaly J. The plasminogen activator inhibitor "paradox" in cancer. Immunology Letters. 2008;118(2):116-24.

[164] Bajou K, Noel A, Gerard RD, Masson V, Brunner N, Holst-Hansen C, et al. Absence of host plasminogen activator inhibitor 1 prevents cancer invasion and vascularization. Nat Med. 1998;4(8):923-8.

[165] Romer MU, Larsen L, Offenberg H, Brunner N, Lademann UA. Plasminogen activator inhibitor 1 protects fibrosarcoma cells from etoposide-induced apoptosis through activation of the PI3K/Akt cell survival pathway. Neoplasia. 2008;10(10):1083-91.

[166] Mathiasen L, Dupont DM, Christensen A, Blouse GE, Jensen JK, Gils A, et al. A Peptide Accelerating the Conversion of Plasminogen Activator Inhibitor-1 to an Inactive Latent State. Molecular Pharmacology. 2008;74(3):641-53.

[167] Hennan JK, Elokdah H, Leal M, Ji A, Friedrichs GS, Morgan GA, et al. Evaluation of PAI-039 [{1-Benzyl-5-[4-(trifluoromethoxy)phenyl]-1H-indol-3-yl}(oxo)acetic Acid], a Novel Plasminogen Activator Inhibitor-1 Inhibitor, in a Canine Model of Coronary Artery Thrombosis. Journal of Pharmacology and Experimental Therapeutics. 2005;314(2):710-6.

[168] Dupont DM, Madsen JB, Kristensen T, Bodker JS, Blouse GE, Wind T, et al. Biochemical properties of plasminogen activator inhibitor-1. Frontiers in bioscience (Landmark edition). 2009;14:1337-61.

[169] Madsen JB, Dupont DM, Andersen TB, Nielsen AF, Sang L, Brix DM, et al. RNA Aptamers as Conformational Probes and Regulatory Agents for Plasminogen Activator Inhibitor-1. Biochemistry. 2010;49(19):4103-15.

8

Relationship of Breast Cancer with Ovarian Cancer

Ayşe Çelik, Muradiye Acar, Catherine Moroski Erkul, Esra Gunduz and Mehmet Gunduz

1. Introduction

Cancer is perhaps the cruelest of deadly diseases in our era. So many factors play a role in cancer and these features were characterized in 2011 as belonging to eight categories: evasion of apoptosis, excessive growth signalling, insensitivity to anti-growth signals, maintained angiogenesis, endless replicative potential, metastasis, reprogramming of energy metabolism and avoidance of immune destruction. Types of cancer may be put in different categories (or combinations of these) according to symptoms and pathogenesis, therefore revealing many relationships.

Breast cancer is the most commonly diagnosed cancer type among women. There are similarities between breast and ovarian cancer such as similar mutations (tumor suppressors, protooncoges), changes in hormone regulation and microenvironment, etc. In 2014, approximately 235,030 new cases are expected, and it is estimated that 40,430 deaths from breast cancer will occur. Also, an estimated 21,980 new cases of ovarian cancer will be diagnosed in 2014, with an estimated 14,270 deaths. Statistical results and similarities raise the question of whether metastasis of breast cancer is related to the occurrence of ovarian cancer.

Several mutations in growth control genes can trigger the development of tumors in the body. The specific causes of the mutations that lead to cancer are not fully known. Recent studies have tried to uncover these unknown relationships between breast and ovarian cancer. Understanding of the correlations between different types of cancers provide knowledge to us about the disease process. Recent studies focus on common mutations, tumor microenvironment, receptor inactivation, Trastuzumab resistance, etc. Thanks to these studies, new therapeutic techniques have been developed such as using miRNA as therapeutic targets or improvement of nanodrug delivery systems. Also, mathematical modeling has been used in attempts to understand changes in metabolic pathways and metastasis.

Briefly, understanding of the associations between breast and ovarian cancers provide opportunities for the prevention of metastasis and allow development of new ways to cure cancer.

2. Hereditary Breast and Ovarian Cancer (HBOC)

Despite intense studies about breast and ovarian cancer, these cancer types are the most significant cause of death in women in our century. Recent studies have tried to identify different types of mutations for certain genes and determine changes in copy numbers, expression profiles, etc. by using high-throughput technologies [1]. Identifying variations among breast and ovarian cancers will hopefully uncover associations between them, thus possibly revealing methods for early disease screening and allow understanding of the mechanism(s) of metastasis between these two cancer types.

Several studies have continued to find a common point for breast and ovarian cancer; all studies have defined certain mutations in BRCA1/BRCA2 for these types of cancer. The statistics show that 60-80% of BRCA1/BRCA2 gene mutation carriers will develop breast cancer and 20-40% will develop ovarian cancer. Some cases of HBOC indicate a connection with constitutive epimutations or other susceptibility genes such as several gene clusters including the Fanconi anemia (FA) cluster (FANCD2, FANCA and FANCC), mismatch repair (MMR) cluster (MLH1, MSH2, PMS1, PMS2 and MSH6), NA repair cluster (ATM, ATR and CHK1/2), and tumor suppressor cluster (TP53, SKT11 and PTEN). If a patient does not have any mutations in the BRCA genes but their cancer has a phenotype characteristic of those with BRCA mutations and a dysfunction in a DNA repair system, it is known as 'BRCAness';[1]. In conclusion,mutations that occur in some DNA repair mechanisms can increase the risk of developing breast and ovarian cancer.

3. Identification of high penetrance of genes

The inactivation of BRCA1 and BRCA2 genes are germline mutations and trigger breast and ovarian cancer. This phenomenon was confirmed by high throughput technologies used for molecular diagnostics such as next generation sequencing (NGS). By using NGS, the DNA of 59 patients harbouring SNVs that include indels or large genomic rearrangements of BRCA1 or BRCA2 was analyzed. Also, 168 patients were used as blind study to compare NGS versus Sanger sequencing or MLPA analyses of BRCA1 and BRCA2. Then, by using three different capture methods, 708 consecutive patients were monitored. A total of 69 deleterious germline alterations within BRCA1 and BRCA2, and 4 TP53 mutations were detected in 468 patients. In addition to this, 36 variations that include either a premature codon stop or a splicing defect among other genes were found (*5/708 in CHEK2, 3/708 in RAD51C, 1/708 in RAD50, 7/708 in PALB2, 3/708 in MRE11A, 5/708 in ATM, 3/708 in NBS1, 1/708 in CDH1, 3/468 in MSH2, 2/468 in PMS2, 1/708 in BARD1, 1/468 in PMS1 and 1/468 in MLH3)*. This study shows the efficiency of NGS in performing molecular diagnosis of HBOC [2].

In the past, full coding exon sequencing was challenging, because researchers had to analyse dozens of coding genes using the traditional method of Sanger sequencing. It is a very time consuming and labor intensive method. Thus, complicated genetic analysis was not possible. However, new techniques have made such research easy. Also, parallel sequencing allows for complicated genetic analysis in a short time. This technique is now reliable for genomic research, but applying this in the clinic is still difficult due to the requirement of complex equipment and highly trained staff [3]. In clinical applications, several library preparation methods have been used to demonstrate a novel capture method. Targeting coding sequences of genes have high coverage in every captured region. In order to streamline the number of germline mutation variants, further whole exon sequencing studies and confirmations are required in order to provide a gold standard for the investigation of germline variants.Nowadays, clinical decisions that include molecular diagnoses have a significant impact on the determination of treatments such as chemotherapy and prophylactic surgery. The association between breast and ovarian cancer try to depend on high or low penetrance of genes that are observable in both cancer types. The most common susceptibility genes in this field are BRCA1/ BRCA2. If any mutations are present in either of these genes, it translates to a 60-85% lifetime risk of developing breast or ovarian cancer [4].

Germline mutations in BRCA1 and BRCA2 can be inherited by offspring and thus are known as constitutional mutations. The mutations may have complete or partial gene deletions, large insertions, duplications, splicing, frameshifts, missense and nonsense mutations. Insertions and deletions may occur at the same position in the sequence and induce gene shuffling, which in turn leads to abnormal gene structure, function,etc. The rate of these mutations changes from population to population. According to data from the Breast Cancer Information Core website, approximately 3500 mutations have been reported for both genes. For instance, female breast cancer patients of Ashkenazi Jewish descent have a 10 – 12 % frequency of mutations in these genes. Frequency of this mutation is higher than in the rest of the Caucasian population, because the female Ashkenazi Jewish population harbors ancient BRCA1 / BRCA 2 mutant alleles. The 5266dup, BRCA2999del5 and BRCA1delexon17 mutations have been defined in some populations such as Slavic, Finnish, Icelandic and German [4].

In addition, the penetrance of mutations is important for genomic rearrangements to develop into a detectable trait. Detection of high penetrance genes is easier than lower ones, because they form symptoms and are always apparent in an individual carrying the allele. However, several variations in low penetrance alleles are more common, and these low penetrance alleles could increase risk to develop cancer and its progression [5]. Some researchers have focused on identification of new genes to explain the missing heritability in BRCA negative cancer patients, including targeted genes that may interact with BRCA pathways and proteins.

Nowadays, several studies have focused on finding these candidate genes and mutations using NGS technologies. According to these studies, additional high penetrance alleles have been found for breast/ovarian cancers; for instance, TP53, STK11,etc. Also, moderate penetrance alleles such as PALB2, BRIP1, RAD51C have a role in cancer via their alteration in pathways like Fanconi Anemia [6],[7]. In addition, ATM and CHEK2 have the same penetrance level and are involved in the homologous recombination repair pathway [8]. Detection of mutations and penetrance within genes other than BRCA1 and BRCA2 has shed light on the genetic heterogeneity of HBOC.

3.1. BRCA1 and BRCA2 genes

BRCA1 and BRCA2 genes are expressed in epithelial cells of breast and ovarian tissues. They regulate the repair of some types of DNA damage and are involved in cell fate decision; if DNA damage is too excessive and cannot be repaired efficiently, the cell will be directed to be destroyed. Briefly, BRCA1 and BRCA2 genes are tumor supressor genes that are essential in homologous recombination repair of double strand breaks [9], [10]. If any mutations or damage occurs in BRCA1/BRCA2, DNA damage cannot be properly repaired and this increases the risk of developing breast cancer [11]. However, BRCA1/2 are not oncogenes.They are normal but their mutations are abnormal and cause formation of breast cancer. Chromosomal arrangements may result from errors in the DNA damage response mechanism. It might lead to genomic instability. If genomic rearrangements are large, they may escape detection. The problem is that standard genetic testing is not capable of identifying large rearrangements and therefore next generation and whole exon sequencing technologies must be used to detect these gene modifications/changes [12].

Some studies have focused on solving the mechanisms of BRCA1 and BRCA2. According to biochemical, genetic and cytological studies, the lack of BRCA1 results in cell death because BRCA1 regulates stem/progenitor cell proliferation and differentiation. Apicobasal polarity is regulated by BRCA1 and RHAMM (hyaluronan-mediated motility receptor), AURKA (aurora kinase A) and TPX2 (microtubule-associated, homolog). This gene complex can change the miotic spindle promoting activity of RHAMM which may control tumor progression. In addition to this, BRCA1 binds and regulates AURKA which plays a role in the cell cycle as a kinase and appears to be strongly involved in centrosome regulation. Therefore, variations of the AURKA gene may contribute to breast cancer progression [13]. BRCA1 causes an accumulation of TPX2 and is required for mitotic spindle- pole assembly. Not only DNA damage response and repair, but also cell differentiation requires the BRCA core complex proteins for functional integrity.

BRCA1 interacting protein or complex	Function of interacting protein	Interacting domain(a.a. residues)	Ref.
RAD51	DSB repair	Exon 11 (758-1064)	[14]
RAD50	DSB repair	Exon 11(341- 748)	[15]
BRCA2	DSB repair	BRCT domain (1314-1863)	[14]
BASC (QTM,BLM,MSH2,MSH6,MLH1,RCF)	Mismatch repair	BRCA part of complex	[16]
p53	Transcription Factor, tumor supressor	Exon 11 and BRCT domain (224 – 500 and 1760-1863)	[17], [18]

BRCA1 interacting protein or complex	Function of interacting protein	Interacting domain(a.a. residues)	Ref.
pRB	Cell cycle regulator	Exon 11 and BRCT domain (304-394 and 15336-1863)	[19]
c-Myc	TF,oncogene	N-terminus and exon11 (175-303 and 433-511)	[20]
ZBRK1	TF,represses GADD45	Exon 11 (341-748)	[21]
ATF	TF	RING (1-101)	[22]
STAT1	Signal transducer,TF	Exon 11(502-802)	[23]
E2F	TF, cell cycle regulator	N-terminus (1-76)	[24]
RNA Pol II holoenzyme *(RPH)	Transcription	BRCT domain (1650-1800)	[25], [26]
RNA helicase A	Component of RPH	BRCT domain (1650-1800)	[27]
Estrogen receptor	Ligand responsive TF	N-terminus (1-300)	[28, 29]
Androgen receptor	Ligand responsive TF	Exon 11;BRCT domain (758-1064 and 1314-1863)	[30]
CtIP	Transcriptional co-repressor	BRCT domain (1651-1863)	[31, 32]
p300/CBP	Transcriptional coactivator	RING and BRCT domain (1-303 and 1314-1863)	[33]
HDAC1 and 2	Histone deacetylation; chromation remodeling	BRCT domain (1563 - 1863)	[34]
Centrosome (p53,Prb,Nm23)	Chromosome segregation	*BRCA1 part of the complex	[35]
BRAP2	Cytoplasmic retention	NLS (303-701)	[36]
Vasolin- containing protein, VCP	ATPase	Exon 11 (303- 625)	[37]
BARD1	Ubiquitination	RING (1-101)	[38]
BAP1	Deubiquitinating enzyme	RING (1-100)	[39]
Importin α	Nuclear transport	NLS (303-701)	[40]
BRCA2 interacting protein or complex	-	Interacting domain (a.a. residues) on BRCA2	[41]

Table 1. BRCA interacting proteins

Many biochemical studies have shed light on a multitude of proteins with defined interactions with BRCA1 and BRCA2. These proteins are involved in control mechanisms of DNA double strand breaks. Within several minutes after damage, H2AX, a member of the histone H2A family of proteins, becomes phosphorylated and foci form at the site of DNA double strand breaks [42]. BRCA1 is recruited with this area within several hours. Subsequently, RAD50 and RAD51 interact with the strand breaks. This situation shows that BRCA1 and H2AX can initiate repair mechanisms of local chromatin structure, thus DNA repair proteins can access damaged sites.

If BRCA1 and BRCA2 genes are absent from the cell, chromosomal abnormalities, breaks, aneuploidy and centrosome amplification occurs. The pathogenic tumor formation in breast and ovarian tissue may depend on chromosomal instability that is the result of deficiency of BRCA1 and BRCA2 genes. In order to reveal this relation, researchers monitored sporadic breast and ovarian tumors. 50 – 70 % of them were found to have lost an BRCA1 allele and 30 – 50 % were found to have lost an BRCA2 allele [43],[44].

Genomic instability of BRCA1 and BRCA2 genes result from the repetitive DNA elements that are of high density. 42% of BRCA1 consists of Alu sequences and 5% non-Alu repeats. The genomic region of BRCA2 consists of 47% repetitive DNA [45]. BRCA1 and BRCA2 are rare genes that include high density repetitive DNA regions. Multiple diseases are mediated by genetic rearrangements of Alu sequences. According to the given density of repeat elements in BRCA1 and BRCA2, careful analysis of these genes can reveal the risk of breast and ovarian cancer due to these susceptibility genes.

The source of the large deletions depends on repetitive regions on genes. One mechanism that manages the large deletions observed around the BRCA1 and BRCA2 that are inherited and sporadic tumors in breast and ovarian cancer (Figure1). These repeat regions may be far apart from the linear DNA but physically close in the nucleus. For instance, if a chromosome break occurs near a replication fork during replication, it might be repaired by HR to a replication fork at a nearby anchorage point.

3.2. Association between DNA damage and BRCA1-BRCA2 genes

Double strand breaks such as exposure to ionizing radiation or certain kinds of DNA-damaging agents. Genetic defects in DNA damage response genes and/or down-regulation of the DNA repair mechanisms induces genomic instability, and this can lead to carcinogenesis [46]. Among the many DNA repair pathways available in mammalian cells are homologous repair, non-homologous end-joining and single-strand annealing [47]. There are several ways that cells can repair double strand breaks. A number of signaling pathways are involved in the detection of DSBs and regulate DNA repair or apoptotic cell death. The main DNA damage recognition molecule is ATM [48], a checkpoint kinase that phosphorylates a number of proteins in response to DNA damage, including p53 and BRCA1 [Figure2].

p53 plays a critical role in preventing cancer development. Generally, p53 gene is mutated in cancer tissue, so it cannot protect the genetic integrity of cells. In physiological conditions, p53 is activated when DNA damage occurs. The failure of DNA damage response results in p53

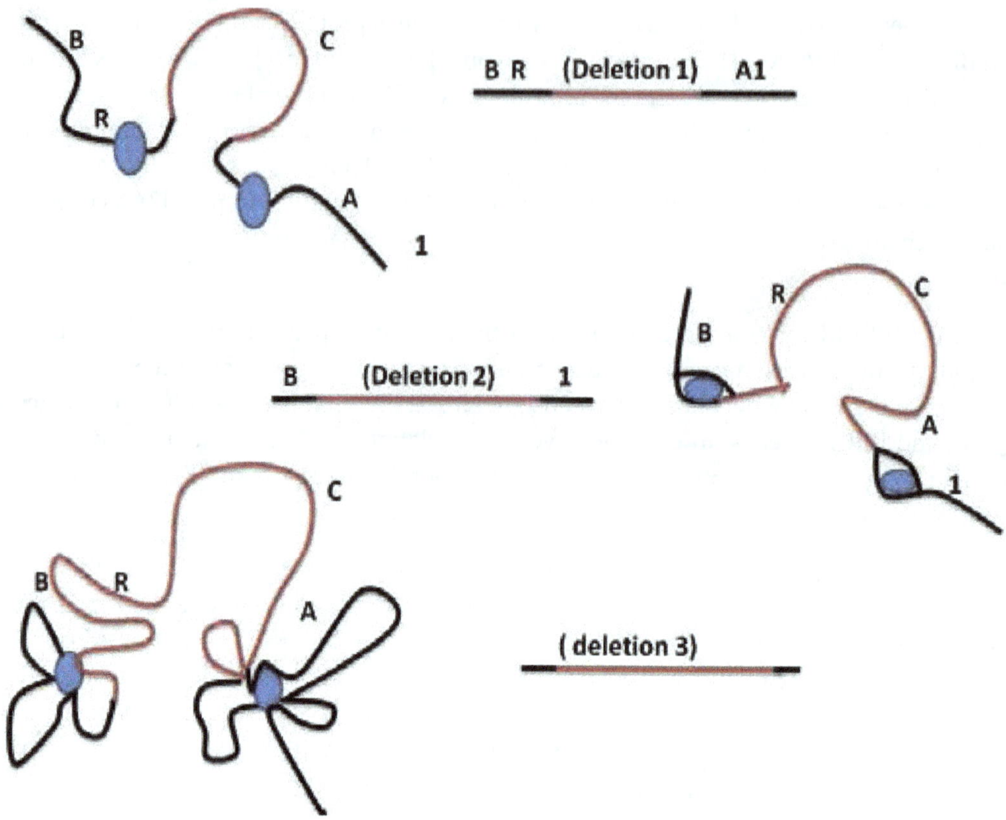

Figure 1. A mechanism for the formation of deletion by loss of a chromatin loop at different stages. Deletions of phase 1 occur in S phase, when the same repetitive sequences are physically brought together by MAR (blue ellipse). Breaks in DNA, and their repair, might lead to deletion of a chromatin loop (red). Deletions of type 2 and 3 occur by the same mechanism but occur later during DNA synthesis in the replication cycle. (Adapted from Piri et al [11])

mediated cell apoptosis [49]. Several mechanisms regulate p53 activity. p21WAF-1 has been shown to play an important role in both p53-dependent [50] and -independent pathways [51]. p21WAF-1 prevents cell cycle progression via interaction with the cyclin-dependent kinase (CDK) complex. Therefore, p53 plays a role in the most important part of providing stability to the genome by using cell cycle checkpoints, DNA repair and apoptosis.

BRCA1 also involves a gold standard for a tumor suppressor gene that is needed to prevent cancer development and progression. BRCA1 / BRCA2 related breast and ovarian cancers are have defects in a DNA repair pathway [52]. Studies have shed light on the functional roles of BRCA1/BRCA2 genes in DNA repair, cell cycle checkpoints and DNA damage signaling pathways [53]. BRCA1 interacts with several cyclins and CDKs, triggers the activation of the CDK inhibitor, p21WAF-1, and p53, thus it can control the cell cycle. The main function of BRCA1 depends on its phosphorylation status, so if the gene becomes hyper-phosphorylated following any damage or exposure to DNA damaging agents, it becomes non-functional[54].

Also, BRCA1 and BRCA2 genes are not only responsible for DNA damage response but also their proteins interact with the estrogen and androgen receptors [55]. These genes inhibit

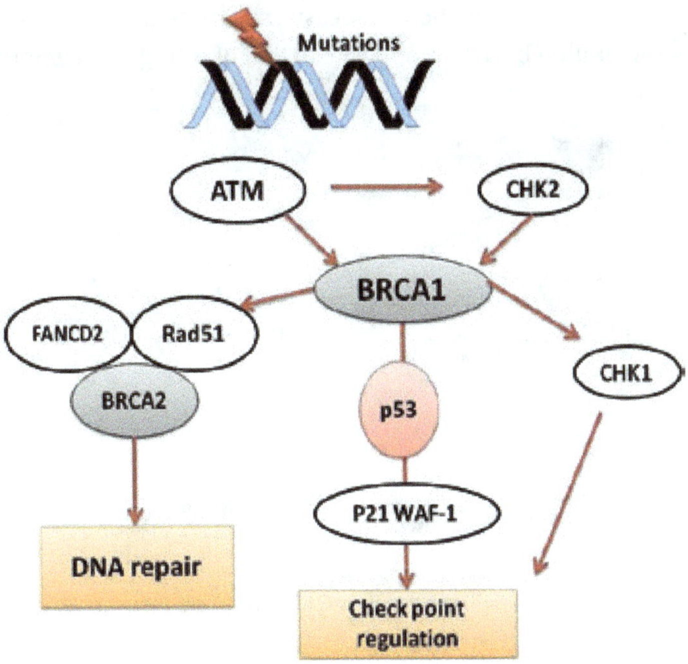

Figure 2. Schematic representation and overview of the DNA repair and checkpoint regulation of cell cycle

estrogen receptor-α activity and stimulate androgen receptors. In this way, BRCA1 mutations are associated with hormone responsive cancer. In other words, the cancer risk of BRCA1 mutation carriers will increase via hormonal factors.

3.3. Association of estrogens — Estrogen receptors with BRCA genes

Estrogen, progesterone and androgen hormones control the initiation of carcinogenesis by using special hormone receptors. Moreover, hormonal therapies frequently regulate hormone-mediated diseases such as cancer. A number of candidate genes have been identified as biomarkers for ovarian and breast cancers [56].

Frequently, damage in the DNA repair system induce growth arrest and cell death. BRCA deficient mice die in the early stages of embryogenesis. The first question that arises is why BRCA deficient breast or ovarian epithelial cells develop tumors instead of undergoing apoptosis? What is special to breast and ovarian epithelial cells that allows them to escape apoptosis or response to the DNA damage response system? Finally, how are BRCA1 and BRCA2 genes associated with estrogen levels?

The transition of the hormone independence induces the progression of breast and ovarian cancer because of DNA repair defects. The estrogen-bound receptor dimerizes and associates with chromatin. The estrogen response elements that are present on a DNA sequence motif bind directly to the receptor dimers. There are two kind of estrogen receptors:estrogen receptor-α and estrogen receptor-β. Estrogen receptor-α plays a role in proliferation, and the activation of estrogen receptor-β controls apoptosis [57]. An increase in estrogen receptor-β levels might be related with a reduction in breast cancer risk [58]. Estrogen receptor-β may prevent cellular proliferation by action opposite to that of estrogen receptor-α.

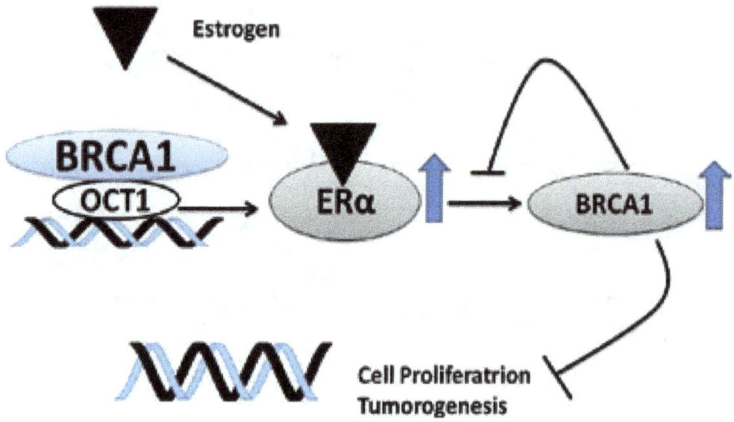

Figure 3. Schematic representation of interaction between BRCA1 and estrogen receptor (ER)-α

A woman exposed to estrogen either endogenously or exogenously, has an increased risk of developing breast or ovarian cancer. BRCA1 and BRCA2 expression levels are highest during pregnancy and puberty, when estrogen levels are increased [59].

If estrogens triggers cell proliferation [60], increased estrogens promotes the probability of developing random genetic rearrangements and errors. Metabolic processes produce reactive oxygen species (ROS) that cause oxidative damage to genomic DNA. In addition, some hormone oxidative metabolites catalyzed by cytochrome p450 enzymes can form unstable adducts in DNA which then leads to mutations [61].

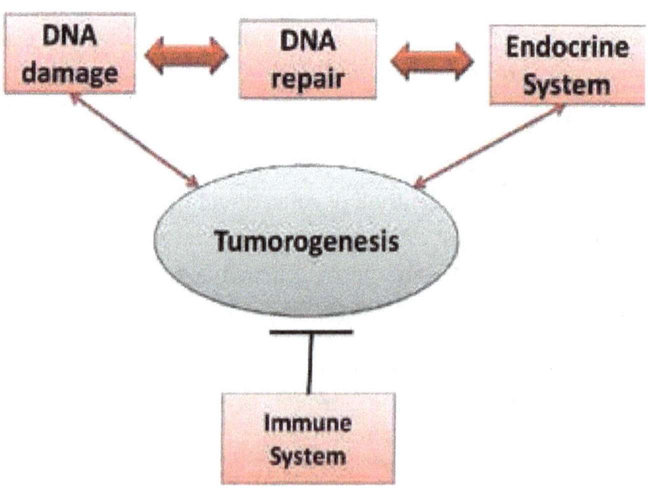

Figure 4. Connection of the hormone endocrine, immune, DNA damage and DNA repair systems in cancer

A long period of exposure to estrogen is strongly associated with an increased risk of developing breast and ovarian cancer. However, activation of DNA damage response mechanisms may be triggered via androgen signaling [62]. The estrogen receptor-mediated pathways are inhibited by BRCA1 and BRCA2 proteins which function as a suppressor in mammary epithelial cell proliferation. Also, the estrogen receptor complex regulates the transcription of BRCA1 and BRCA2 under the condition of estrogen stimulation. In addition, estrogens are not only essential for mammary growth and differentiation, but also enhance the activity of the p53 tumor suppressor protein [63].

4. Biomarkers in breast and ovarian cancer

4.1. The KRAS-variant (A germline microRNA binding site-disrupting variant)

Cancer susceptibility genes increase the risk of malignancy as a result of mutations in tumor suppressor or oncogenes that control different pathways. The KRAS variants are active at the site of the 3′-untranslated region of the complementary site of let-7 miRNA. miRNAs are 22-nucleotide long noncoding RNAs that are conserved regions. They are a novel class of oncogenes and tumor supressors that are upregulated in cancers [64]. Recent studies showed that SNPs that are present in miRNA binding sites can be powerful markers of cancer risk [65]. Ratner et al. reported that KRAS is associated with 61% of cases of breast and ovarian cancer syndrome. In another study, KRAS variants were observed to be increased within women with triple-negative breast cancer [66]. A study at Yale University, involving 58 hereditary breast and ovarian syndrome patients tested for the presence of the KRAS variant. The KRAS-variant was identified in 60% of HBOC patients who lacked BRCA1 or BRCA2 mutations. These findings strongly support the hypothesis that the KRAS-variant is a genetic marker of an increased risk of developing ovarian cancer[67].

The KRAS variant might be a new biomarker for breast and ovarian cancer. Therefore, preventing or identifying cancer in early steps may be possible by using this biomarker.

4.2. Flap Endonuclease 1 (FEN1) as a biomarker in breast and ovarian cancer

FEN1 is a kind of flap structure endonuclease that is critical for DNA repair processing. It is involved in long patch base excision repair (LP-BER) and Okazaki fragment maturation during replication. In addition, it plays a role in rescue delayed in replication forks, managing of telomere stability and apoptotic formation of DNA [68] [69]. Fen1 is also a main actor in posttranslational modifications such as acetylation, phosphorylation, sumoylation, methylation and ubiquitylation which control nuclease activities [68] [69].

FEN1 has a role in tumor formation. A FEN1 E160D mutant mouse model shows alteration in DNA repair [70] [71]. These changes trigger an increased frequency of cancer development. Polymorphic variations of FEN1 in humans may be associated with high frequency cancer susceptibility [72, 73].

FEN1 has an impact on breast tumors. It affects BRCA1, PARP1, XRCC1 and TOP2A genes. There is an association between high FEN1 and ATM expression. FEN1 may regulate the ER-induced transcriptional response with interaction of estrogen response elements [74]. There is a complex network between ER, FEN1 and ATM in breast cancer cells. Similarly, in ovarian cancer, FEN1 expression is linked to an aggressive phenotype and poor survival [75]. Abdel-Fatah et al. demonstrated that FEN1 overexpression is associated with an aggressive phenotype and poor survival in breast and ovarian cancer.

5. Conclusion

Despite the more intense studies about breast and ovarian cancer, these cancer types are the most significant cause of death in women in our century. Recent studies have tried to streamline the number of mutations for specific genes and identify changes in copy number, expression profiles, etc. by using high-throughput technologies for identification of variations. Identification of all kinds of variations will uncover associations between breast and ovarian cancer, and thus reveal potential disease screening methods and provide an understanding of the mechanism of metastasis between these two cancer types. In this chapter, we aimed to gather the current knowledge about susceptibility genes BRCA1 and BRCA2 which are highly connected with breast and ovarian cancer. Also, mechanisms and hormones (estrogen) that induce cancer associated with BRCA1/BRCA2 have been discussed. Finally, new biomarkers including FEN1 and KRAS for breast and ovarian cancer have been discussed.

Author details

Ayşe Çelik, Muradiye Acar, Catherine Moroski Erkul, Esra Gunduz and Mehmet Gunduz*

*Address all correspondence to: mehmet.gunduz@gmail.com

Department of Medical Genetics, Faculty Of Medicine, Turgut Ozal University, Ankara, Turkey

References

[1] Wooster, R. and B.L. Weber, *Breast and ovarian cancer.* N Engl J Med, 2003. 348(23): p. 2339-47.

[2] Castera, L., et al., *Next-generation sequencing for the diagnosis of hereditary breast and ovarian cancer using genomic capture targeting multiple candidate genes.* Eur J Hum Genet, 2014.

[3] Need, A.C., et al., *Clinical application of exome sequencing in undiagnosed genetic conditions.* J Med Genet, 2012. 49(6): p. 353-61.

[4] Dillenburg, C.V., et al., *Prevalence of 185delAG and 5382insC mutations in BRCA1, and 6174delT in BRCA2 in women of Ashkenazi Jewish origin in southern Brazil.* Genet Mol Biol, 2012. 35(3): p. 599-602.

[5] Levy-Lahad, E. and E. Friedman, *Cancer risks among BRCA1 and BRCA2 mutation carriers.* Br J Cancer, 2007. 96(1): p. 11-5.

[6] Catucci, I., et al., *Germline mutations in BRIP1 and PALB2 in Jewish high cancer risk families.* Fam Cancer, 2012. 11(3): p. 483-91.

[7] Gracia-Aznarez, F.J., et al., *Whole exome sequencing suggests much of non-BRCA1/BRCA2 familial breast cancer is due to moderate and low penetrance susceptibility alleles.* PLoS One, 2013. 8(2): p. e55681.

[8] Weischer, M., et al., *CHEK2*1100delC heterozygosity in women with breast cancer associated with early death, breast cancer-specific death, and increased risk of a second breast cancer.* J Clin Oncol, 2012. 30(35): p. 4308-16.

[9] Duncan, J.A., J.R. Reeves, and T.G. Cooke, *BRCA1 and BRCA2 proteins: roles in health and disease.* Mol Pathol, 1998. 51(5): p. 237-47.

[10] Yoshida, K. and Y. Miki, *Role of BRCA1 and BRCA2 as regulators of DNA repair, transcription, and cell cycle in response to DNA damage.* Cancer Sci, 2004. 95(11): p. 866-71.

[11] *Breast and Ovarian Cancer Genetic Screening.* Palo Alto Medical Foundation, 4 October 2008.

[12] Ewald, I.P., et al., *Genomic rearrangements in BRCA1 and BRCA2: A literature review.* Genet Mol Biol, 2009. 32(3): p. 437-46.

[13] Ruan, Y., et al., *Genetic polymorphisms in AURKA and BRCA1 are associated with breast cancer susceptibility in a Chinese Han population.* J Pathol, 2011. 225(4): p. 535-43.

[14] Scully, R., et al., *Association of BRCA1 with Rad51 in mitotic and meiotic cells.* Cell, 1997. 88(2): p. 265-75.

[15] Zhong, Q., et al., *Association of BRCA1 with the hRad50-hMre11-p95 complex and the DNA damage response.* Science, 1999. 285(5428): p. 747-50.

[16] Wang, Y., et al., *BASC, a super complex of BRCA1-associated proteins involved in the recognition and repair of aberrant DNA structures.* Genes Dev, 2000. 14(8): p. 927-39.

[17] Zhang, H., et al., *BRCA1 physically associates with p53 and stimulates its transcriptional activity.* Oncogene, 1998. 16(13): p. 1713-21.

[18] Chai, Y.L., et al., *The second BRCT domain of BRCA1 proteins interacts with p53 and stimulates transcription from the p21WAF1/CIP1 promoter.* Oncogene, 1999. 18(1): p. 263-8.

[19] Aprelikova, O.N., et al., *BRCA1-associated growth arrest is RB-dependent.* Proc Natl Acad Sci U S A, 1999. 96(21): p. 11866-71.

[20] Wang, Q., et al., *BRCA1 binds c-Myc and inhibits its transcriptional and transforming activity in cells.* Oncogene, 1998. 17(15): p. 1939-48.

[21] Zheng, L., et al., *Sequence-specific transcriptional corepressor function for BRCA1 through a novel zinc finger protein, ZBRK1.* Mol Cell, 2000. 6(4): p. 757-68.

[22] Houvras, Y., et al., *BRCA1 physically and functionally interacts with ATF1.* J Biol Chem, 2000. 275(46): p. 36230-7.

[23] Ouchi, T., et al., *Collaboration of signal transducer and activator of transcription 1 (STAT1) and BRCA1 in differential regulation of IFN-gamma target genes.* Proc Natl Acad Sci U S A, 2000. 97(10): p. 5208-13.

[24] Wang, H., et al., *BRCA1 proteins are transported to the nucleus in the absence of serum and splice variants BRCA1a, BRCA1b are tyrosine phosphoproteins that associate with E2F, cyclins and cyclin dependent kinases.* Oncogene, 1997. 15(2): p. 143-57.

[25] Scully, R., et al., *BRCA1 is a component of the RNA polymerase II holoenzyme.* Proc Natl Acad Sci U S A, 1997. 94(11): p. 5605-10.

[26] Schlegel, B.P., et al., *BRCA1 interaction with RNA polymerase II reveals a role for hRPB2 and hRPB10alpha in activated transcription.* Proc Natl Acad Sci U S A, 2000. 97(7): p. 3148-53.

[27] Anderson, S.F., et al., *BRCA1 protein is linked to the RNA polymerase II holoenzyme complex via RNA helicase A.* Nat Genet, 1998. 19(3): p. 254-6.

[28] Fan, S., et al., *BRCA1 inhibition of estrogen receptor signaling in transfected cells.* Science, 1999. 284(5418): p. 1354-6.

[29] Fan, S., et al., *Role of direct interaction in BRCA1 inhibition of estrogen receptor activity.* Oncogene, 2001. 20(1): p. 77-87.

[30] Yeh, S., et al., *Increase of androgen-induced cell death and androgen receptor transactivation by BRCA1 in prostate cancer cells.* Proc Natl Acad Sci U S A, 2000. 97(21): p. 11256-61.

[31] Li, S., et al., *Binding of CtIP to the BRCT repeats of BRCA1 involved in the transcription regulation of p21 is disrupted upon DNA damage.* J Biol Chem, 1999. 274(16): p. 11334-8.

[32] Wong, A.K., et al., *Characterization of a carboxy-terminal BRCA1 interacting protein.* Oncogene, 1998. 17(18): p. 2279-85.

[33] Pao, G.M., et al., *CBP/p300 interact with and function as transcriptional coactivators of BRCA1.* Proc Natl Acad Sci U S A, 2000. 97(3): p. 1020-5.

[34] Yarden, R.I. and L.C. Brody, *BRCA1 interacts with components of the histone deacetylase complex.* Proc Natl Acad Sci U S A, 1999. 96(9): p. 4983-8.

[35] Hsu, L.C. and R.L. White, *BRCA1 is associated with the centrosome during mitosis.* Proc Natl Acad Sci U S A, 1998. 95(22): p. 12983-8.

[36] Li, S., et al., *Identification of a novel cytoplasmic protein that specifically binds to nuclear localization signal motifs.* J Biol Chem, 1998. 273(11): p. 6183-9.

[37] Zhang, H., et al., *VCP, a weak ATPase involved in multiple cellular events, interacts physically with BRCA1 in the nucleus of living cells.* DNA Cell Biol, 2000. 19(5): p. 253-63.

[38] Wu, L.C., et al., *Identification of a RING protein that can interact in vivo with the BRCA1 gene product.* Nat Genet, 1996. 14(4): p. 430-40.

[39] Jensen, D.E., et al., *BAP1: a novel ubiquitin hydrolase which binds to the BRCA1 RING finger and enhances BRCA1-mediated cell growth suppression.* Oncogene, 1998. 16(9): p. 1097-112.

[40] Chen, C.F., et al., *The nuclear localization sequences of the BRCA1 protein interact with the importin-alpha subunit of the nuclear transport signal receptor.* J Biol Chem, 1996. 271(51): p. 32863-8.

[41] Fuks, F., J. Milner, and T. Kouzarides, *BRCA2 associates with acetyltransferase activity when bound to P/CAF.* Oncogene, 1998. 17(19): p. 2531-4.

[42] Paull, T.T., et al., *A critical role for histone H2AX in recruitment of repair factors to nuclear foci after DNA damage.* Curr Biol, 2000. 10(15): p. 886-95.

[43] Futreal, P.A., et al., *BRCA1 mutations in primary breast and ovarian carcinomas.* Science, 1994. 266(5182): p. 120-2.

[44] Cleton-Jansen, A.M., et al., *Loss of heterozygosity in sporadic breast tumours at the BRCA2 locus on chromosome 13q12-q13.* Br J Cancer, 1995. 72(5): p. 1241-4.

[45] Smith, T.M., et al., *Complete genomic sequence and analysis of 117 kb of human DNA containing the gene BRCA1.* Genome Res, 1996. 6(11): p. 1029-49.

[46] Kelly, G.L. and A. Strasser, *The essential role of evasion from cell death in cancer.* Adv Cancer Res, 2011. 111: p. 39-96.

[47] Natarajan, A.T. and F. Palitti, *DNA repair and chromosomal alterations.* Mutat Res, 2008. 657(1): p. 3-7.

[48] Bhatti, S., et al., *ATM protein kinase: the linchpin of cellular defenses to stress.* Cell Mol Life Sci, 2011. 68(18): p. 2977-3006.

[49] Martinez-Rivera, M. and Z.H. Siddik, *Resistance and gain-of-resistance phenotypes in cancers harboring wild-type p53.* Biochem Pharmacol, 2012. 83(8): p. 1049-62.

[50] Gartel, A.L., *p21(WAF1/CIP1) and cancer: a shifting paradigm?* Biofactors, 2009. 35(2): p. 161-4.

[51] Ocker, M. and R. Schneider-Stock, *Histone deacetylase inhibitors: signalling towards p21cip1/waf1.* Int J Biochem Cell Biol, 2007. 39(7-8): p. 1367-74.

[52] Osborne, M.P., *Chemoprevention of breast cancer.* Surg Clin North Am, 1999. 79(5): p. 1207-21.

[53] Roy, R., J. Chun, and S.N. Powell, *BRCA1 and BRCA2: different roles in a common pathway of genome protection.* Nat Rev Cancer, 2012. 12(1): p. 68-78.

[54] Ouchi, T., *BRCA1 phosphorylation: biological consequences.* Cancer Biol Ther, 2006. 5(5): p. 470-5.

[55] Kotsopoulos, J. and S.A. Narod, *Androgens and breast cancer.* Steroids, 2012. 77(1-2): p. 1-9.

[56] Dumitrescu, R.G., *Epigenetic markers of early tumor development.* Methods Mol Biol, 2012. 863: p. 3-14.

[57] Wada-Hiraike, O., et al., *The DNA mismatch repair gene hMSH2 is a potent coactivator of oestrogen receptor alpha.* Br J Cancer, 2005. 92(12): p. 2286-91.

[58] Murphy, L.C. and E. Leygue, *The role of estrogen receptor-beta in breast cancer.* Semin Reprod Med, 2012. 30(1): p. 5-13.

[59] Welcsh, P.L. and M.C. King, *BRCA1 and BRCA2 and the genetics of breast and ovarian cancer.* Hum Mol Genet, 2001. 10(7): p. 705-13.

[60] Mueck, A.O. and R. Sitruk-Ware, *Nomegestrol acetate, a novel progestogen for oral contraception.* Steroids, 2011. 76(6): p. 531-9.

[61] Anaganti, S., et al., *p53-Dependent repression of focal adhesion kinase in response to estradiol in breast cancer cell-lines.* Cancer Lett, 2011. 300(2): p. 215-24.

[62] Comstock, C.E. and K.E. Knudsen, *The complex role of AR signaling after cytotoxic insult: implications for cell-cycle-based chemotherapeutics.* Cell Cycle, 2007. 6(11): p. 1307-13.

[63] Lu, S., et al., *Transcriptional responses to estrogen and progesterone in mammary gland identify networks regulating p53 activity.* Endocrinology, 2008. 149(10): p. 4809-20.

[64] Esquela-Kerscher, A. and F.J. Slack, *Oncomirs - microRNAs with a role in cancer.* Nat Rev Cancer, 2006. 6(4): p. 259-69.

[65] Ratner, E., et al., *A KRAS-variant in ovarian cancer acts as a genetic marker of cancer risk.* Cancer Res, 2010. 70(16): p. 6509-15.

[66] Paranjape, T., et al., *A 3′-untranslated region KRAS variant and triple-negative breast cancer: a case-control and genetic analysis.* Lancet Oncol, 2011. 12(4): p. 377-86.

[67] Weidhaas, J.B., *A KRAS-variant as a biomarker of ovarian cancer risk.* American Society of Clinical Oncology, 2010. Vol 28, No 15.

[68] Shen, B., et al., *Multiple but dissectible functions of FEN-1 nucleases in nucleic acid processing, genome stability and diseases.* Bioessays, 2005. 27(7): p. 717-29.

[69] Zheng, L., et al., *Functional regulation of FEN1 nuclease and its link to cancer.* Nucleic Acids Res, 2011. 39(3): p. 781-94.

[70] Zheng, L., et al., *Fen1 mutations result in autoimmunity, chronic inflammation and cancers.* Nat Med, 2007. 13(7): p. 812-9.

[71] Larsen, E., et al., *Early-onset lymphoma and extensive embryonic apoptosis in two domain-specific Fen1 mice mutants.* Cancer Res, 2008. 68(12): p. 4571-9.

[72] Liu, L., et al., *Functional FEN1 genetic variants contribute to risk of hepatocellular carcinoma, esophageal cancer, gastric cancer and colorectal cancer.* Carcinogenesis, 2012. 33(1): p. 119-23.

[73] Yang, M., et al., *Functional FEN1 polymorphisms are associated with DNA damage levels and lung cancer risk.* Hum Mutat, 2009. 30(9): p. 1320-8.

[74] Schultz-Norton, J.R., et al., *The deoxyribonucleic acid repair protein flap endonuclease-1 modulates estrogen-responsive gene expression.* Mol Endocrinol, 2007. 21(7): p. 1569-80.

[75] Abdel-Fatah, T.M., et al., *DNA polymerase beta deficiency is linked to aggressive* breast cancer: a comprehensive analysis of gene copy number, mRNA and protein expression in multiple cohorts. Mol Oncol, 2014. 8(3): p. 520-32.

9

Genome-Wide Gene Expression Analysis to Identify Epistatic Gene-Pairs Associated with Prognosis of Breast Cancer

I-Hsuan Lin and Ming-Ta Hsu

1. Introduction

Breast cancer is the most common cancer in women in the world [1]. According to the most recent estimates from GLOBOCAN published by the International Agency for Research on Cancer (IARC) [2], there were nearly 1.7 million new breast cancer cases diagnosed in 2012 (25.2% of all cancers in women) and 6.3 millions have been diagnosed with breast cancer in 2007-2012. Breast cancer incidence has been increasing by more than 20% and mortality increased by 14% since 2008 and is the most common cause of cancer death in women in less developed regions (324,000 deaths, 14.3% of total). Breast cancer is less favorable in the under-developed countries due to less advanced medical diagnosis and treatments. Therefore a good diagnosis/prognosis would help to prevent as well as provide effective clinical treatments.

Biomarker testing is an essential step in the evaluation of breast cancer and help medical doctors and patients in deciding the best treatment strategy. There are several commercial products or services developed towards this purpose. The Oncotype DX (Genomic Health) measures the expression levels of 21 genes and is most helpful for patients of early stage breast cancer with estrogen receptor (ER) positivity and no cancer cells in the lymph node. The HERmark assay (Monogram Biosciences) can quantitatively measure the HER2 total proteins with greater sensitivity than immunohistochemistry (IHC) which is an important indicator of predicting response of HER2-positive breast cancer patients to trastuzumab therapy. There are also tests for *BRCA1* and *BRCA2* mutations for the hereditary breast cancer patients. The targeted sequencing-based breast cancer panels such as BreastNext (Ambry Genetics) and BROCA (University of Washington) can be used to screen for mutations and copy number variants in genes implicated in breast cancer, including *BRCA1* and *BRCA2*.

Despite the relative success of these tests, there is a need for more efficient biomarkers in specific groups of breast cancer, such as lobular carcinoma [3, 4], triple-negative breast cancer [5] and early-onset breast cancers [6, 7] for diagnostic and/or prognostic application. We believe the discovery of more useful markers using the wealth of gene expression data available publicly nowadays would help medical doctors in the decision of the best way to help breast cancer patients, especially if the markers are correlated with specific therapeutic interventions. In the past decade, the high throughput microarray technique has been widely used to identify potential biomarkers for various cancers [8-12]. Recent years, the employment of RNA sequencing (RNA-seq) allows researchers to obtain transcriptome information and differential gene expression profiling at a much higher resolution. With the huge amount of data generated by these technologies, we are able to study the association of genes with cancer survival and identify novel potentially prognostic biomarkers for cancers with improved estimation. Traditionally, genetic search identifies genes that correlate with poor or good prognosis of patients. However, it is important to consider the epistatic gene-gene interactions underlying gene expression in complex diseases such as cancer. The epistatic (second or higher order) information would allow more refined prognostic evaluation that may help clinical treatments. Furthermore, epistatic analysis could be useful for identifying hub genes involved in prognosis and help to identify the major genetic risk factors and pathways in breast cancer.

In this work, we utilized the breast tumor RNA-seq data from The Cancer Genome Atlas (TCGA) as well as microarray-based expression datasets from Gene Expression Omnibus (GEO) to detect differentially expressed genes in various subsets of breast cancer patients, to identify genes whose expression profile is associated with survival of breast cancer patients and to examine the influence of co-expression of a second gene in the survival of patients. This analysis identifies specific gene groups differentially expressed between early-onset vs. late-onset breast cancer, between ductal vs. lobular carcinoma, between early vs. advanced stage breast tumors and tumor of various receptor status. Furthermore, epistatic interactions among these genes demonstrate the gene-gene interactions in patient survival and identify several hub genes that may be important determinants of breast cancer.

2. Statistical analysis of gene expression data

A global change in gene expression is a common theme in many human cancers. High-throughput techniques such as microarrays and next generation sequencing allow investigators to observe and compare the transcriptional landscapes of tumor cells in different biological states [13-18]. In this work, we integrated multiple gene expression data from several large-scale breast cancer studies to improve the assessment of differential gene expression in breast tumor cells and to effectively increase statistical power.

We collected 3,188 breast cancer related Affymetrix expression microarray data from GEO (http://www.ncbi.nlm.nih.gov/geo) from the following 16 series: GSE2603, GSE4922, GSE2990, GSE3494, GSE6532, GSE9195, GSE7390, GSE20194, GSE20271, GSE20685, GSE25066, GSE16391, GSE19615, GSE42568, GSE45255 and GSE50948. We also obtained 1,172 breast invasive carcinoma (BRCA) RNA-seq Level 3 data from TCGA Data Portal (http://tcga-data.nci.nih.gov/). The demographic and clinicopathological characteristics of the breast cancer patients from each study were also retrieved.

2.1. Processing of gene expression data and differential gene expression analysis

The CEL files obtained from microarray experiments were pre-processed by subjecting to quality check using Bioconductor in the R environment to ensure comparability between the different series and microarray platforms. The following quality measurements from the *simpleaffy* and *affy* packages were performed: average background (avbg), scale factor (sfs), percent present (percent.present), and possible RNA Degradation (AffyRNAdeg) of the array. Additionally, the relative log expression (RLE) and normalized unscaled standard error (NUSE) was also estimated using the *affyPLM* package. 466 arrays that did not pass the quality control tests were removed. For the 2,722 arrays that had sufficient quality, the quantile normalization and background correction were performed using the justRMA (robust multi-array average) algorithm of the *affy* package and the gene (probe set)-level log2-transformed expression values were summarized with Custom CDF file annotations (version 18.0.0. ENSG) [19]. Lastly, the COMBAT method available in the *inSilicoMerging* package was used to remove batch effect when combining the final expression data from the HG-U133A and HG-U133 Plus 2.0 arrays [20]. The RMA-normalized expression values from microarrays and the raw count data from RNA-seq datasets were then analyzed using the *edgeR* package [21]. The differentially expressed genes were selected with a threshold of FDR adjusted P-value < 0.05.

2.2. Chinicopathological characteristics of breast cancer patients

We include 2,722 breast cancer patients from various microarray-based studies (referred as GEO cohort) and 1,052 breast cancer patients from the TCGA project (referred as TCGA cohort) following differential gene expression analyses (Table 1). All patients were women in the GEO cohort with a median age of 53 years. The patients from the TCGA cohort were older with a median age of 58 years and approximately 96% of patients were women. There was a significant amount of clinicopathological data not available from the GEO cohort as noted in Table 1. In both cohorts, there were more stage I/II breast cancer cases than advanced stage cases, and invasive ductal carcinoma (IDC) being the major histological subtype diagnosed. The data also contained status of tumor receptors such as the estrogen receptor (ER), progesterone receptor (PR) and HER2 which are frequently used prognostic factors to aid therapeutic decisions. Many patients were positive for the ER and/or PR, and/or negative for the HER2 receptor.

Characteristic	No. of Patients			
	Microarray (n = 2722), %		RNA-seq (n = 1052), %	
Sex				
Male	0	0.0%	11	1.0%

Characteristic	No. of Patients			
	Microarray (n = 2722), %		RNA-seq (n = 1052), %	
Female	2722	85.4%	1005	95.5%
Missing data	0	0.0%	36	3.4%
Median Age (range)	53 (24-93)		58 (26-90)	
Younger than 40	300	11.0%	71	6.7%
40 to 55	1184	43.5%	365	34.7%
Older than 55	1224	45.0%	580	55.1%
Missing data	14	0.5%	36	3.4%
Stage				
Early (Stage I and II)	1236	45.4%	751	71.4%
Late (Stage III and IV)	370	13.6%	246	23.4%
Missing data	1116	41.0%	55	5.2%
Histologic Subtype				
IDC	500	18.4%	754	71.7%
ILC	32	1.2%	168	16.0%
Mixed	47	1.7%	29	2.8%
Others	6	0.2%	64	6.1%
Missing data	2137	78.5%	37	3.5%
ER Status				
ER positive	1710	62.8%	749	71.2%
ER negative	647	23.8%	222	21.1%
Missing data	365	13.4%	81	7.7%
PR Status				
PR positive	1017	37.4%	650	61.8%
PR negative	684	25.1%	318	30.2%
Missing data	1021	37.5%	84	8.0%
HER2 Status				
HER2 positive	202	7.4%	150	14.3%
HER2 negative	946	34.8%	524	49.8%
Missing data	1574	57.8%	378	35.9%
Female patients with a least one type of survival data	2294	84.3%	999	36.7%

Table 1. Patient characteristics of the GEO and TCGA cohorts.

2.3. Differentially expressed genes in patients from different age groups

Differential gene expression analysis was performed to identify over- and under-expressed genes specific to tumors derived from young, middle-aged and elderly breast cancer patients. As presented in Figure 1, there were very few middle-aged-specific expression signatures, indicating that the gene expression pattern of middle-aged patients was not significantly different from the young adults and/or elderly patients. In contrast, the elderly breast cancer patients possessed a high number of differentially expressed genes specific to this age group. IPA analysis of the differentially expressed genes from tumor cells obtained from older patients have decreased cell proliferation, movement, migration and cell cycle progression (activation z-score between -2.677 and -1.611) and increased cell death (activation z-score = 1.321). On the contrary, tumor cells from young patients were predicted to have increased proliferation of cells and DNA synthesis (activation z-score between 2.000 and 2.117) and decreased cell death and apoptosis (activation z-score between -0.586 and -0.299).

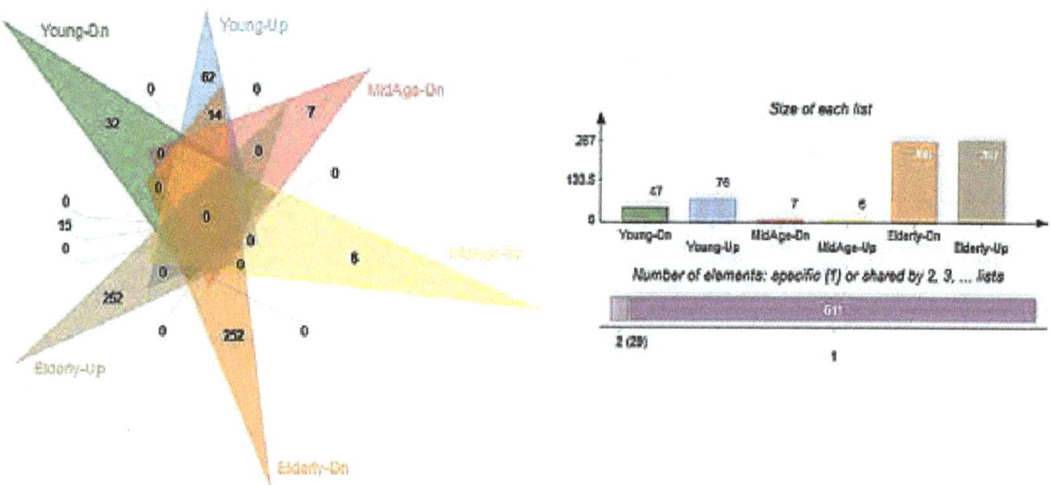

Figure 1. Number of significantly over- and under-expressed genes in the three age groups presented with the jvenn Venn diagram viewer [22].

It is interesting to note that 14 genes that were over-expressed in young patients were under-expressed in elderly patients, and conversely, 15 genes under-expressed in young patients were over-expressed in elderly patients (Table 2). Several of these genes such as *BIRC5* (survivin), *KPNA2*, *PLAC8* (onzin), *TFPI2*, *CITED2*, *NKX3-1*, *PIP* and *ZNF395* have been found to play a role in cancer cell proliferation and cancer progression [23-28].

Type	Symbol	Entrez Gene Name	Location	Type(s)
Young-Up Elderly-Dn	*BIRC5*	baculoviral IAP repeat containing 5	Cytoplasm	Other
	DCX	doublecortin	Cytoplasm	Other
	GAL	galanin/GMAP prepropeptide	Extracellular Space	Other

Type	Symbol	Entrez Gene Name	Location	Type(s)
	HN1	hematological and neurological expressed 1	Nucleus	Other
	KPNA2	karyopherin alpha 2	Nucleus	Transporter
	NOL11	nucleolar protein 11	Nucleus	Other
	NUP85	nucleoporin 85kDa	Cytoplasm	Other
	PLAC8	placenta-specific 8	Nucleus	Other
	POLR3G	polymerase (RNA) III (DNA directed) polypeptide G	Nucleus	Enzyme
	PSMA4	proteasome alpha 4 subunit isoform 1	Cytoplasm	Peptidase
	RAPGEFL1	Rap guanine nucleotide exchange factor	Other	Other
	TFPI2	tissue factor pathway inhibitor 2	Extracellular Space	Other
	UCHL1	ubiquitin carboxyl-terminal esterase L1	Cytoplasm	Peptidase
	XDH	xanthine dehydrogenase	Cytoplasm	Enzyme
Young-Dn Elderly-Up	*ABCC6*	ATP-binding cassette, sub-family C, member 6	Plasma Membrane	Transporter
	ACAA1	acetyl-CoA acyltransferase 1	Cytoplasm	Enzyme
	CCDC28A	coiled-coil domain containing 28A	Other	Other
	CITED2	Cbp/p300-interacting transactivator	Nucleus	Transcription regulator
	CLMN	calmin (calponin-like, transmembrane)	Cytoplasm	Other
	CTDSPL	small CTD phosphatase 3 isoform 1	Nucleus	Other
	CTSF	cathepsin F	Cytoplasm	Peptidase
	FMO5	flavin containing monooxygenase 5	Cytoplasm	Enzyme
	GPC4	glypican 4	Plasma Membrane	Transmembrane receptor
	KIF13B	kinesin family member 13B	Cytoplasm	Other
	NDST1	N-deacetylase/N-sulfotransferase (heparan)	Cytoplasm	Enzyme
	NKX3-1	NK3 homeobox 1	Nucleus	Transcription regulator
	PIP	prolactin-induced protein	Extracellular Space	Peptidase
	ZNF385D	zinc finger protein 385D	Nucleus	Other
	ZNF395	zinc finger protein 395	Cytoplasm	Other

Table 2. Concordant differentially expressed genes identified in the young and elderly breast cancer patients.

2.4. Differentially expressed genes in patients with early stage versus advanced stage breast cancer

We compared the gene expression profile of patients diagnosed with early stage (stage I and II) breast cancer with those with advanced stage (stage III and IV) breast cancer. We identified 79 over-expressed and 140 under-expressed genes in early stage breast cancer. IPA analysis showed 121 of the total 219 differentially expressed genes were associated with cancer (*P*-value = 4.81E-02), and 24 were specifically associated with breast cancer (*P*-value = 3.25E-03, Table 3). Also, there were 17 under-expressed genes in early stage breast cancer (i.e. over-expressed in advanced stage tumors) that were found to be cancer recurrence-associated (*ADORA3, FLT4, GSR, HSP90AA1, TEK* and *TXNRD1*) and metastasis-associated (*ACP5, FLT4, FTL, GSR, HSP90AA1, MAPK11, MMP9, NRAS, PGF, SCD* and *TEK*). Interestingly, we detected over-expression of the DNA methyltransferase *DNMT1* in early stage tumors. In cancer cells, the over-expression of this gene can lead to hypermethylation of CpG islands and epigenetically silences multiple tumor suppressor genes and hence promotes tumorigenesis in early stage cancers [29-31].

Symbol	Entrez Gene Name	Location	Type(s)	DE Status
ACP5	acid phosphatase 5, tartrate resistant	Cytoplasm	phosphatase	Down
APOE	apolipoprotein E	Extracellular Space	transporter	Down
ARRB1	arrestin, beta 1	Cytoplasm	other	Down
CDKN1A	cyclin-dependent kinase inhibitor 1A	Nucleus	other	Down
ETV1	ets variant 1	Nucleus	transcription regulator	Down
FLT4	fms-related tyrosine kinase 4	Plasma Membrane	transmembrane receptor	Down
GPC3	glypican 3	Plasma Membrane	other	Up
GPR126	G protein-coupled receptor 126	Plasma Membrane	G-protein coupled receptor	Down
HBB	hemoglobin, beta	Cytoplasm	transporter	Down
HIC1	hypermethylated in cancer 1	Nucleus	transcription regulator	Down
HSP90AA1	heat shock protein 90kDa alpha (cytosolic)	Cytoplasm	enzyme	Down
HSPB7	cardiovascular heat shock protein	Cytoplasm	other	Down
MMP15	matrix metalloproteinase 15 preproprotein	Extracellular Space	peptidase	Down
MMP28	matrix metalloproteinase 28 isoform 1	Extracellular Space	peptidase	Down
MMP9	matrix metalloproteinase 9 preproprotein	Extracellular Space	peptidase	Down
NOS3	nitric oxide synthase 3 (endothelial cell)	Cytoplasm	enzyme	Down
PPM1D	protein phosphatase 1D	Cytoplasm	phosphatase	Down
PSIP1	PC4 and SFRS1 interacting protein 1	Nucleus	other	Up
PXN	paxillin	Cytoplasm	other	Down
S100A2	S100 calcium binding protein A2	Nucleus	other	Down
SELL	selectin L	Plasma Membrane	transmembrane receptor	Down
TAL1	T-cell acute lymphocytic leukemia 1	Nucleus	transcription regulator	Down
TEK	TEK tyrosine kinase, endothelial	Plasma Membrane	kinase	Down
TNC	tenascin C	Extracellular Space	other	Up

Table 3. The 25 differentially expressed genes associated with breast cancer in the early versus advanced stage analysis.

2.5. Differentially expressed genes in patients with Invasive Ductal Carcinoma (IDC) versus Invasive Lobular Carcinoma (ILC)

The invasive ductal carcinoma (IDC) and invasive lobular carcinoma (ILC) are the two major histological subtypes of breast cancer. They also represented the main types of breast cancer cases gathered in this study. We compared the gene expression profiles of patients with IDC and ILC and identified 216 over-expressed and 126 under-expressed genes in IDC as compared to patients with ILC. IPA analysis showed 66 genes were related to breast cancer (Table 4), including 12 transcription regulators (*ATF3, BTG2, EGR1, EZH2, FOS, FOSB, JUN, JUNB, MTDH, STAT1, ZFP36* and *ZNF423*) and a translation regulator (*EIF4EBP1*). There were also 12 genes annotated as tumor suppressor genes in the TSGene database [32], where *CDH1, DKK1* and *S100A2* were over-expressed in IDC and *BTG2, CAV1, EGR1, GPC3, MUC1, NR4A1, SLIT2, TGFBR2* and *ZFP36* were under-expressed in IDC. IPA predicted common upstream regulators *KDM5B, STUB1, CDKN1A, HIF1A* and *TGFB1* to be inhibited whereas *FOXM1, IFNB1, IFNG* and *PPARG* were in activated states. Additionally, the activities of several disease functions such as cell proliferation, invasion and DNA replication were predicted to be increased in IDC (activation z-score between 1.342 and 3.092).

Symbol	Entrez Gene Name	Location	Type(s)	DE Status
ACACB	acetyl-CoA carboxylase beta	Cytoplasm	enzyme	Down
ALDH1A1	aldehyde dehydrogenase 1 family, member A1	Cytoplasm	enzyme	Down
APOBEC3B	apolipoprotein B mRNA editing enzyme, catalytic	Cytoplasm	enzyme	Up
ATF3	activating transcription factor 3	Nucleus	transcription regulator	Down
BIRC5	baculoviral IAP repeat containing 5	Cytoplasm	other	Up
BTG2	BTG family, member 2	Nucleus	transcription regulator	Down
CAV1	caveolin 1, caveolae protein, 22kDa	Plasma Membrane	transmembrane receptor	Down
CCL21	chemokine (C-C motif) ligand 21	Extracellular Space	cytokine	Down
CD34	CD34 molecule	Plasma Membrane	other	Down
CD69	CD69 molecule	Plasma Membrane	transmembrane receptor	Down
CDC20	cell division cycle 20	Nucleus	other	Up
CDH1	cadherin 1, type 1, E-cadherin (epithelial)	Plasma Membrane	other	Up
CDH3	cadherin 3, type 1, P-cadherin (placental)	Plasma Membrane	other	Up
CDH5	cadherin 5, type 2 (vascular endothelium)	Plasma Membrane	other	Down
CDK1	cyclin-dependent kinase 1	Nucleus	kinase	Up

Symbol	Entrez Gene Name	Location	Type(s)	DE Status
CXCL14	chemokine (C-X-C motif) ligand 14	Extracellular Space	cytokine	Down
CXCL2	chemokine (C-X-C motif) ligand 2	Extracellular Space	cytokine	Down
CYR61	cysteine-rich, angiogenic inducer, 61	Extracellular Space	other	Down
DKK1	dickkopf WNT signaling pathway inhibitor 1	Extracellular Space	growth factor	Up
DSCC1	DNA replication and sister chromatid cohesion 1	Nucleus	other	Up
DUSP1	dual specificity phosphatase 1	Nucleus	phosphatase	Down
EGR1	early growth response 1	Nucleus	transcription regulator	Down
EIF4EBP1	eukaryotic translation initiation factor 4E	Cytoplasm	translation regulator	Up
EZH2	enhancer of zeste homolog 2 (Drosophila)	Nucleus	transcription regulator	Up
FABP7	fatty acid binding protein 7, brain	Cytoplasm	transporter	Up
FOS	FBJ murine osteosarcoma viral oncogene homolog	Nucleus	transcription regulator	Down
FOSB	FBJ murine osteosarcoma viral oncogene homolog B	Nucleus	transcription regulator	Down
GPC3	glypican 3	Plasma Membrane	other	Down
GRB7	growth factor receptor-bound protein 7	Plasma Membrane	other	Up
HSPB8	heat shock 22kDa protein 8	Cytoplasm	kinase	Up
IER2	immediate early response 2	Cytoplasm	other	Down
IGF1	insulin-like growth factor 1 (somatomedin C)	Extracellular Space	growth factor	Down
IGFBP6	insulin-like growth factor binding protein 6	Extracellular Space	other	Down
ITIH5	inter-alpha trypsin inhibitor heavy chain	Other	other	Down
JUN	jun proto-oncogene	Nucleus	transcription regulator	Down
JUNB	jun B proto-oncogene	Nucleus	transcription regulator	Down
KPNA2	karyopherin alpha 2	Nucleus	transporter	Up
KRT6B	keratin 6B	Cytoplasm	other	Up
MMP1	matrix metalloproteinase 1 preproprotein	Extracellular Space	peptidase	Up
MMP9	matrix metalloproteinase 9 preproprotein	Extracellular Space	peptidase	Up
MRPL13	mitochondrial ribosomal protein L13	Cytoplasm	other	Up
MRPL15	mitochondrial ribosomal protein L15	Cytoplasm	other	Up
MTDH	metadherin	Cytoplasm	transcription regulator	Up

Symbol	Entrez Gene Name	Location	Type(s)	DE Status
MUC1	mucin 1, cell surface associated	Plasma Membrane	other	Down
NR4A1	nuclear receptor subfamily 4, group A, member 1	Nucleus	ligand-dependent nuclear receptor	Down
ORM1	orosomucoid 1	Extracellular Space	other	Up
PCNA	proliferating cell nuclear antigen	Nucleus	enzyme	Up
PDK4	pyruvate dehydrogenase kinase, isozyme 4	Cytoplasm	kinase	Down
PGK1	phosphoglycerate kinase 1	Cytoplasm	kinase	Up
RFC4	replication factor C (activator 1) 4, 37kDa	Nucleus	other	Up
RRM2	ribonucleotide reductase M2	Nucleus	enzyme	Up
S100A2	S100 calcium binding protein A2	Nucleus	other	Up
SLIT2	slit homolog 2 (Drosophila)	Extracellular Space	other	Down
SPP1	secreted phosphoprotein 1	Extracellular Space	cytokine	Up
SQLE	squalene epoxidase	Cytoplasm	enzyme	Up
STAT1	signal transducer and activator of transcription	Nucleus	transcription regulator	Up
TCP1	t-complex 1	Cytoplasm	other	Up
TGFBR2	transforming growth factor, beta receptor II	Plasma Membrane	kinase	Down
TIMP4	TIMP metallopeptidase inhibitor 4	Extracellular Space	other	Down
TOP2A	topoisomerase (DNA) II alpha 170kDa	Nucleus	enzyme	Up
TPD52	tumor protein D52	Cytoplasm	other	Up
TYMS	thymidylate synthetase	Nucleus	enzyme	Up
UBE2C	ubiquitin conjugating enzyme E2C	Cytoplasm	enzyme	Up
VEGFA	vascular endothelial growth factor A	Extracellular Space	growth factor	Up
ZFP36	ZFP36 ring finger protein	Nucleus	transcription regulator	Down
ZNF423	zinc finger protein 423	Nucleus	transcription regulator	Down

Table 4. The 66 differentially expressed genes associated with breast cancer in the IDC versus ILC analysis.

2.6. Differentially expressed genes in patients with different receptor status

In the last part of the differential gene expression analysis, we sought to examine the differentially expressed genes of breast cancer patients of different receptor status: (1) estrogen receptor positive (ER+) versus ER negative (ER–), (2) progesterone receptor positive (PR+) versus PR negative (PR–), (3) HER2 receptor positive (HER2+) versus HER2 negative (HER2–), and (4) triple-negative breast cancer (TNBC, also known as basal-like breast cancer) versus non-TNBC. The Venn diagram in Figure 2 summarized the intersections between the differentially expressed genes identified in the four assays. There were 57% and 65% of breast cancer patients that were both ER+ and PR+ in the GEO and TCGA cohorts respectively; hence the patient pools divided by the ER positivity for gene expression assays are similar to that divided by the PR positivity. Because of this fact, it is not surprising to observe genes that were found over- or under-expressed in the ER assay were also differentially expressed in the same direction in the PR assay. Likewise, genes that were over-expressed in TNBC were under-expressed in the ER and PR assays (n = 74) and ER, PR and HER2 assays (n = 35), and vice versa for the under-expressed genes in TNBC (n = 87 and 2 respectively).

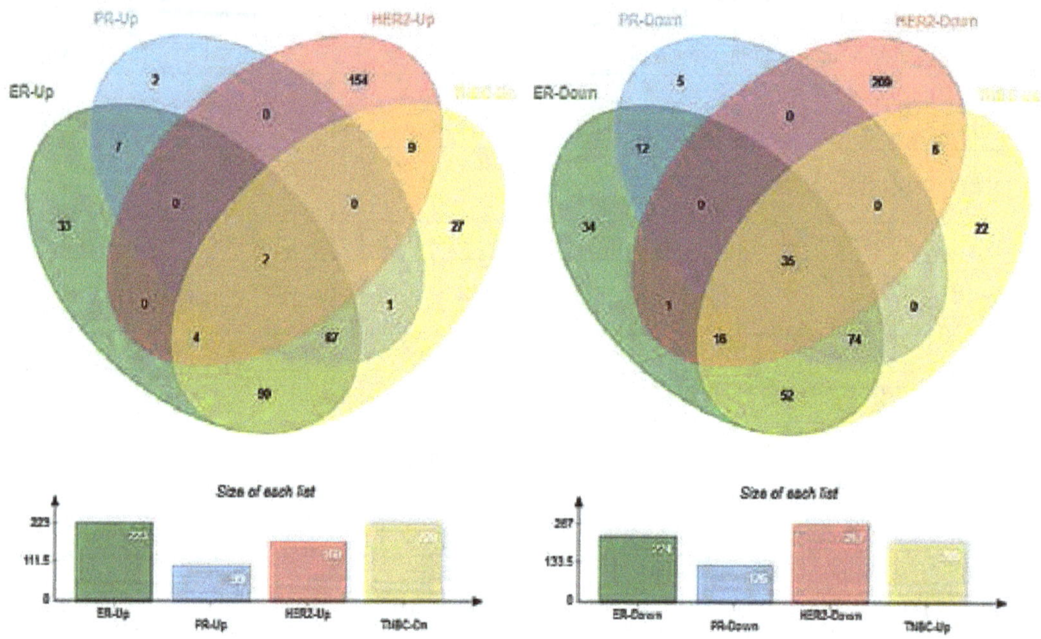

Figure 2. Number of differentially up- and down-regulated genes in the ER, PR, HER2 or TNBC receptor status assays.

The *GALNT6* (polypeptide N-acetylgalactosaminyltransferase) and *SCGB2A2* (secretoglobin) are the two genes consistently over-expressed in ER+, PR+, HER2+ breast tumors but under-expressed in TNBC. There were also 87 genes over-expressed in ER+ and PR+ breast tumors and under-expressed in TNBC, including seven transcription regulators (*EGR3, FOXA1, GATA3, INSM1, NRIP1, TBX3* and *XBP1*) and 11 breast cancer associated genes (*ABAT, AGR2, CXCL14, GSTM3, HSPB8, MUC1, NR4A2, PGR, PIP, PLAT* and *PSD3*). On the other hand, there were more under-expressed genes (n = 35) shared among ER+, PR+ and HER2+ breast tumors that were over-expressed in TNBC. Among these are four transcription regulators (*ELF5, EN1, FOXC1* and *ZIC1*) and 12 extracellular proteins (*CHI3L1, CHI3L2, COL2A1, COL9A3, CRLF1, KLK6, KLK7, MMP12, MMP7, PTX3, SERPINB5* and *SOSTDC1*), and some of these genes are known TNBC-associated markers [33-37].

3. Identifying survival-related genes of patients with breast cancer

In cancer survival analysis, survival time is often defined as the period of time from the beginning of the medical process (treatment, surgery, etc.) until the death (or some other events such as development of a particular symptom or to relapse after the remission of disease) of the observed patient or until the end of observation. The goal of such analysis is to link the time to event (i.e. survival time) to certain explanatory variables. New methodologies were developed for calculating the survival probabilities using gene expression profiles when genome-wide expression data becomes increasingly available in the past two decades [38-42].

In this work, we analyzed associations between breast cancer patient survival and gene expression of breast tumors from published microarray and the RNA-seq datasets, denoted as the GEO and TCGA cohorts respectively. Survival analysis was performed separately for each cohort and the median times from diagnosis to death or last follow-up were 99.5 and 21.4 months in the GEO and TCGA cohorts respectively. We transform the expression values into gene expression status (i.e. 0 for low expression and 1 for high expression) using the modified auto_cutoff function of the R script available from the Kaplan Meier-plotter website (http://kmplot.com/). The survival probability is calculated using the "survival" package and modified *kmplot* function (http://biostat.mc.vanderbilt.edu/wiki/Main/TatsukiRcode#kmplot) is used to plot Kaplan-Meier curves. The hazard ratio with 95% confidence intervals and log-rank *P*-value are estimated using the Cox proportional hazards model. All analyses were conducted within the R statistical environment.

3.1. Univariate gene selection and survival analysis

We extract the gene expression profiles of 1,694 genes that were found differentially expressed (consistently in microarray and RNA-seq datasets) in any one type of the assays discussed in section 2.3 to 2.6. We calculated the overall survival (OS), relapse-free survival (RFS) and the distant metastasis-free survival (DMFS) of breast cancer patients with respect to the expression status. DMFS is not calculated for the TCGA cohort due to unavailability of the time to distant metastases information from patients in this cohort. The log-rank *P*-values were adjusted for multiple comparisons using the Benjamini-Hochberg false discovery rate (FDR) method and were used to select genes expression profiles significantly associated with survival.

We summarized the survival statistics, including the hazard ratios (an estimate of the ratio of the hazard rate in the highly versus the lowly expressed patient group) and the estimated 2- and 10-year survival rates in Table 5. There were about 24% OS-associated, 48% RFS-associated and 51% DMFS-associated genes that have adjusted log-rank *P*-value < 0.01 in the GEO cohort. There were 23% OS-associated genes but only 1.3% RFS-associated genes in the TCGA cohort, due to much fewer relapse/recurrence information in this cohort (adjusted log-rank *P*-value < 0.05). The breast cancer patients in the TCGA cohorts have lower overall survival (10-year) than those from the GEO and both cohorts have similar RFS rates. In the DMFS analysis, 51% of the differentially expressed genes were significant predictor of DMFS.

Statistics	GEO	TCGA
Adjusted log-rank *P*-value cutoff	0.01	0.05
Overall survival (OS)		
No. of genes associated with OS	414 (24.4%)	386 (22.8%)
Hazard Ratio > 1		
No. of genes	192	134
2-year survival (low / high expression)	0.969, 0.923	0.968, 0.947
10-year survival (low / high expression)	0.798, 0.658	0.562, 0.369
Hazard Ratio < 1		
No. of genes	222	252
2-year survival (low / high expression)	0.918, 0.968	0.945, 0.970
10-year survival (low / high expression)	0.654, 0.787	0.382, 0.558
Relapse-free survival (RFS)		
No. of genes associated with RFS	811 (47.8%)	22 (1.3%)
Hazard Ratio > 1		
No. of genes	344	7
2-year survival (low / high expression)	0.901, 0.840	0.949, 0.829
10-year survival (low / high expression)	0.685, 0.586	0.754, 0.555
Hazard Ratio < 1		
No. of genes	467	15
2-year survival (low / high expression)	0.845, 0.900	0.826, 0.946
10-year survival (low / high expression)	0.588, 0.684	0.538, 0.749
Distant metastasis-free survival (DMFS)		
No. of genes associated with DMFS	856 (50.5%)	NA
Hazard Ratio > 1		
No. of genes	384	
2-year survival (low / high expression)	0.923, 0.863	NA
10-year survival (low / high expression)	0.755, 0.663	
Hazard Ratio < 1		
No. of genes	472	
2-year survival (low / high expression)	0.858, 0.926	NA
10-year survival (low / high expression)	0.667, 0.754	

Table 5. Survival statistics according to gene expression profiles of breast cancer patients.

3.2. Cox regression analysis using the expression profiles of two genes

From the three survival data, i.e. OS, RFS and DMFS, we selected the top 500 most significantly survival associated gene expression profiles consistent in both cohorts to generate 124,750 two-gene combinations and perform Cox regression analysis with two covariates (i.e. using the expression status of each gene as a covariate).

There were 81,902 (65.7%) and 78,136 (62.6%) pairs whose expression signatures of both genes remained predictors of OS in the GEO and TCGA cohorts respectively (*P*-value of the coefficient estimates < 0.05). Of these, 31,189 pairs were mutual in the two cohorts and 234 gene-pairs (consisting of 131 genes) had survival probability patterns greatly shifted compared with the previous single-gene model. The strongest predictor pairs were *COL16A1-ARHGEF3, IGF1R-LTB, IGF1R-PTGDS, NPY1R-ARHGEF3* and *SERPINA1-ACADSB,* where the lower expression of both genes in each pair was associated with lowest survival probabilities in all five cases. The results were presented as Kaplan Meier plots in Figure 3A to E.

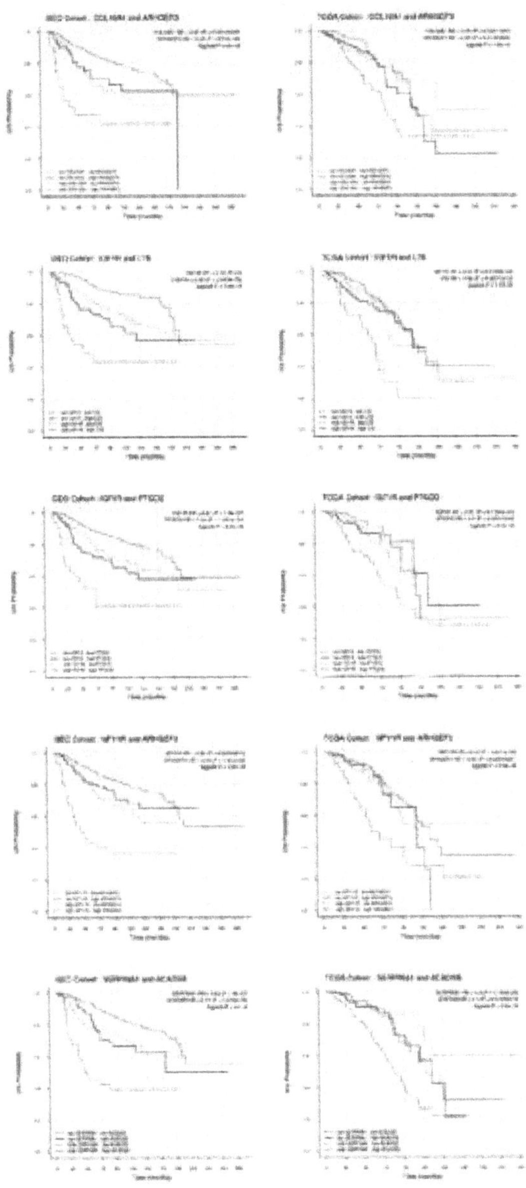

Figure 3. The Kaplan Meier plots of five OS-associated gene-pairs that also gained most changes in survival probabilities compared to the matching univariate approach.

The same analysis was also performed for RFS in the GOE and TCGA cohorts, and 85,244 (68.3%) and 64,049 (51.3%) pairs were significant predictors of RFS respectively (*P*-value of the coefficient estimates < 0.05). We found 22,165 significant pairs common in the two cohorts and 1,130 gene-pairs (consisting of 276 genes) whose survival probability patterns had greatly shifted compared with the single-gene model. The most significant RFS-associated pairs were *ADM-MYBPC1, DIRAS3-TANC2, KIFC1-ADORA3, PDSS1-DIRAS3, STMN1-ADORA3* (Figure 4).

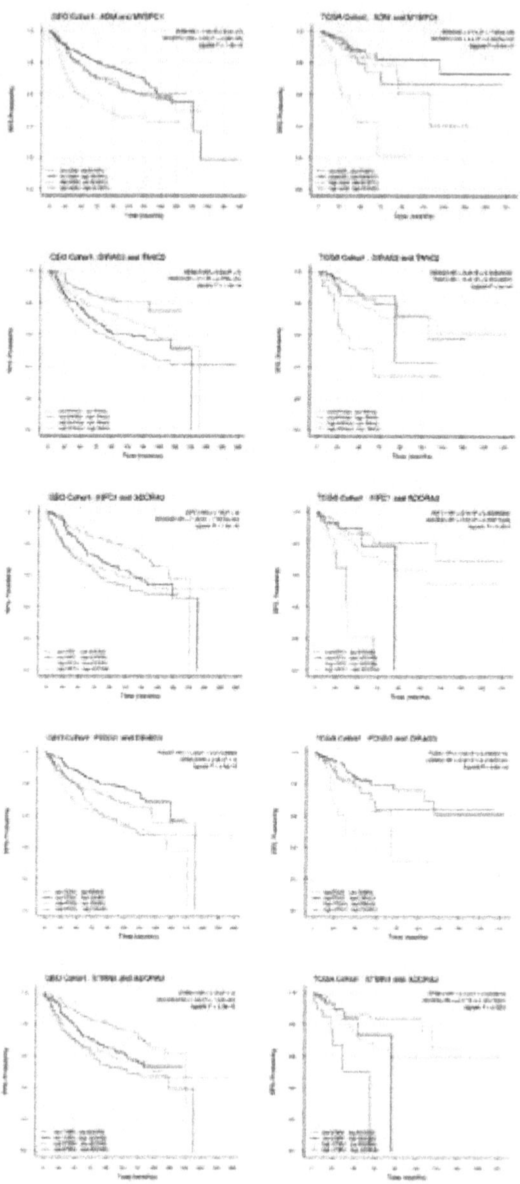

Figure 4. The Kaplan Meier plots of five RFS-associated gene-pairs that also gained most changes in survival probabilities compared to the matching univariate approach.

Lastly, we also make use of the DMFS data available from the GEO cohort to demonstrate the improvement of epistatic gene-pair approach in predicting survival probabilities. Of the 124,750 two-gene combinations, 122,751 (98.4%) were significant predictors of DMFS in breast cancer patients. The high percentage of strong two-gene predictors derived from the DMFS analysis was most likely due to the already high numbers of strong single-gene predictors as shown in Table 5. We further distinguished 228 gene-pairs (consisting of 138 genes) whose survival probability patterns had greatly shifted compared with the single-gene model. Six most significantly improved DMFS-associated pairs were *MMP15-SPDEF, TRIB3-ETV1, TRIB3-PLD1, TRIB3-TRIM2, TRIM2-KRT14* and *XBP1-TRIB3* (Figure 5).

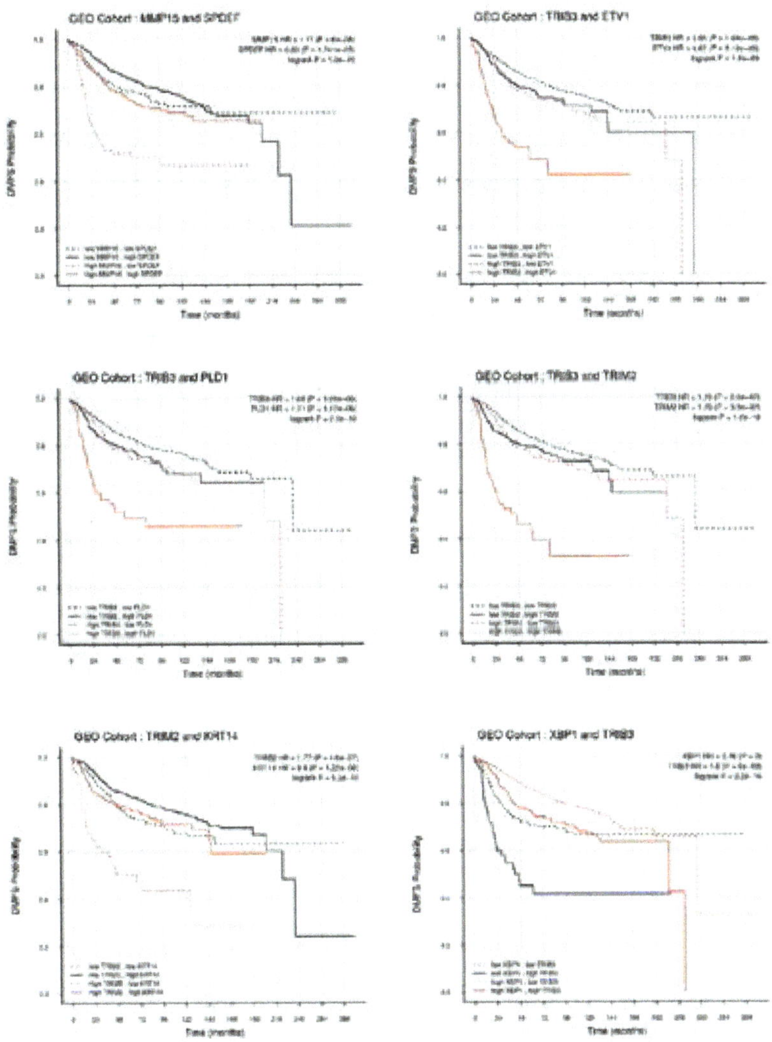

Figure 5. The Kaplan Meier plots of six DMFS-associated gene-pairs that also gained most changes in survival probabilities compared to the matching univariate approach.

3.3. Differentially expressed survival-associated hub genes and gene-pair candidates

As mentioned in the section 3.2, we have identified 234, 1,130 and 228 OS-, RFS- and DMFS-associated gene-pairs (consisting of 131, 276 and 138 genes respectively) that showed improved predictive performance. Some of these genes may be paired with many partners while remaining highly significant. In Table 6, we list five genes that have high number of pairing possibilities and also common in OS, RFS and DMFS analysis.

Genes	No. of Gene-pairs			GEO RFS log-rank *P*	
	OS	RFS	DMFS	single covariate	multiple covariates
MEOX1	6	18	0	4.94E-08	3.43E-11 (C3orf18) ~ 4.02E-08
PPAP2B	37	14	0	1.27E-04	1.07E-10 (ADM) ~ 7.17E-05
PRPF38B	8	49	0	3.41E-02	1.04E-12 (DIRAS3) ~ 1.17E-02
SERPINA1	7	20	22	3.21E-05	2.30E-12 (CDT1) ~ 2.34E-05
XBP1	0	11	5	1.97E-03	2.47E-13 (DIRAS3) ~ 1.11E-03

Table 6. Five hub genes that associated with more than one type of survival data.

Gene-Pairs	OS		RFS		DMFS		DE Status of Gene 1	DE Status of Gene 2
	HR1	HR2	HR1	HR2	HR1	HR2		
C3orf18-PPAP2B	0.51	0.51	0.66	0.64	–	–	Her2+ Down	Elderly Down
IGF1R-KLRB1	0.39	0.60	0.72	0.73	–	–	ER+ Up / TNBC Down	IDC Down
NME5-PPAP2B	0.51	0.56	0.77	0.67	–	–	ER+ Up / PR+ Up / Her2+ Down / TNBC Down	Elderly Down
PRPF38B-RAMP3	0.56	0.58	0.80	0.62	–	–	Early Stage Up (i.e. Advanced Stage Down)	ER+ Up / PR+ Up / Her2+ Down / TNBC Down
GATA3-SERPINA1	0.62	0.41	–	–	0.56	0.56	ER+ Up / PR+ Up / TNBC Down	Young Down / ER+ Up / PR+ Up / Her2+ Down / TNBC Down
PSAT1-SERPINA1	1.61	0.44	–	–	1.53	0.56	Elderly Down / ER+ Down / PR+ Down / TNBC Up	Young Down / ER+ Up / PR+ Up / Her2+ Down / TNBC Down
MMP15-SLC44A4	–	–	1.29	0.75	1.69	0.60	Early Stage Down (i.e. Advanced Stage Up)	ER+ / TNBC Down

Table 7. The gene-pairs that associated with more than one type of survival data.

There were also seven gene-pairs that were significantly associated with more than one type of survival data (Table 7). By incorporating the differential expression information we derived previously, we may observe that the TNBC patients were noticeably having worse survival outcomes than non-TNBC patients as TNBC is known to be an aggressive breast cancer subtype [43, 44]. For example, both *GATA3* [45, 46] and *SERPINA1* were found significantly under-expressed in TNBC cases and the low expressions of both genes were correlated with poor OS and DMFS. Additionally, the over-expression of *PSAT1* and the under-expression of *SERPINA1* in TNBC patients also correlated with poor OS and DMFS. Moreover, the over-expression of *MMP15* relating to advanced stage breast cancer and the under-expression of *SLC44A4* associated with TNBC are predictors of cancer recurrence as well as distant metastases.

4. Conclusion and perspectives

In section 2 of this chapter, we identified 1,694 genes that were differentially expressed in breast cancer patients of three age groups, early versus advanced stage breast cancers, invasive ductal versus invasive lobular breast cancers, and patients of various receptor status. While some of these genes are known to participate in the biological and genetic pathways that lead to breast cancer and many are novel findings. In section 3, we showed that more than 20% the differentially expressed genes were associated with at least one type of survival data. Our data indicated improved predictive performance when using a multivariate approach of combining the expression of two genes in the assessment of survival data. Perceivably, the gene pairs found in the epistatic analysis could provide useful pictures in gene interactions in breast carcinogenesis.

Breast cancer is a heterogeneous and complex disease where researchers and doctors have implemented different classifications (be it molecular, pathological, genetic or prognostic) to aid disease diagnosis and treatment decision. In the future, we hope to use the gene expression profiles of multiple survival-associated biomarkers to sub-classify patients of different types of breast cancer, and ultimately allow medical practitioners to derive better disease assessment and treatment decision.

Acknowledgements

The authors acknowledge financial support from the Ministry of Science and Technology, Taiwan (MOST 103-2811-B-010-020), and from the Ministry of Education, Taiwan (Aim for the Top University Plan; 103AC-T903). The funders had no role in study design, data collection and analysis, decision to publish, or preparation of the manuscript.

Author details

I-Hsuan Lin and Ming-Ta Hsu*

*Address all correspondence to: mth@ym.edu.tw

Institute of Biochemistry and Molecular Biology, School of Life Science, National Yang-Ming University, Taipei, Taiwan

References

[1] Breast cancer: prevention and control. World Health Organization (WHO) Web site. http://www.who.int/cancer/detection/breastcancer/en/. Accessed June 2014. [http://www.who.int/cancer/detection/breastcancer/en/]

[2] Breast Cancer - Estimated Incidence, Mortality and Prevalence Worldwide in 2012. GLOBOCAN 2012 Fact Sheets. http://globocan.iarc.fr/Pages/fact_sheets_cancer.aspx?cancer=breast. Accessed June 2014. [http://globocan.iarc.fr/Pages/fact_sheets_cancer.aspx?cancer=breast]

[3] Cristofanilli M, Gonzalez-Angulo A, Sneige N, Kau SW, Broglio K, Theriault RL, Valero V, Buzdar AU, Kuerer H, Buchholz TA, Hortobagyi GN: Invasive lobular carcinoma classic type: response to primary chemotherapy and survival outcomes. *J Clin Oncol* 2005, 23:41-48.

[4] Reis-Filho JS, Simpson PT, Turner NC, Lambros MB, Jones C, Mackay A, Grigoriadis A, Sarrio D, Savage K, Dexter T, et al: FGFR1 emerges as a potential therapeutic target for lobular breast carcinomas. *Clin Cancer Res* 2006, 12:6652-6662.

[5] Lehmann BD, Pietenpol JA: Identification and use of biomarkers in treatment strategies for triple-negative breast cancer subtypes. *J Pathol* 2014, 232:142-150.

[6] Fredholm H, Eaker S, Frisell J, Holmberg L, Fredriksson I, Lindman H: Breast cancer in young women: poor survival despite intensive treatment. *PLoS One* 2009, 4:e7695.

[7] Assi HA, Khoury KE, Dbouk H, Khalil LE, Mouhieddine TH, El Saghir NS: Epidemiology and prognosis of breast cancer in young women. *J Thorac Dis* 2013, 5 Suppl 1:S2-8.

[8] Clarke PA, te Poele R, Workman P: Gene expression microarray technologies in the development of new therapeutic agents. *European journal of cancer* 2004, 40:2560-2591.

[9] Midorikawa Y, Makuuchi M, Tang W, Aburatani H: Microarray-based analysis for hepatocellular carcinoma: from gene expression profiling to new challenges. *World journal of gastroenterology : WJG* 2007, 13:1487-1492.

[10] Lacroix L, Commo F, Soria JC: Gene expression profiling of non-small-cell lung cancer. *Expert review of molecular diagnostics* 2008, 8:167-178.

[11] Nannini M, Pantaleo MA, Maleddu A, Astolfi A, Formica S, Biasco G: Gene expression profiling in colorectal cancer using microarray technologies: results and perspectives. *Cancer treatment reviews* 2009, 35:201-209.

[12] Sorensen KD, Orntoft TF: Discovery of prostate cancer biomarkers by microarray gene expression profiling. *Expert review of molecular diagnostics* 2010, 10:49-64.

[13] Oostlander AE, Meijer GA, Ylstra B: Microarray-based comparative genomic hybridization and its applications in human genetics. *Clinical genetics* 2004, 66:488-495.

[14] Shih Ie M, Wang TL: Apply innovative technologies to explore cancer genome. *Current opinion in oncology* 2005, 17:33-38.

[15] Dupuy A, Simon RM: Critical review of published microarray studies for cancer outcome and guidelines on statistical analysis and reporting. *Journal of the National Cancer Institute* 2007, 99:147-157.

[16] Morozova O, Hirst M, Marra MA: Applications of new sequencing technologies for transcriptome analysis. *Annual review of genomics and human genetics* 2009, 10:135-151.

[17] Marguerat S, Bahler J: RNA-seq: from technology to biology. *Cellular and molecular life sciences : CMLS* 2010, 67:569-579.

[18] Costa V, Aprile M, Esposito R, Ciccodicola A: RNA-Seq and human complex diseases: recent accomplishments and future perspectives. *European journal of human genetics : EJHG* 2013, 21:134-142.

[19] Dai M, Wang P, Boyd AD, Kostov G, Athey B, Jones EG, Bunney WE, Myers RM, Speed TP, Akil H, et al: Evolving gene/transcript definitions significantly alter the interpretation of GeneChip data. *Nucleic Acids Res* 2005, 33:e175.

[20] Johnson WE, Li C, Rabinovic A: Adjusting batch effects in microarray expression data using empirical Bayes methods. *Biostatistics* 2007, 8:118-127.

[21] Robinson MD, McCarthy DJ, Smyth GK: edgeR: a Bioconductor package for differential expression analysis of digital gene expression data. *Bioinformatics* 2010, 26:139-140.

[22] Bardou P, Mariette J, Escudie F, Djemiel C, Klopp C: jvenn: an interactive Venn diagram viewer. *BMC Bioinformatics* 2014, 15:293.

[23] Chou YT, Wang H, Chen Y, Danielpour D, Yang YC: Cited2 modulates TGF-beta-mediated upregulation of MMP9. *Oncogene* 2006, 25:5547-5560.

[24] Sohn DM, Kim SY, Baek MJ, Lim CW, Lee MH, Cho MS, Kim TY: Expression of survivin and clinical correlation in patients with breast cancer. *Biomedicine & pharmacotherapy = Biomedecine & pharmacotherapie* 2006, 60:289-292.

[25] Naderi A, Meyer M: Prolactin-induced protein mediates cell invasion and regulates integrin signaling in estrogen receptor-negative breast cancer. *Breast cancer research : BCR* 2012, 14:R111.

[26] Noetzel E, Rose M, Bornemann J, Gajewski M, Knuchel R, Dahl E: Nuclear transport receptor karyopherin-alpha2 promotes malignant breast cancer phenotypes in vitro. *Oncogene* 2012, 31:2101-2114.

[27] Xu C, Wang H, He H, Zheng F, Chen Y, Zhang J, Lin X, Ma D, Zhang H: Low expression of TFPI-2 associated with poor survival outcome in patients with breast cancer. *BMC cancer* 2013, 13:118.

[28] Li C, Ma H, Wang Y, Cao Z, Graves-Deal R, Powell AE, Starchenko A, Ayers GD, Washington MK, Kamath V, et al: Excess PLAC8 promotes an unconventional ERK2-dependent EMT in colon cancer. *The Journal of clinical investigation* 2014, 124:2172-2187.

[29] Vertino PM, Yen RW, Gao J, Baylin SB: De novo methylation of CpG island sequences in human fibroblasts overexpressing DNA (cytosine-5-)-methyltransferase. *Molecular and cellular biology* 1996, 16:4555-4565.

[30] Sun L, Hui AM, Kanai Y, Sakamoto M, Hirohashi S: Increased DNA methyltransferase expression is associated with an early stage of human hepatocarcinogenesis. *Japanese journal of cancer research : Gann* 1997, 88:1165-1170.

[31] Damiani LA, Yingling CM, Leng S, Romo PE, Nakamura J, Belinsky SA: Carcinogen-induced gene promoter hypermethylation is mediated by DNMT1 and causal for transformation of immortalized bronchial epithelial cells. *Cancer Res* 2008, 68:9005-9014.

[32] Zhao M, Sun J, Zhao Z: TSGene: a web resource for tumor suppressor genes. *Nucleic Acids Res* 2013, 41:D970-976.

[33] Bauer JA, Chakravarthy AB, Rosenbluth JM, Mi D, Seeley EH, De Matos Granja-Ingram N, Olivares MG, Kelley MC, Mayer IA, Meszoely IM, et al: Identification of markers of taxane sensitivity using proteomic and genomic analyses of breast tumors from patients receiving neoadjuvant paclitaxel and radiation. *Clinical cancer research : an official journal of the American Association for Cancer Research* 2010, 16:681-690.

[34] Ray PS, Wang J, Qu Y, Sim MS, Shamonki J, Bagaria SP, Ye X, Liu B, Elashoff D, Hoon DS, et al: FOXC1 is a potential prognostic biomarker with functional significance in basal-like breast cancer. *Cancer Res* 2010, 70:3870-3876.

[35] Rody A, Karn T, Liedtke C, Pusztai L, Ruckhaeberle E, Hanker L, Gaetje R, Solbach C, Ahr A, Metzler D, et al: A clinically relevant gene signature in triple negative and basal-like breast cancer. *Breast cancer research : BCR* 2011, 13:R97.

[36] Umekita Y, Ohi Y, Souda M, Rai Y, Sagara Y, Tamada S, Tanimoto A: Maspin expression is frequent and correlates with basal markers in triple-negative breast cancer. *Diagnostic pathology* 2011, 6:36.

[37] Beltran AS, Graves LM, Blancafort P: Novel role of Engrailed 1 as a prosurvival transcription factor in basal-like breast cancer and engineering of interference peptides block its oncogenic function. *Oncogene* 2013.

[38] Jenssen TK, Kuo WP, Stokke T, Hovig E: Associations between gene expressions in breast cancer and patient survival. *Hum Genet* 2002, 111:411-420.

[39] Gordon GJ, Richards WG, Sugarbaker DJ, Jaklitsch MT, Bueno R: A prognostic test for adenocarcinoma of the lung from gene expression profiling data. *Cancer Epidemiol Biomarkers Prev* 2003, 12:905-910.

[40] Huang E, Cheng SH, Dressman H, Pittman J, Tsou MH, Horng CF, Bild A, Iversen ES, Liao M, Chen CM, et al: Gene expression predictors of breast cancer outcomes. *Lancet* 2003, 361:1590-1596.

[41] Sotiriou C, Neo SY, McShane LM, Korn EL, Long PM, Jazaeri A, Martiat P, Fox SB, Harris AL, Liu ET: Breast cancer classification and prognosis based on gene expression profiles from a population-based study. *Proc Natl Acad Sci U S A* 2003, 100:10393-10398.

[42] Zhao H, Ljungberg B, Grankvist K, Rasmuson T, Tibshirani R, Brooks JD: Gene expression profiling predicts survival in conventional renal cell carcinoma. *PLoS Med* 2006, 3:e13.

[43] Bernardi R, Gianni L: Hallmarks of triple negative breast cancer emerging at last? *Cell Res* 2014, 24:904-905.

[44] Al-Ejeh F, Simpson PT, Sanus JM, Klein K, Kalimutho M, Shi W, Miranda M, Kutasovic J, Raghavendra A, Madore J, et al: Meta-analysis of the global gene expression profile of triple-negative breast cancer identifies genes for the prognostication and treatment of aggressive breast cancer. *Oncogenesis* 2014, 3:e100.

[45] Yoon NK, Maresh EL, Shen D, Elshimali Y, Apple S, Horvath S, Mah V, Bose S, Chia D, Chang HR, Goodglick L: Higher levels of GATA3 predict better survival in women with breast cancer. *Human pathology* 2010, 41:1794-1801.

[46] Chu IM, Michalowski AM, Hoenerhoff M, Szauter KM, Luger D, Sato M, Flanders K, Oshima A, Csiszar K, Green JE: GATA3 inhibits lysyl oxidase-mediated metastases of human basal triple-negative breast cancer cells. Oncogene 2012, 31:2017-2027.

Permissions

All chapters in this book were first published in ACRMPBC, by InTech Open; hereby published with permission under the Creative Commons Attribution License or equivalent. Every chapter published in this book has been scrutinized by our experts. Their significance has been extensively debated. The topics covered herein carry significant findings which will fuel the growth of the discipline. They may even be implemented as practical applications or may be referred to as a beginning point for another development.

The contributors of this book come from diverse backgrounds, making this book a truly international effort. This book will bring forth new frontiers with its revolutionizing research information and detailed analysis of the nascent developments around the world.

We would like to thank all the contributing authors for lending their expertise to make the book truly unique. They have played a crucial role in the development of this book. Without their invaluable contributions this book wouldn't have been possible. They have made vital efforts to compile up to date information on the varied aspects of this subject to make this book a valuable addition to the collection of many professionals and students.

This book was conceptualized with the vision of imparting up-to-date information and advanced data in this field. To ensure the same, a matchless editorial board was set up. Every individual on the board went through rigorous rounds of assessment to prove their worth. After which they invested a large part of their time researching and compiling the most relevant data for our readers.

The editorial board has been involved in producing this book since its inception. They have spent rigorous hours researching and exploring the diverse topics which have resulted in the successful publishing of this book. They have passed on their knowledge of decades through this book. To expedite this challenging task, the publisher supported the team at every step. A small team of assistant editors was also appointed to further simplify the editing procedure and attain best results for the readers.

Apart from the editorial board, the designing team has also invested a significant amount of their time in understanding the subject and creating the most relevant covers. They scrutinized every image to scout for the most suitable representation of the subject and create an appropriate cover for the book.

The publishing team has been an ardent support to the editorial, designing and production team. Their endless efforts to recruit the best for this project, has resulted in the accomplishment of this book. They are a veteran in the field of academics and their pool of knowledge is as vast as their experience in printing. Their expertise and guidance has proved useful at every step. Their uncompromising quality standards have made this book an exceptional effort. Their encouragement from time to time has been an inspiration for everyone.

The publisher and the editorial board hope that this book will prove to be a valuable piece of knowledge for researchers, students, practitioners and scholars across the globe.

List of Contributors

Yunus A. Luqmani and Maitham A. Khajah
Faculty of Pharmacy, Kuwait University, Safat, Kuwait

Nawal Mahfoudh and César Lozano-López
Departamento de Química Farmacéutica y Orgánica, Facultad de Farmacia, Universidad de Granada, Campus de Cartuja s/n, Granada, Spain

Joaquín M. Campos and M. Eugenia García-Rubiño
Departamento de Química Farmacéutica y Orgánica, Facultad de Farmacia, Universidad de Granada, Campus de Cartuja s/n, Granada, Spain
Departamento de Química Farmacéutica y Orgánica, Instituto de Investigación Biosanitaria ibs.GRANADA, Universidad de Granada, Granada, Spain

Somaira Nowsheen and Khaled Aziz
Medical Scientist Training Program, Mayo Graduate School, Mayo Medical School, Mayo Clinic, Rochester, MN, USA

Asef Aziz
Baylor University, Waco, TX, USA

Alexandros G Georgakilas
Department of Physics, School of Applied Mathematical and Physical Sciences, National Technical University of Athens, Zografou Campus, GR, Athens, Greece

Hacer Esra Gurses, Omer Faruk Hatipoğlu, Mehmet Gunduz and Esra Gunduz
Department of Medical Genetics, Faculty of Medicine, Turgut Ozal University, Ankara,Turkey

Majed S. Alokail
Biomarker Research Group, Biochemistry Department, College of Science, King Saud University, Riyadh, Saudi Arabia

Amal M. Alenad
School of Biological Sciences, Life Science Building, University of Southampton, Southampton, UK

Beyzanur Yigitoglu, Eyyup Uctepe, Esra Gunduz and Mehmet Gunduz
Department of Medical Genetics, Faculty of Medicine, Turgut Ozal University, Ankara, Turkey

Ramazan Yigitoglu
Medical Biochemistry, Faculty of Medicine, Turgut Ozal University, Ankara, Turkey

Catherine Leurer and Shafaat Ahmed Rabbani
Department of Medicine, McGill University Health Center, Canada

Ayşe Çelik, Muradiye Acar, Catherine Moroski Erkul, Esra Gunduz and Mehmet Gunduz
Department of Medical Genetics, Faculty Of Medicine, Turgut Ozal University, Ankara, Turkey

I-Hsuan Lin and Ming-Ta Hsu
Institute of Biochemistry and Molecular Biology, School of Life Science, National Yang-Ming University, Taipei, Taiwan

Index

www.ingramcontent.com/pod-product-compliance
Lightning Source LLC
LaVergne TN
LVHW080609210926
848485LV00003B/125

* 9 7 8 1 6 3 9 8 7 3 7 5 3 *